To my wife, Arlene, and our children,
Janet Bracha and David Pesach,
and to *Shalom Ba'it*.

The intellect of the rational soul, which is the faculty that conceives any thing is given the appellation of *chochmah* — the "potentiality" of "what is." When one brings forth this power from the potential into the actual, that is, when (a person) cogitates with his intellect in order to understand a thing truly and profoundly as it evolves from the concept which he has conceived in his intellect, this is called *binah* . . . *Da'at* implies attachment and union.

Schneur Zalman of Liadi, *Tanya*

Contributors

Paul S. Appelbaum, MD
Co-Director, Law and Psychiatry
  Program
Western Psychiatric Institute and
  Clinic
Assistant Professor of Psychiatry
University of Pittsburgh School
  of Medicine
Adjunct Associate Professor of
  Law
University of Pittsburgh School
  of Law
Pittsburgh, Pennsylvania

Jerrold G. Bernstein, MD
Associate Medical Director
Human Resource Institute
Assistant Psychiatrist
Massachusetts General Hospital
Assistant Attending Psychiatrist
McLean Hospital
Assistant Clinical Professor of
  Psychiatry
Harvard Medical School
Boston, Massachusetts

Mamoun Dabbagh, MD
Fellow in Psychiatry
Lafayette Clinic
Wayne State University School
  of Medicine
Detroit, Michigan

Irl Extein, MD
Medical Director
Falkirk Hospital
Central Valley, New York

Samuel Gershon, MD
Director
Lafayette Clinic
Professor and Chairman
Department of Psychiatry
Wayne State University School
  of Medicine
Detroit, Michigan

Rachel Gittelman, PhD
Director of Psychology
New York State Psychiatric
  Institute
Professor of Clinical Psychology
Columbia University College of
  Physicians and Surgeons
New York, New York

Mark S. Gold, MD
Director of Research
Psychiatric Diagnostic
  Laboratories of America
Summit, New Jersey

Ernest Hartmann, MD
Director, Sleep Research
  Laboratory
West-Ros-Park Mental Health
  Center
Professor of Psychiatry
Tufts University School of
  Medicine
Boston, Massachusetts

Andres Kanner, MD
Child Psychiatry Research Fellow
Department of Psychiatry
Columbia University College of
  Physicians and Surgeons
New York, New York

Gerald L. Klerman, MD
Director, Stanley Cobb Psychiatric
  Research Laboratories
Massachusetts General Hospital
Harrington Professor of Psychiatry
Harvard Medical School and
  Harvard School of Public Health
Boston, Massachusetts

Aurelio Ortiz, MD
Fellow in Psychiatry
Lafayette Clinic
Wayne State University School
  of Medicine
Detroit, Michigan

A. Carter Pottash, MD
Medical Director
Fair Oaks Hospital
Summit, New Jersey

Mai-Lan Rogoff, MD
Staff Psychiatrist
Developmental Evaluation Clinic
Childrens Hospital Medical
  Center
Instructor in Psychiatry
Harvard Medical School
Boston, Massachusetts

Alan F. Schatzberg, MD
Co-Director, Affective Disease
  Program
McLean Hospital
Associate Professor of Psychiatry
Harvard Medical School
Boston, Massachusetts

David V. Sheehan, MD
Director, Psychosomatic Unit
Massachusetts General Hospital
Assistant Professor of Psychiatry
Harvard Medical School
Boston, Massachusetts

Contents

Foreword

During my residency in psychiatry at the Johns Hopkins Hospital just over 20 years ago, a greatly loved and respected psychiatrist was found hanging. He was known to have had mood swings, and had access to the best help that the resources of a great medical center could offer. His death saddened all, and his Quaker memorial service served to teach us to accept fate. The following year I went to Seymour Kety's Laboratory of Clinical Science at the National Institute of Mental Health. There, Richard Green had somehow learned of the use of lithium in manic-depressive illness and introduced it into our clinical work. Lithium's introduction in the United States came 17 years after Cade's work in Australia, and seven years after Schou's convincing demonstration of its effectiveness. Several more years were to elapse before it became more widely used in American psychiatry.

My teacher's dying of an illness untreated by a medicine that was available, but unfamiliar, has been a central stimulus to my interest in sharing knowledge about the benefits of psychotropic medications. In helping to found a psychiatric hospital, the Human Resource Institute, I wanted one cornerstone of each patient's care to be the skillful and enlightened use of psychotropic medication.

I have been most fortunate in having Dr Bernstein join our staff. He has served as a constant resource for scientific knowledge about developments in psychopharmacology, and as a wise and experienced consultant to us all. He has led the development of our annual psychopharmacology symposia. These conferences have served to inform our psychiatric community of the spectrum of use of medications, as well as their biologic and psychologic basis. The chapters of this book are drawn from some of the participants in our most recent symposia.

Dr Bernstein's credentials for his contributions to psychopharmacology are outstanding. He is well trained in internal medicine, clinical pharmacology, and psychiatry. To my mind, foremost is his clinical commitment to patients. His expertise comes from their continuing care over a period of many years. While he has access to studies and shares experiences with colleagues at Massachusetts General Hospital and McLean Hospital, he has the first hand knowledge of following the life history of his patients in seeing how much medication can and cannot do. He has chosen authors wisely for each subject, so that the information presented is clinically balanced and up to date.

The recent textbook authored by Dr Bernstein, *Handbook of Drug Therapy in Psychiatry*, is an outstanding contribution to the literature. It is scientifically rigorous and clinically wise. It is comprehensive and serves as a companion piece to the present volume.

The future of psychopharmacology is partly new drugs and partly the recognition of those patients who will benefit from our present medications. In my area of interest, affective illness, when to use antidepressants in adolescents and which borderlines respond to lithium still need further research. There is much more than even our present medications can do.

We are fortunate to have this new edition of *Clinical Psychopharmacology*, which presents some of the most current information in this rapidly advancing field of clinical practice.

Bernard Levy, MD
Medical Director
Human Resource Institute
Assistant Clinical Professor of Psychiatry
Harvard Medical School
Consultant in Psychiatry
Massachusetts General Hospital

Preface

Since the publication of the first edition of *Clinical Psychopharmacology* in 1978, there have been many advances in this young and burgeoning field. As in other areas of scientific endeavor, the more we learn, the better we understand the incompleteness of our knowledge. Although relatively few new psychotropic medications have been marketed since 1978, there have been some useful additions to our armamentarium, most notably among the antidepressants. More importantly, we have learned from investigative studies and clinical experience how to more effectively utilize available pharmaceutical products in the treatment of psychiatric illness. More is now known about the limitations and adverse effects, as well as the beneficial effects, of this useful group of therapeutic agents.

Psychotherapy remains a widely employed and useful treatment technique that increasingly must be viewed in light of our knowledge of neurochemistry and pharmacology. Dr Klerman has elucidated the interactions of these therapeutic approaches in a most practical and interesting fashion. He has pointed out those areas in which psychological techniques are not therapeutic, and has discussed those conditions in which medication treatment is not indicated.

Despite advances in the medical treatment of psychiatric illness, many patients remain reluctant to accept the benefits of these advances. Therefore, numerous legal and ethical issues emerge in the clinical practice of psychopharmacology, which are ably discussed by Dr Appelbaum.

Specialized laboratory techniques are becoming available to aid in psychiatric diagnosis and in monitoring the response to pharmacotherapy. Dr Gold and his colleagues have reviewed this topic in a manner that will help clinicians understand the rationale and proper application of these tests in the practice of modern clinical psychiatry.

In view of the increasingly apparent connection between neurotransmitters and the etiology and treatment of mental disorders, a basic understanding of this interaction is central to the practice of clinical psychopharmacology. I have attempted to integrate scientific and clinical information about neurotransmitters and how they interact with receptors and drugs without becoming enmired in excessively technical details of biochemistry and physical chemistry.

Despite the powerful therapeutic action of antidepressant drugs, not all patients respond adequately to simple drug regimens. Thus, Dr Schatzberg has presented some approaches to help those patients who fail to respond as quickly and dramatically to conventional treatment modalities as we would like.

Anxiety disorders differ in their clinical presentations, mechanisms, and response to treatment. Proper assessment of the patient and avoidance of the routine administration of conventional antianxiety drugs are the mark of the sophisticated clinician. As discussed by Dr Sheehan, use of more specialized therapeutic agents, such as the monoamine oxidase inhibitors, can spell the difference between a functional person with a history of panic disorder and an individual literally crippled by panic attacks.

Dr Samuel Gershon, who helped to introduce lithium into the practice of psychiatry in the United States, has presented, along with his colleagues, a detailed overview of the mechanisms of action, complications, and therapeutic applications of this amazing ion. His discussion of lithium addresses potential therapeutic uses beyond manic-depressive illness and, with the help of a voluminous bibliography, gives the reader the necessary tools for further study.

Although antipsychotic drugs have been in use for 30 years, their efficacy and safety is dependent on a thorough understanding of their pharmacology and the proper techniques of dosage titration in individual clinical situations. Since the latter issue has been of great interest to me over a number of years, I have emphasized both clinical techniques and pharmacology in discussing these drugs that are the cornerstone of psychopharmacology.

Disturbances of sleep are a common cause of medical and psychiatric consultation. The ability to differentiate abnormal sleep patterns is essential to appropriate treatment. Physicians and patients must recognize the limitations as well as the potential safe use of medications that may reduce the discomfort of insomnia.

Although the concerned physician must see each patient as "special," the last three chapters of the present volume examine some special types of patients who frequently require psychotropic medication: children, the developmentally disabled, and the elderly. In each of these groups, application of the standard techniques and dosages employed in adult psychopharmacology is likely to result in therapeutic misadventures. The clinician must recognize those patients and the drug-related factors that may predispose these "special patients" to adverse drug reactions or inadequate therapeutic responses. Willingness to start slowly with lower than conventional doses and to titrate dosage with adequate periods of observation, is the most likely way to improve the response to treatment and avoid unwanted effects.

As I have stated many times previously, a guiding principle in the practice of psychopharmacology is that the physician prescribing medication must adequately discuss the treatment program with the patient. Patients entrusted to us for care have a right to know the nature, benefits, and adverse effects of the medications they will be receiving. This educational process will enhance the therapeutic alliance and improve patient compliance and, therefore, increase the chance of favorable response to treatment. Even if the correct medication is properly prescribed, active participation of the patient is essential to a favorable therapeutic outcome. Not only physicians, but all clinicians working with patients must understand psychotropic medications. It is indeed my hope that this book will be of value in achieving this goal.

This second edition of *Clinical Psychopharmacology*, as was the first, is the outgrowth of a series of psychopharmacology symposia sponsored by the Human Resource Institute. Each of the chapters, however, was written for the express purpose of the present volume. I am indebted to the knowledgeable and distinguished authors for the thoroughness, practicality, and readability of their individual contributions.

My colleagues at the Human Resource Institute have aided me immeasurably in conducting the symposia and in bringing this book to fruition. I am ever appreciative of my good friend and colleague, Dr Bernard Levy, for his constant support and encouragement. I wish to thank Mrs Jane Dolph and Miss Donna Cummings for their help over a number of years in the organization and smooth running of these symposia and Miss Lucia Messina for her help in typing a considerable portion of this manuscript.

I appreciate the help I have received from the staff of John Wright • PSG Inc; most notably, Ms Bette J. Aaronson, Managing Editor. Finally, as always, I am thankful for the understanding and support of my wife, Arlene, and our children, who have allowed this book and all else that I attempt to come forth from the potential into the actual.

Jerrold G. Bernstein, MD

1

Psychotherapy
and Pharmacotherapy

Gerald L. Klerman

This chapter reviews issues related to decisions that clinicians and patients make about the selection of treatment for depression, particularly the relationship between psychotherapy and pharmacotherapy.

The process by which the patient selects a consultant or psychotherapist guarantees that the patient arrives with preconceptions as to the nature of his/her illness and treatment(s) he/she feels would be best. Psychotherapists, whether they be psychologists, psychiatrists, or nurses, have reputations in the community. Patients learn through the grapevine whether a psychotherapist is drug oriented. There is no way this process can be avoided.

We, in psychiatry, may not have the level of knowledge that other fields of medicine have, but controversy as to choice of treatment is not restricted to psychiatry. For example, in the field of cardiology there is a dispute regarding the value of coronary bypass surgery for arteriosclerotic heart disease. Before patients get to the surgeon, they have gone through a comparable but less explicit process.

THE CLINICAL PHENOMENA

Figure 1-1 illustrates the point to be made. The caption is, "I do like you. *You* don't like you." It is not necessary to have a PhD or an MD to know that the patient is the female. That is understood by nonverbal

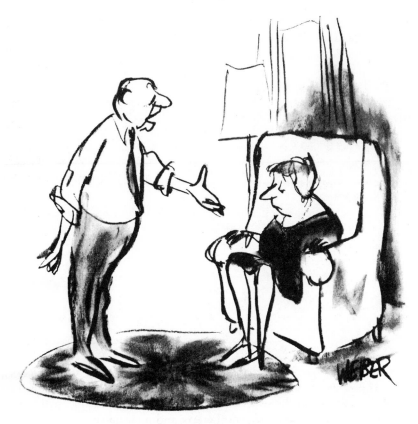

"I do like you. You don't like you."

Figure 1-1   Drawing by Weber. Copyright © 1965 The New Yorker Magazine, Inc.

cues; anyone who reads *The New Yorker* can immediately make the clinical diagnosis. First, she is a woman. Depression occurs more frequently in women than in men, at about the ratio of two to one. This is reflected in the fact that the majority of patients in therapy, whether pharmacotherapy or psychotherapy for depression, are women.

The changes in facial expressions, the flattening of the nasolabial folds, the furrowing of the brow, and the downcast gaze were first described by Darwin. Those are the characteristic nonverbal facial cues of depression that occur in all mammals, including monkeys and dogs. She is dressed in black, depressed patients take less interest in their grooming. She has psychomotor retardation as manifested by her being slumped in the chair. She feels she has no place in life. She complains of backache, and worries that she is going through the "change of life." He (the husband, I presume) has attempted to apply the psychotherapy and pharmacotherapy of everyday life: he has taken her out to dinner, given her wine, or taken her on a trip, but nothing has worked.

There are four possible responses to this situation. If there was a drawing of her in a classic psychoanalytic situation, the analyst would tell her that her problem is dependency — she is still tied to her mother. He would diagnose her as borderline and an oral dependent personality, and conclude that this depression is a recurrence of her unresolved fixations at the breast and recommend that she undergo five years of intensive psychoanalysis.

Another drawing would show her in the office of a psychopharmacologist. He would say her problem does not lie at the breast but in the diencephalon. She is suffering from an imbalance of her neurotransmitters, her norepinephrine is down, her acetylcholine is sideways. She needs to have a combination of amoxapine and lithium.

A third drawing would show her with a family therapist who would say that the problem is not "in" her, but it is "in" the transaction with her husband. They have had a longstanding marital schism, in which he has had the dominant role and she has passively accepted the position of female. Therefore, her depression is a reflection of her unresolved rage at having accepted this passive position through life. The husband has to change and acknowledge her individuality.

In the fourth drawing, she would go to a feminist therapist who would say, "she is not depressed but is oppressed." She has low self-esteem, and feels that there is no place for her in the world. She is confused and oppressed in a society where women are dominated by male sexism. She does not need therapy. The very fact of giving her a diagnosis reinforces her learned helplessness and treats her like a victim. What she needs to do is have her consciousness raised and to march for the ERA.

These hypothetical vignettes illustrate how the same clinical situation can be responded to by different therapists, depending on their ideological and theoretical backgrounds.

Are we completely without data? Is the only thing that we in clinical psychiatry can do is to throw up our hands in frustration and acknowledge the medical splits in our field and conclude that all treatments are equally effective? It is not possible in a situation like this to be equally right. The choices that clinicians and patients make have consequences in the rate at which patients improve. There is a growing body of evidence that is pertinent to treatment decisions, which concerns the efficacy of combining drugs and psychotherapy for the management of the acute depressive episode and for long-term treatment to prevent relapses and to enhance the social and familial adjustment of patients.

In approaching this problem, the main stumbling block to decision-making and to making use of the body of knowledge is not intellectual-cognitive. It is the ideological and theoretical background that clinicians and patients bring to the decision-making process.

4

COMMON MISCONCEPTIONS

There are some misconceptions that interfere with decision making. A commonly held view is that all patients should have psychotherapy. In my residency training 25 years ago, the common view was that everyone was a candidate for psychotherapy. That view is still held throughout the practicing community, and it is also held by many parts of the public sector, particularly the better educated, middle-class community who have come to accept a psychologically oriented value system. There are at least four groups of depressed patients that should not receive psychotherapy alone, and for whom the evidence indicates that psychotherapy alone is ineffective and possibly harmful.[1,2]

In the first group are patients who have a psychotic or delusional depression. They may have delusions of bodily change, stating that their bowels are rotting or that they have cancer. They may present with mild hypochondriacal complaints, but if pursued carefully, they will have a fixed belief in their illness, that they are not looking for psychiatric treatment, but for some medical diagnosis, and they are convinced that their situation is hopeless. Psychotherapy alone is not useful for such patients, nor are tricyclics. The evidence indicates that the presence of delusions and other psychotic features contraindicates the use of tricyclics alone.[1] For such patients, the best treatment is the combination of a tricyclic and a neuroleptic such as haloperidol or perphenazine.

One study of delusional depression assigned patients randomly to either amitriptyline alone, perphenazine alone or a combination of both. The patient group that received the combination achieved an 80% improvement rate in ten weeks, which was twice that of the group that received amitriptyline or perphenazine alone.[3] Psychotherapy may be useful in combination with drug treatment, particularly for people who have delusions involving concurrent life events.

A case in point is a 72-year-old high school teacher who retired to Cape Cod after having served as head of the music department in a high school. Soon after retiring, he lost 20 pounds and developed the delusion that the telephone was tapped and that the FBI was after him. He also had the delusion that he had committed a horrible sin on his income tax and that he was about to be sent to jail, which he felt was his just punishment.

As it developed, there was a secret in this family based around sin. The man had been a bisexual for many years and had been engaged in open homosexual activities with some of his associates on the high school faculty. It had been known to his children and to his wife, but they had never talked about it.

One of the consequences of his retiring was the separation from some of his homosexual partners. In a situation like this, he was initially treated intensively with a combination of haloperidol (Haldol) and amitriptyline (Elavil). Then he was engaged with the family in a series of meetings to uncover the family secret and to deal with the issue that everyone in the family had known about. The interpretation was that his sense of guilt and conflict over the secret sin was displaced from his sexuality to his income tax return. That is one common example.

A second group of patients who should not receive psychotherapy alone are bipolar, or manic-depressive, patients. There are not many psychotherapists who recommend psychotherapy for the acute manic episode, but there are a larger number of patients who present with cyclothymia and hypomania. Many of these people are quite successful; the cyclothymic or hypomanic personality is often adaptive in our society. They have a high energy level and a sense of mission; they are often "workaholics." These people are good candidates for lithium. Recently, there has been a number of interesting reports regarding the value of combining lithium with couples groups for patients with manic bipolar disease. These are patients who are on lithium, but without lithium it would not be possible for them to engage in the psychotherapeutic process.[1]

A third group are patients with the endogenous or melancholic symptom complex. The classic endogenous symptom complex is called "melancholia" in the DSM-III classification.[4] It consists of the characteristic pattern of sleep difficulty, particularly early morning awakening, weight loss, loss of appetite, loss of energy, decrease in sexual interest and activity, and either psychomotor retardation or psychomotor agitation. This symptom complex is very pervasive, and occurs in about 50% to 70% of hospitalized depressives and 25% to 30% of outpatient depressives.[1] This combination of symptoms is highly predictive of a good response to tricyclic antidepressants and a poor response to psychotherapy alone, except in the presence of a situational ongoing life crisis. The decision to use medication for patients with this symptom complex should be based upon the presenting manifest symptoms complained of by the patient and the degree to which they are impairing the patient's usual social, occupational and family functioning. There are presently three excellent studies, including one in which Dr Weissman of Yale and I are participating, which indicate that psychotherapy alone for these patients is not beneficial and, in fact, they do worse than if they were treated with placebo alone.[2]

The fourth group of patients for whom psychotherapy alone is not useful are patients with severe agoraphobia. Agoraphobia is not usually discussed in relationship to depression. Patients with agoraphobia have periods of panic attacks, with sweating, palpitations, and fearfulness. They feel that they cannot go out of their home, except when accompanied by a companion. In the presence of a companion, family member or otherwise, they can go shopping or attend social events. They develop anticipatory anxiety and a reactive depression. Both the tricyclic antidepressants and the MAO inhibitors are effective in treating agoraphobia as are certain forms of behavioral therapy, such as desensitization and exposure in vivo. However, dynamically oriented individual psychotherapy is not useful for such patients except after they have had their panic attacks brought under control by either medication or more behaviorally oriented therapy.[1]

Thus, there are several common misconceptions around the decision of who should receive psychotherapy. A second set of misconceptions is that all depressed patients should be medicated. Just as psychotherapists are at fault for their blanket prescription of psychotherapy, the advocates of biological psychiatry are potentially at fault for advocating that all forms of depression should be treated with medication. Particularly in the nonendogenous, nonpsychotic, nonbipolar forms of depression, the patient can do equally well with some form of psychotherapy as with medication.[1]

Bipolar or manic depressive illness accounts for approximately 10% of all depression.[5] Its lifetime prevalence throughout the population is somewhere between 1% and 2%; that is, overall, about 1% or 2% of the population will at some point during their adult life manifest some form of bipolar illness. As we learn more about the value of lithium and the epidemiology of that disorder, its prevalence will rise to 2% or 3%. It is more common in middle class and better educated families; it is more common in whites as compared to blacks. It is common in people of Scandinavian descent, and it seems that there are very important genetic components of the predisposition to this illness. It is more likely to be seen in a hospital than in an ambulatory setting.

Delusional depression is also relatively uncommon, at most 10% to 15% in hospitalized series.[1] It is less common in outpatient samples, but the presence of delusions has important consequences for the choice of treatment. The endogenous pattern is more common, about 40% to 50% of hospitalized patients and about 25% of ambulatory patients are afflicted.[1]

These three diagnostic groupings are not mutually exclusive. Bipolar patients can have endogenous features and endogenous patients can have delusions. In ambulatory settings, including private practice, mental health clinics and outpatient clinics, about 70% of the depressed patients will be nonendogenous, nonpsychotic, and nonbipolar.[1] In DSM-II, they were diagnosed as psychoneurotic depressive reaction (300.4). They would be termed major depressive disorder, nonmelancholic without mood congruent delusions in DSM-III.[4]

THE ROLE OF PSYCHOTHERAPY

The clinician has a wide variety of effective treatments available. In addition to the MAO inhibitors and the new tricyclic and tetracyclics, there are now at least four forms of psychotherapy for depression whose efficacy has been established through randomized controlled trials. In at least 20 randomized controlled trials, a group of patients were assigned to either the psychotherapy or control group or to medication with or without the psychotherapy. These trials demonstrated some degree of efficacy of psychotherapy over and above the control group.[1]

The randomized clinical trial was first developed for the evaluation of drugs and is now being used increasingly for the evaluation of surgical procedures, radiation therapy as well as psychotherapy. It provides the most rigorous and definitive type of evidence that we have for the efficacy of any treatment.

The four forms of psychotherapy for which there is some evidence of efficacy are: cognitive therapy, interpersonal therapy, social learning, and marital therapy. Cognitive therapy is the most widely known; it was developed by Beck and his associates at the University of Pennsylvania and is based on the assumption that patients who are depressed come to their illness with marked negative self-evaluations, and they view the world in a pessimistic distorted manner, interpreting every event in a negative way.[6]

It is difficult to describe cognitive psychotherapy without making it appear like a version of Norman Vincent Peale's "positive thinking." There are four randomized trials in which this treatment fares better than placebo, including a recent one in the *British Journal of Psychiatry* by the Medical Research Counsel Unit in Edinburgh. Interestingly enough, the Brain Research Unit at Edinburgh undertook a study in which they showed, as a number of other studies had shown previously, that cognitive therapy was as effective as a tricyclic for nonpsychotic, non-bipolar patients.[7]

The second form of psychotherapy is known as interpersonal therapy. It is based on the presumption that the main problem depressed patients have is their interpersonal relations.

Women are more prone to depression than men. It is an alternative to the explanation of the feminist — sociological interpretation that the reason women are depressed is because they are oppressed by a male-dominated, discriminating society. The psychotherapeutic consequences of this view is that most women get depressed in the context of a disruption or threatened disruption in their interpersonal relations, most usually with a member of the opposite sex, either their husband or other significant male in their lives. The New Haven studies found that 40% of depressed women who applied for outpatient treatment reported that the precipitating event of their depression was some unresolved issue with the "man in their life."[8]

There are interesting differences between men and women with respect to the way they handle marital disputes. Given a heterosexual dispute, women come into treatment for depressive symptoms during the height of the impasse, when they feel hopeless, helpless, and powerless to alter the course of events. They feel threatened with the disruption of the relationship of the attachment bond. In contrast, men come into treatment not at the impasse stage but after there has been a separation or disruption of the bond, when the man is confronted with his loneliness, absence of the children, and has a sense of contrition and guilt. He often will report an increase in alcohol consumption or development of some bodily compliant such as backache or headache. There is good epidemiologic evidence that women are more prone to depression. Whatever the reason, the facts substantiate that they are more likely to come into treatment, particularly when there has been a threat to the attachment bond, or the threat of an impending loss. Interpersonal psychotherapy deals with this situation by clarifying the mutual expectations of the two parties, either through individual or couples therapy. There is good evidence as to the efficacy of this treatment, particularly for nonendogenous, nonpsychotic depression.[1]

The third form of treatment is social learning therapy; it has been developed mainly in Pittsburgh and on the West Coast, particularly in Oregon by Peter Lewisohn.[9] The basic ideas of this approach began with the ideas of B. F. Skinner, Professor of Psychology at Harvard. The Skinnerians propose that depressed individuals lack the social skills needed to elicit positive reinforcement from their environment. The normal person has gained these skills through learning and childhood experiences. He/she knows how to elicit from the environment forms of positive reinforcement, the equivalent of "M&M's." The most valued reinforcement for adult humans is approval, affection, nurturing, and loving. Normal persons know how to mingle in groups and participate in the various social behaviors of reaching out to people, sometimes even participating in small talk, which has, in turn, reciprocal positive social reinforcement such as in smiling and saying, "My, how nice your tie is," "Your hair looks good," "How are the children?" or "How did you enjoy your summer?" Depressives do not have sustained relationships that provide reinforcement. Furthermore, they often elicit negative reinforcement which further depresses their self-esteem and reinforces their sense of worthlessness.

The majority of clinicians in the psychiatric community are not trained in any of the above techniques. The most valued form of psychotherapy in this community is some variant of individual dynamic psychotherapy, usually derived from the teachings of Freud or his psychoanalytic followers. There is no evidence for the efficacy of this treatment for depression.

There is a form of psychotherapy for which the evidence is negative, and that is Rogerian or nondirective therapy. There are studies which indicate that depressed patients treated with nondirected, Rogerian-type therapy do not do as well as a control group.[10] The reason seems to be that the patients interpret the nondirective, passive, behavior of the therapist as a lack of personal interest and as a form of further self-deprecation. They feel they are uninteresting, that nobody cares, and they experience the passive therapeutic intervention as a worsening of their condition. My interpretation of that situation is that in clinical work, particularly during an acute episode, the therapist should avoid the extensive use of nondirective techniques, should be active, even at times expressing optimism and reassurance, and should engage in active inquiry as to not only the past history of the patient's life but a careful inventory of the patient's current relations, particularly interpersonal and social relations.

A common misconception is that neurotic depression should not be treated with medication. The term "neurotic" does not appear in DSM-III. Recent research has indicated that there is ambiguity in the use of the term "neurotic depression." Sometimes it refers to depression that is nonpsychotic, without delusions. Sometimes, neurotic refers to depression that involves a precipitating life event, also called "reactive" or "situational" depression. Sometimes the term neurotic depression is used to refer to depressions that arise as a consequence of the character or personality maladjustments of the patient and, in that sense, are not precipitated, but arise because of the patient's longstanding character or personality conflicts. Sometimes neurotic depression is used to refer to less severe depressions. There is very good evidence that neurotic depressions do respond to medication, as well as to psychotherapy.[1]

There are two bodies of evidence that refute the misconception that neurotic depression should not be treated with medication. First, a fair percentage of patients with endogenous or melancholic symptom patterns report life events that precipitate the current depression. The relationship between adverse life events as precipitants and this particular symptom pattern is not as the textbook would have it. The decision to use medication should not be based on the presence or absence of precipitating life events, but on the characteristic symptoms and their intensity. Do they distress the patient? Do they impair his or her usual level of social functioning at work or at home? For the patient who has both the symptom complex and the adverse life event, as is the case in the majority of outpatients, the combination of drugs and psychotherapy is highly successful.

The second misconception has to do with characterological depression. There is an expectation not to use medication in patients whose depressions are chronic or who have long-term character problems.[11] The common diagnostic term is "borderline character disorder."[1,12] Currently, it is the most widely misused and abused diagnostic category in the psychiatric community. It does significant harm to depressed patients. Many psychotherapeutically oriented psychiatrists, particularly those who have been influenced by Otto Kernberg and by Kohut, see everyone who comes into their office as having borderline or narcissistic character features. Aside from the issue of whether or not that is true, it has a very significant adverse consequence. A high percentage of patients with character pathology present with affective symptoms, usually a mild to severe depression. These patients, who have been in psychotherapy for a long time, often have been told that they have borderline features, and sometimes their therapist says he or she does not believe in medication. And, if the patient asks for medication, they are told they should stop treatment because they are just seeking a "crutch." The combination of excessive preoccupation with the patient's character pathology combined with a negative attitude toward the use of medication still occurs in certain parts of the psychotherapeutic community and does a profound disservice to the patient.

In an ongoing unpublished study done at Yale, the research team reviewed the case records of 25 patients diagnosed as "borderline personality disorders" and assessed the patients utilizing the SADS and RDC.[12,13] Over one-half of them met the criteria for either bipolar affective disorder or for major depressive disorder. Eleven patients were placed on lithium with dramatic improvement of their clinical picture within six weeks. Another study at the University of Tennessee described 70 patients diagnosed as borderline, of whom approximately 40% met the criteria for major depressive disorder.[14,15] Focus on the character pathology led the clinician to miss, or not inquire about, matters such as sleep disturbance or appetite loss, to not take advantage of the availability of medication, and to discount the patients' complaints and request for relief of their distress. The presence or absence of character pathology, whether borderline, narcissistic, or passive-dependent, does not in itself preclude the value of medication.[14] In my opinion, the psychotherapy that is directed towards uncovering and dealing with longstanding character issues is best conducted after the resolution of the acute episode.

SUMMARY

This chapter has reviewed some of the theoretical and practical issues involved in decisions as to whether to use medication alone, psychotherapy alone, or a combination of both. Also discussed were some common misconceptions: 1) all patients who are depressed should have psychotherapy, 2) all patients who are depressed should be medicated, 3) neurotic patients should not receive drug therapy, 4) precipitating life events predict a poor response to drugs, and 5) drug therapy is not useful in people with character problems.

REFERENCES

1. Klerman GL: Overview of affective disorders, in Kaplan HI, Freedman A, Sadock BJ (eds): *Comprehensive Textbook of Psychiatry*. Baltimore, Williams & Wilkins, 1980, pp 1305–1319.
2. Rounsaville BJ, Klerman GL, Weissman MM: Do psychotherapy and pharmacotherapy for depression conflict? *Arch Gen Psychiatry* 1981;38:24–29.
3. Spiker DG, Hanin I, Coxsky JE, et al: *Pharmacological Treatment of Delusional Depressives*. Presented at the American College of Neuropsychopharmacology, San Juan, Puerto Rico, December, 1980.
4. American Psychiatric Association: *Diagnostic and Statistical Manual of Mental Disorders*. Washington, DC, American Psychiatric Association, 1980.
5. Krauthammer C, Klerman GL: The epidemiology of mania, in Shopsin B (ed): *Manic Illness*. New York, Raven Press, 1979, pp 11–28.
6. Beck AT, Ward CH, Mendelson M, et al: An inventory of measuring depression. *Arch Gen Psychiatry* 1963;4:561–571.
7. Blackburn IM, Bishop S, Glen AI, et al: The efficacy of cognitive therapy and pharmacotherapy. *Br J Psychiatry* 1981;139:181–189.
8. Weissman MM, Prusoff BA, DiMascio A, et al: The efficacy of drugs and psychotherapy in the treatment of acute depression episodes. *Am J Psychiatry* 1979;136:555–558.
9. Lewisohn PM, Hoberman HM: Depression, in Bellack L, Hersen M, Kasdin M (eds): *International Handbook of Behavior Modification and Therapy*. New York, Plenum Press, 1982.
10. Shaw BF: Comparisons of cognitive therapy and behavior therapy in the treatment of depression. *J Consult Clin Psychol* 1977;45:543–551.
11. Akiskal HS: Dysthymic disorder: Psychopathology of proposed chronic depressive subtypes. *Am J Psychiatry* 1983;140:11–21.
12. Spitzer RL, Endicott J, Robins E: Research diagnostic criteria. *Arch Gen Psychiatry* 1978;35:773–782.
13. Klerman GL: Neurotic and psychotic depression—A re-evaluation. *Bull Neuroinformation Laboratory* 1981;8:71–89.
14. Akiskal HS: Subaffective disorders: Dysthymic, cyclothymic, and bipolar II disorders in the "borderline" realm. *Psychiatr Clin North Am* 1981; 4:25–46.
15. Akiskal HS, Rosenthal TL, Haykal RF, et al: Characterological depressions—Clinical and sleep EEG findings separating "subaffective dysthymias" from "character-spectrum disorders." *Arch Gen Psychiatry* 1980;37:777–783.

2

Legal and Ethical Aspects
of Psychopharmacologic Practice

Paul S. Appelbaum

As little as two decades ago, a chapter dealing with legal and ethical considerations would have seemed peculiarly out of place in a book about clinical psychopharmacology. To the generation that witnessed the introduction of effective psychotropic medications into psychiatric practice, their selection and prescription would have appeared to be a quintessentially clinical matter. The role of clinical acumen, of course, is still paramount in the treatment process, but the responsible clinician can no longer afford to act in ignorance of the legal rules that govern psychopharmacologic practice. This chapter will consider the evolution and current status of these legal regulations and their related ethical maxims. It will do so from the perspective of the clinician, whose primary concern is not legal theory, but effective patient care.

THE DOCTRINE OF INFORMED CONSENT

The basis for the revolution in legal regulation of psychiatric practice is the doctrine of informed consent. As perplexing as informed consent law appears to many clinicians, it is in reality the logical outgrowth of several centuries of Anglo-American precedent.[1] This common law tradition had long held that every person had the right to give or to withhold consent for bodily intrusions, whether or not they were motivated by therapeutic intent. In its purest form, this early version of consent law held that a surgical procedure performed without a person's consent (or over a person's objections) constituted a battery – an unconsented touching – for which damages could be claimed. For many years, however, the physician's demonstration that the patient's consent had been obtained prior to the procedure acted as an effective counter to any legal action.

In a series of malpractice cases that began in the late 1950s, this defense was shattered.[2,3] Courts began to insist that the patient's simple acquiescence in the procedure was an insufficient basis for physician immunity should harm occur to the patient. The requirement for simple consent was replaced by the need for *informed* consent. As the courts elaborated this concept, informed consent had three required components: 1) that the patient be presented with sufficient information to make an informed decision; 2) that the patient's consent be uncoerced; and 3) that the patient be legally competent to offer a consent.[4]

Before considering how the courts have elaborated on these requirements, it may be useful to examine the basis for this relatively sudden shift in the legal approach to medical care. The requirement for an informed consent reflects an intensified emphasis on patients' right of autonomous decision making. It reflects the concern that, unless the law acts to redress the balance, the individual confronted by an increasingly complicated world will cede the power to control his future to a variety of more knowledgeable professionals. An effort has therefore been made to reinforce individual autonomy by requiring medical professionals to share their specialized knowledge with their patients, thereby facilitating patients' participation in the decision process. Although some may question the legitimacy of using the law to promote a particular moral perspective, there is little doubt that our judiciary has traditionally, if at times unconsciously, used tort law (the law of civil wrongs) to effect similarly sweeping changes in the conception of individual responsibility.

The clinician, however, is less concerned with debates about jurisprudence than with the implications for clinical practice of the court decisions and state statutes dealing with informed consent. Although some aspects of the doctrine differ across jurisdictions, three central components – information, voluntariness, and competency – are always present.

Information

The need for some clarification of the requirement that information be provided to patients was apparent from the inception of informed consent law. In response to the question, "What should I tell my patients?" a number of possible standards of disclosure were proposed: "complete" information (although almost everyone recognized the impossibility of meeting such a standard); all information that *this patient* might want to know (which appeared to require some mind reading on the part of the physician); whatever information a "reasonable patient" might want to know; and whatever information a "reasonable practitioner" would ordinarily divulge. The legal standard varies from state to state, but almost all jurisdictions have selected one of the latter two options.[5]

In practical terms, these standards have tended to converge in a widely accepted set of guidelines. Whether measured according to the practice of the "reasonable practitioner," or the desires of the equally mythical "reasonable patient," most courts agree that the physician must convey the nature of the treatment proposed, its potential risks and benefits, and the presence of any alternatives (including the alternative of no treatment) and their risks and benefits. The risks to be disclosed are often conceptualized as those risks that a reasonable patient or practitioner would find material to decision making. As a rule of thumb, risks that are either exceptionally common (eg, extrapyramidal symptoms with neuroleptic medications) or serious, even if rare (eg, death following electroconvulsive therapy), ought to be disclosed. The only exceptions to these disclosure requirements are in emergencies, when the time taken to obtain a consent might endanger the patient or others; when the patient waives the right to be informed; when the disclosure itself might directly harm the patient; and, as will be discussed below, when the patient is incompetent to decide about treatment.[6]

The usual objections of psychiatrists to the requirement for disclosure is that the mentally ill are especially prone to misinterpret this information. Paranoid patients, it is argued, are particularly likely to seize on an enumeration of risks as confirmatory evidence that the proposed treatment is part of a diabolical scheme to cause them harm. Others, including depressed patients, may be put off by an outpouring of information, and by the expectation that they will act on the data they receive, at a time when passive acquiescence is the most they can offer and a dependent posture would be comforting.

Without denying the validity of these objections (while recognizing that they have yet to be proven empirically), we must note that our society has chosen to take the chance that the treatment of some patients may suffer for the potential gain of greater participation by all patients in decisions about their care. The task of the clinician, therefore, is to meet the legal requirements while advancing patients' treatment. This can best be done by individualized disclosure — a process that demands the active involvement of the psychiatrist in the consent transaction. As the required information is being conveyed, the clinician should be monitoring the patient's responses to the disclosure. If unrealistic fears are being evoked, they should be undercut. If the patient feels overwhelmed by the data and uncertain what to do with it, the basis for that feeling of helplessness should be explored, just as it is in any other therapeutic encounter. In essence, instead of being seen as a legal formality superimposed on the patient's treatment, the informed consent disclosure should be seen as part of the treatment itself.

There are a number of implications of this approach to disclosure. Given the need to assess patients' reactions as the information is conveyed, the use of written consent forms as the sole means of disclosure should be shunned. (Of course, they may have a useful adjunctive role in allowing patients to reflect on what they were told and to formulate questions that can be answered subsequently.) Similarly, the informed consent transaction should not be relegated to a member of the treatment team who is unlikely to be sensitive to patients' idiosyncratic areas of concern. If a patient's primary therapist is the prescribing psychiatrist, then the psychiatrist should obtain the consent directly. If the therapist is a nonpsychiatric clinician, the consent transaction should take place with both the primary therapist and the psychiatrist present.

Empirical studies of the informed consent process in psychiatry and general medicine have suggested that patients often have a great deal of difficulty absorbing the information provided to them.[7] Although most of these studies were seriously flawed (they tended not to monitor disclosure, thus raising questions as to whether patients were actually told about the material on which they were later tested,[8] they do point to another area of concern for the clinician. Informed consent law does not require that patients actually understand what they are told in order for a consent to be considered valid. At most, the law asks that the disclosure be made in such a manner that a reasonable person would understand it and that any obvious misunderstanding be corrected.[9] If the consent transaction is to be turned to therapeutic advantage, however, and if subsequent noncompliance on the basis of erroneous knowledge is to be prevented, there would appear to be adequate clinical grounds to insist that understanding, and not merely disclosure, is the goal.

To that end, psychiatrists should attempt to monitor patients' cognitive understanding in the same way that they tune in to the emotional effects of the information. A few questions about salient elements of the disclosure can quickly reveal to the clinician whether the patient in fact understands. If he does not, every effort should be made to present the data again in a manner that the patient can assimilate. Just this kind of feedback process has been lacking in most studies of informed consent, which suggests that optimism is still warranted about the potential of patients to learn about their treatment, if a genuine attempt is made to teach them.

The issue of documentation of the disclosure often arises. The desire for legally binding proof that an informed consent transaction has taken place has led many facilities to adopt written consent forms, which are signed by the patient (and sometimes by the therapist) at the conclusion of the disclosure. Unfortunately, since they are seen as legal documents, these forms are often devised largely by the facilities' lawyers. The product is a complex tangle of clinical information and legal boilerplate that is often impenetrable for patients. Further, once the forms exist, there is a tendency for clinicians to rely on them as the exclusive source of disclosure. As a result, the fears of all sides in the informed consent controversy are realized: patients do not achieve a real understanding of the proposed treatment and thus are not able to participate in the selection of alternative forms of care; and the information they do receive, compounded as it is with legalisms, is likely to arouse unjustified fears and discourage compliance.

Nor is a signed consent form an ironclad protection against suit. It may merely constitute evidence that a crucial datum was *not* disclosed, or that everything was conveyed in a form unintelligible to the average person. A far better alternative is for the psychiatrist to make a handwritten note in the patient's chart shortly after informed consent has been obtained, briefly outlining the scope of the discussion and the nature of the patient's response. This is likely to provide just as adequate legal documentation of the disclosure, without the liabilities of written consent forms.

A final consideration relates to the temporal nature of disclosure. Although the law's view of the consent process is basically cross-sectional — that is, at one point in time patient and psychiatrist come together, information is provided, questions are asked, and consent is obtained — the reality of clinical care is that information is often provided over a period of time. In place of an informed consent *event*, most patients experience an informed consent *process*.[10] Attempts to deny the reality, and even the desirability, of this structure of the consent process, in order to conform to legal suppositions, should be resisted. Information provided over time allows patients to consider options carefully, discuss them with others, raise questions, and to become comfortable with their ultimate decision in a way that is not possible when disclosure and consent all take place on the same day. One moment in time may be seen, for formal purposes, as the day on which consent occurred, but patients should be encouraged to consider the question well before that day, as well as to raise questions and to continue the dialogue even after an initial consent has been obtained.

Voluntariness

The requirement that consent be uncoerced is usually the least discussed aspect of the doctrine of informed consent. In part, this reflects the complexity of the concept. It may seem straightforward that coercion has occurred when a patient is threatened with termination of welfare benefits for refusing to take medication, but such situations rarely occur. In fact, therapists frequently bemoan their impotence in exercising any leverage over their patients' decisions about complying with recommendations for treatment. Nonetheless, some mentally ill persons may be particularly susceptible to less overt forms of coercion that may raise cause for concern.

Patients with marked passivity and dependency, whether as a result of personality disorders or such illnesses as chronic schizophrenia, and patients with impaired intellectual functioning may accede to pressures from their therapists or families to consent to treatment that they would otherwise have refused. The key here (although it constitutes an extraordinarily difficult task) is to distinguish between legitimate exhortation and illegitimate coercion. A psychiatrist certainly has the right — even the obligation — to encourage a patient to comply with treatment that will be in his/her best interests. That encouragement crosses the border of coercion only when there is an implied or explicit threat that the patient will be punished in some way for a failure to comply.

The sorts of punishments involved can range from overt to quite subtle. A patient might be told, for example, that the therapist will not support the application for disability benefits if he/she fails to take the medication prescribed. The evidence of coercion here is rather gross. More subtly, however, the therapist's tone may imply a withdrawal of interest and psychological support should the patient refuse an alteration in medication. Both of these examples represent coercion, although in the second case the law would be hard put to prove that the patient's voluntary choice had been impaired. Thus, coercion is as much an ethical as a legal matter. Therapists must examine their own feelings about the patient and the implicit messages they convey to ensure that there is no threat of retaliation for a disfavored choice. There are, of course, circumstances in which a psychiatrist may be justified in terminating treatment of a patient who repeatedly refuses to take medications that are considered essential, a complex subject discussed at length elsewhere.[6]

Competency

The law requires that a patient be legally competent to decide about treatment before a consent can be considered binding. Conversely, the consent of an incompetent, should adverse effects occur, may provide no protection from an allegation of negligence. Given that many psychiatric patients suffer from serious impairment of their cognition, psychiatrists are rightly concerned about their obligations in this area.

Unfortunately, the law of competency suffers from a great deal of imprecision. Competency is undefined in most states or is described in such vague terms as "able to care for his person and property."[11] Further, even when statutory descriptions of competency exist, they tend to refer to global conceptions of competency, that is, competency to function in society in general, rather than to the specific question of competency to consent to treatment. Suggestions for dealing with potential incompetency, therefore, must take into account the uncertainties of the current state of the law.

In general, all adult patients are presumed to be competent to manage their own affairs. (The definition of an adult for the purpose of consent to psychiatric treatment, however, may vary and in some states it may be as low as age 12.) This presumption falls in two circumstances: 1) when a court has declared the person legally incompetent, in which case a substituted consent must be obtained regardless of the person's functional capacity at that moment; and 2) when the psychiatrist has reason to believe that the patient's ability to participate in the informed consent process may be impaired. In the latter case, it is incumbent on the psychiatrist to evaluate the patient further and to take appropriate measures.

A problem is immediately apparent. Since the states have not clearly defined competency, the psychiatrist may be at a loss to know how to begin his evaluation. The author (in collaboration with Loren Roth, MD) has elsewhere suggested a model of evaluating competency that might be useful in such circumstances.[11] In increasing order of stringency, one can ask whether the patient can: 1) evidence a choice concerning treatment; 2) achieve a factual understanding of the issues at stake; 3) rationally manipulate the information that is provided to him or her; and 4) appreciate the nature of the situation and the consequences of the decision. The failure to meet any of these standards raises sufficient doubt about the patient's competency that a judicial determination may be called for.

Should the court find a patient incompetent, it can then appoint a guardian with the power to consent to treatment in his stead. Alternatively, the court itself can grant authorization for treatment to proceed. (One state supreme court has decided that *only* a court has the power to offer a substitute consent for treatment with neuroleptics.[12]) The clinician then engages in the informed consent process with the substitute decision maker rather than with the patient.

Although this is the theory of how to deal with an incompetent patient, the practice is often quite different. A competency hearing is a legal proceeding that usually requires the assistance of counsel. Its cost may range up to $1000. Many families are unable to afford this magnitude of legal fees and alternative legal services may be unavailable. For older, chronic patients, it is likely that no family exists to pursue a competency determination.[13] The onus may then fall on the facility, which may also lack the resources to pursue the issue. Further, even if a court hearing is obtained, there may be no one willing to serve as the guardian of an indigent incompetent. (Some states overcome this problem by establishing guardianship services that accept responsibility for indigents.[14])

Because of these problems, the question of competency for the consenting patient is usually ignored. Only when the patient refuses, in most cases, is the question of competency raised, and then only if the refusal is likely to have significant, deleterious consequences. Since the likelihood is miniscule that an indigent incompetent will ever sue for adverse consequences resulting from treatment, most practitioners feel secure in this approach to the problem.

The practical difficulties in living up to the expectations of informed consent law concerning competency are troubling. When a legally authorized, substituted consent is not obtained, the individual therapist should not take sole responsibility for the decision to ignore a patient's apparent incompetency. The issue should be raised with the facility's administration and a decision should be made, preferably after consultation with legal counsel, as to the proper procedures to follow. If the decision is to proceed with treatment of the incompetent consenter, an extra burden falls on the therapist. Ordinarily, competent persons can afford themselves some measure of protection from unwanted adverse effects of treatment. That may not be the case for the incompetent patient. It therefore devolves on the therapist to weigh treatment decisions with an extra measure of care, taking into account as much as possible what a competent patient's view of potential side effects would be. With no one else to protect the patient's interests, the clinician must assume the role.

The Special Question of Tardive Dyskinesia

For psychiatrists, no aspect of informed consent has been as troubling as discussing the risk of tardive dyskinesia (TD) with patients. It is widely assumed that mention of TD when neuroleptics are first prescribed, particularly if patients are acutely disturbed, will induce patients disproprotionately and unreasonably to reject treatment. The literature reflects this anxiety, as a number of authors have suggested waiting periods of up to several months before the question of TD is raised.[15-16] The justification that usually is offered for this practice is that TD is unlikely to occur soon after the implementation of neuroleptic therapy and therefore does not constitute a risk at the time that consent is first obtained. It is reasoned that after some months of treatment, patients more rationally will be able to decide whether the risk of TD is worth the benefits of continued treatment.

Despite the appeal that this practice has for psychiatrists, its adoption is problematic. Fear that a patient may reject treatment if information about risks is provided has never been a legally accepted justification for withholding those data. To the contrary, allowing patients to make their own decisions about which risks they wish to take is precisely the point of informed consent law. If the fear is that the patient will be likely to distort the meaning of the information, on the other hand, then he may well not be competent to decide about treatment and a substitute decision maker should be appointed. In addition, for a large number of patients who have been treated previously with neuroleptics, it is *not* true that the period of risk does not begin until several months after the initiation of treatment. The risk of TD is now believed to be (at least in part) a function of the total lifetime dose of neuroleptic medication. Even the first dose, therefore, in someone who has been treated previously, incrementally increases the risk. Finally, there is something inherently deceptive about treating someone with an effective medication on which they may come to rely, only to reveal to them, after stabilization has occurred, a new set of risks of which they were previously ignorant.

The strongest justification for initially withholding information about TD probably comes from the realities of the treatment of incompetent patients discussed earlier. As long as these patients are being treated without the consent of a substitute decision maker, with the psychiatrist presumably acting in their best interests, some delay in discussing TD may be acceptable. But clinicians who employ this widely heralded practice should be aware that its ethical basis is tenuous and that there is little legal support.

THE RIGHT TO REFUSE PSYCHIATRIC TREATMENT

Legal Aspects of Refusal

One who was otherwise ignorant of the history of mental health care in the United States might assume, on the basis of the previous discussion of the law of consent, that psychiatric patients have always had the right to decide whether to accept or to reject proffered care. For a variety of reasons, however, this has not been the case. In many states, until the middle of this century, commitment to a mental hospital resulted in an automatic declaration of incompetency; superintendents were frequently appointed as guardians and thereby gave nominal consent for patients' care.[17] Even when this formal finding of incompetency was not made, it was generally assumed that the mentally ill were unable to decide rationally about their care, and that commitment (or perhaps even voluntary admission) was all the predicate that was needed to proceed with treatment. This rationale was reinforced by the generally accepted assumption that the purpose of commitment was to treat the mentally ill.

In recent years, however, in response to the dictates of the judiciary, which has had difficulties accepting the constitutional validity of commitment solely for the purpose of treatment, involuntary hospitalization has come to assume a function closer to that of preventive detention. Commitment laws now almost uniformly require that patients be dangerous to themselves or to others before they can be hospitalized involuntarily.[18] Many judges and lawyers, consequently, have come to view the purpose of commitment as preventing the predicted danger from materializing, rather than as treating the underlying illness. If protection is the goal, and that goal can be realized in many cases simply by quarantining the patient within the walls of a mental hospital, they ask: Should not patients have a right to refuse treatment that does not further advance the state's interest?

Augmenting this argument, which in effect calls for an extension of the law of informed consent to the mentally ill, were some very realistic concerns about the quality of care in many state institutions. Documentation exists of instances in which psychotropic medications were used inappropriately, for purposes of punishment or sedation, rather than as components of an integrated plan of care. When combined with the risk of substantial side effects from neuroleptic drugs, particularly tardive dyskinesia, state hospital conditions provided a powerful impetus for the mental health bar to press their claims that involuntary medication violates patients' constitutional rights. [19]

The legal issues at stake are complex. In various cases across the country, it has been argued that patient's constitutional rights to refuse treatment derive from the right to privacy, the right to liberty guaranteed by the fourteenth amendment, the right to equal protection of the laws, the right to generate thoughts freely, and the right to be free from cruel and unusual punishment. In general, federal and state courts have looked favorably on these arguments (particularly the first two) and the number of states is growing in which a judicially sanctioned right to refuse exists. [20]

On the other hand, no court has found that involuntary mental patients have an absolute right, under all circumstances, to refuse medication. (Voluntary patients probably do have an absolute right to refuse, although they can be discharged if their refusal stymies effective treatment.) All involved agree that in emergencies, when a patient's behavior threatens his/her own life or safety or that of others, medication can be administered. The courts, however, have differed on other circumstances in which the right to refuse can be abridged, and on the procedures to be followed in those instances. The federal Third Circuit Court of Appeals, ruling in the New Jersey case of *Rennie v. Klein*, has held that patients' refusals can be overridden when an internal review by the department of mental health concludes that treatment is warranted. [21] In contrast, the federal First Circuit Court of Appeals in the Massachusetts case of *Rogers v. Mills* supports the position that only a judicial hearing at which the patient is found to be incompetent provides justification for ignoring patients' wishes in regard to medication. [22]

Complicating this situation are statutes in many states that grant patients some degree of decision-making power about their treatment, or that provide alternative means of dealing with refusals. In Utah, for example, competency is decided at the time of commitment and the psychiatrist is thereafter empowered to prescribe treatment as he thinks appropriate. [23] A similar procedure in Florida was deemed to violate the state's constitution. [24] In New York, administrative regulations established a review process within the Office of Mental Health that closely resembles the procedures endorsed by the court in *Rennie*.[25]

As of this writing, there is little uniformity in either law or practice from jurisdiction to jurisdiction. Clinicians are advised to keep up to date on developments in their state, to ensure that their facility has a clearly defined policy for dealing with refusal, and to follow that policy. In the absence of any state law on the matter, it seems advisable to require, at a minimum, that a psychiatrist not directly involved in the care of a refusing patient evaluate the situation and concur in the wisdom of the proposed treatment before it is administered over a patient's objections.

There is some hope for clarification of this issue in the next several years. Although the Supreme Court ducked two chances in 1982 to decide whether there was a constitutional basis for the right to refuse treatment, its actions in one of those cases, *Rennie v. Klein*, suggested its views on the issue. The Supreme Court remanded *Rennie* for reconsideration by the Third Circuit in light of the Supreme Court's opinion in another mental health case, *Youngberg v. Romeo*.[26] In *Romeo*, the court indicated that it was willing to give great deference to the decisions of mental health professionals concerning the necessity for limiting the liberty interests of patients. (The case addressed, in relevant part, the use of bodily restraints.) No particular procedures were found to be constitutionally required. The remand of *Rennie* appears to give the court's approval to a fairly liberal use of physician discretion in dealing with refusals, although many years of litigation lie ahead before the court's stance is likely to be clarified.

Clinical Aspects of Refusal

The preceding discussion should provide ample evidence of the law's inadequacies in dealing with patients' refusal of treatment. To look to the law for a solution when confronted by a refusal is to invite confusion, prolonged court proceedings, neglect of patients' clinical needs, and a rupture of the therapeutic alliance between patients and psychiatrists. Rather than asking how a patient's refusal can be overridden, therefore, it makes more sense for the clinician to inquire how refusals can be prevented in the first place, and how they can be managed clinically once they have occurred.[27]

Unfortunately, the empirical data with which to answer these questions are largely lacking.[28] Only a few studies have assessed the reasons psychiatric patients refuse treatment. Appelbaum and Gutheil found that refusal was a common occurrence in the inpatient setting, that it was often provoked by a combination of intrapsychic and environmental factors, and that the vast majority of refusals were self-limited.[29] Marder et al have correlated refusal in a small sample with severity of psychotic illness.[30] There have been no studies on the clinical management of refusal.

Thus, we are forced to rely upon clinical experience and the related literature on patient noncompliance in medical and psychiatric settings to formulate an approach to this problem.[31]

The message of the existing literature is that refusal is not a unitary phenomenon. Patients refuse for a wide variety of reasons, some related to their illnesses and some not related to them. Thus, when attempting to deal with a patient's refusal, the clinician must again individualize the approach. An initial effort must be made to uncover *this patient's* reasons for refusal and to deal with them accordingly.

The first area that should be explored is the patient's understanding of the purpose, benefits, and risks of the medication. Many psychiatric patients are grossly uninformed about their treatment.[32-33] Research with medical patients has demonstrated that anger over the failure of caregivers to inform patients about their treatment, or the mistaken impressions that flourish in the absence of facts can precipitate patients' refusal of treatment.[34] In essence, the first step for the psychiatrist is to ask: Has an adequate informed consent process been undertaken with this patient? Conversely, some refusal may be aborted entirely by the provision of information, and the ascertainment that the patient in fact understands what has been conveyed at the very beginning of treatment may be the most effective prophylactic measure.

Part of the inquiry into patients' understanding of prescribed treatment must transcend factual issues. Patients may have idiosyncratic views of their medication which exist alongside otherwise appropriate understandings of the usual risks and benefits.[35] Many patients, for example, are concerned with the possibility of addiction to neuroleptics. Others see acceptance as an acknowledgment of their chronicity, a conclusion they feel compelled to resist. Not infrequently, patients are concerned to demonstrate that *they* and not the medication are the "cause" of their improvement. All of these issues are susceptible to therapeutic exploration, but only if they are first uncovered by careful questioning of the patient.

If the patient has a reasonable grasp of the facts of treatment, one must next consider whether reality-based concerns are motivating refusal. The psychiatrist should inquire about the existence of unpleasant side effects, particularly those whose presence the patient might not spontaneously report. These include akinesia and akathisia, the latter of which has been linked to failure to take medications,[36] or a generally dysphoric response to the drug.[37] Sexual dysfunction, about which patients may be reluctant to talk, must be sought after specifically. Side effects experienced with similar medications in the past may also lead patients to refuse medication. The provision of an antiparkinsonian drug, or the substitution of another medication less likely to cause the side effect in question, can preclude the necessity of a lengthy court proceeding.

In addition to side effects, one must consider the dynamic setting of the psychiatrist-patient relationship.[38] Patients' transference to psychiatrist or other staff members may inhibit acceptance of treatment. An agreement to take medication may be seen as a sign of submission to or merger with the therapist. Or refusal may recreate an early, unresolved struggle with a primary object in the patient's life. In either event, the refusal should be seen as part of the treatment process and should be dealt with as any other transference phenomenon. Even if it were possible to override the patient's decision in a case like this, the effect would only be to bury information about the state of transference that the refusal has brought to light — information which may only be uncovered laboriously at a later point in the therapy.

In exploring the underlying bases of refusal, it is important to recognize that patients' views about the desirability of treatment are not always congruent with those of their psychiatrists. Patients may see primary gains in remaining ill, including a somewhat pleasurable grandiose state,[39] and the defenses against depression and anger that their psychosis may represent. Unless recognized and addressed, this difference in values can undermine the therapeutic alliance and vitiate efforts at treatment. In many cases, of course, there are also secondary gains involved. These may include the bed and board available in the hospital as long as one is sick enough to warrant inpatient treatment, or for outpatients, the promise of the continued attentions of one's therapist. Patients can also use refusal, and the associated deterioration, as a way of getting back at family members, perhaps by provoking guilt.

Finally, when investigating the roots of a patient's refusal of treatment, the role of family and close friends should not be ignored. Family members may encourage refusal, often covertly, as an element of their own denial about the severity of the patient's illness or as an angry means of retaliating at the patient. On the other hand, family members who are sympathetic to the goals of treatment can be enlisted to undercut patients' fears of treatment and to support them during the decision-making process. Friends may play similar roles. If they share an organized belief system with the patient that is antagonistic to the use of medications (eg, macrobiotic food enthusiasts), they may undermine the patient's trust in the treating psychiatrist. In other circumstances, they can be enlisted to persuade the patient to cooperate in his/her care.

There are hints from several courts, including the U.S. Supreme Court, that the more radical decisions concerning the right to refuse treatment may give way to a position that recognizes some rights in this area, but allows them to be overcome by professional discretion. At its worst, such an outcome could mean a return to an automatic rejection of patients' attempts to shape their treatment and a corresponding reliance on involuntary medication. If psychiatrists see treatment refusal as strictly a legal issue, and if their concern is solely with the extent of the powers granted to them by the courts, this will undoubtedly occur in some institutions. In contrast, the clinical approach to refusal suggested here holds out the possibility of a different outcome.

Treating patients' refusals as uniquely motivated acts conveys to patients a measure of respect for their opinions. It is also consistent with the ethical principles that underlie informed consent law in general: a respect for patients as persons and a recognition of the desirability of maximizing their responsible, autonomous functioning. It is unfortunate that the law, rather than psychiatry, has been seen as the champion of these values, given that they inhere in good clinical practice. Any retreat by the courts from an endorsement of a comprehensive right to refuse treatment should be viewed as an opportunity for psychiatrists to espouse and implement these values, without the clumsy overlay of legalisms and endless judicial procedures.

The approach to psychopharmacologic practice advocated by this chapter reflects the belief that it is desirable on both practical and ethical grounds for patients to be well-informed participants in decision making about their treatment. The law sometimes facilitates that process and sometimes hinders it, but the opportunity is always present for psychiatrists to advance this collaborative approach to patient care.

REFERENCES

1. Meisel A: The expansion of liability for medical accidents: From negligence to strict liability by way of informed consent. *Nebraska Law Review* 1977; 56:51–152.
2. *Salgo v. Leland Stanford Jr. University Board of Trustees*, 154 Cal.App.2d 560, 317 P.2d 170 (1957).
3. *Natanson v. Kline*, 186 Kan. 393, 350 P.2d 1093; *rehearing denied* 187 Kan. 186, 354 P.2d 670 (1960).
4. Meisel A, Roth LH, Lidz CW: Toward a model of the legal doctrine of informed consent. *Am J Psychiatry* 1977;134:285–289.
5. Miller LJ: Informed consent: I. *JAMA* 1980;244:2100–2103.
6. Gutheil TG, Appelbaum PS: *Clinical Handbook of Psychiatry and the Law.* New York, McGraw-Hill, 1982.
7. Appelbaum PS, Mirkin SA, Bateman AL: Competency to consent to psychiatric hospitalization: An empirical assessment. *Am J Psychiatry* 1981;138: 1170–1176.
8. Meisel A, Roth LH: What we do and do not know about informed consent. *JAMA* 1981;246:2473–2477.
9. Simpson RE: Informed consent: From disclosure to patient participation in medical decisionmaking. *Northwestern University Law Review* 1981;76: 172–207.
10. Lidz C, Meisel A, Zerubavel E, et al: *Informed Consent: A Study of Psychiatric Decisionmaking.* New York, Guilford Press, 1983.
11. Appelbaum PS, Roth LH: Competency to consent to research: A psychiatric overview. *Arch Gen Psychiatry* 1982;39:951–958.
12. *In the Matter of Guardianship of Richard Roe III*, 421 N.E.2d 40 (Mass. 1981).
13. Gutheil TG, Shapiro R, St. Clair RL: Legal guardianship in drug refusal: An illusory solution. *Am J Psychiatry* 1980;137:347–352.
14. Axilbund MT: *Exercising Judgment for the Disabled: Report of an Inquiry into Limited Guardianship, Public Guardianship, and Adult Protective Services in Six States.* Washington, DC, Commission on the Mentally Disabled, American Bar Association, 1979.
15. DeVeaugh-Geiss J: Informed consent for neuroleptic therapy. *Am J Psychiatry* 1979;136:959–962.
16. Sovner R, DiMascio A, Berkowitz D, et al: Tardive dyskinesia and informed consent. *Psychosomatics* 1978;19:172–177.
17. Brakel S, Rock R: *The Mentally Disabled and the Law* (revised edition). Chicago, University of Chicago Press, 1971.
18. Schwitzgebel RK: Survey of state commitment statues, in McGarry AL, Schwitzgebel RK, Lipsett PD, et al: *Civil Commitment and Social Policy: An Evaluation of the Massachusetts Mental Health Reform Act of 1970*, Rockville, MD, National Institute of Mental Health, 1981.
19. Appelbaum PS, Gutheil TG: The right to refuse treatment: The real issue is quality of care. *Bull Am Acad Psychiatry Law* 1981;9:199–202.
20. Brooks AD: The constitutional right to refuse antipsychotic medications. *Bull Am Acad Psychiatry Law* 1980;8:179–221.
21. *Rennie v. Klein*, 462 F. Supp. 1131 (D.N.J. 1978), 476 F. Supp. 1294 (D.N.J. 1979), *aff'd in part*, 653 F.2d 836 (3rd Cir. 1981), *vacated and remanded* 102 S.Ct. 3506 (1982).
22. *Rogers v. Okin*, 478 F. Supp. 1342 (D. Mass. 1979), *aff'd in part*, 634 F.2d 250 (1st Cir. 1980), *vacated and remanded* sub nom *Mills v. Rogers*, 102 S.Ct. 2442 (1982).

23. Appelbaum PS: *A.E. & R.R.*: Utah's compromise on the right to refuse treatment. *Hosp Community Psychiatry* 1981;32:167–168.
24. *Bentley v. State ex. rel. Rogers*, 398 So.2d 992 (Fla. App. 1981).
25. 14 N.Y.C.R.R. 27.8.
26. *Romeo v. Youngberg*, No. 76-3429 (E.D. Pa. 1978), 644 F.2d 147 (3d Cir. 1980), *vacated and remanded*, 102 S.Ct. 24 (1982).
27. Appelbaum PS, Gutheil TG: Clinical aspects of treatment refusal. *Comp Psychiatry* 1982;23:560–566.
28. Roth LH, Appelbaum PS: What we do and do not know about treatment refusals in mental institutions, in Doudera AE, Swazey JT (eds): *Refusing Treatment in Mental Institutions: Values in Conflict*. Ann Arbor, AUPHA Press, 1982.
29. Appelbaum PS, Gutheil TG: Drug refusal: A study of psychiatric inpatients. *Am J Psychiatry* 1980;137:340–346.
30. Marder SR, Mebane A, Chien CP, et al: A comparison of patients who refuse and consent to neuroleptic treatment. *Am J Psychiatry* 1983;140:470–472.
31. Blackwell B: Treatment adherence. *Br J Psychiatry* 1976;129:513–531.
32. Geller JL: State hospital patients and their medication — Do they know what they take? *Am J Psychiatry* 1982;139:611–615.
33. Soskis DA: Schizophrenic and medical inpatients as informed drug consumers. *Arch Gen Psychiatry* 1978;35:645–647.
34. Appelbaum PS, Roth LR: Treatment refusal in medical hospitals, in *Making Health Care Decisions, Vol 2: Appendix*. Washington, DC, President's Commission for the Study of Ethical Problems in Medicine and Biochemical and Behavioral Research, 1982.
35. Stimson GV: Obeying doctor's orders: A view from the other side. *Soc Sci Med* 1974;8:97–104.
36. Van Putten T: Why do schizophrenic patients refuse to take their drugs? *Arch Gen Psychiatry* 1974;31:67–72.
37. Van Putten T, May PRA, Marder SR, et al: Subjective response to antipsychotic drugs. *Arch Gen Psychiatry* 1981;38:187–190.
38. Havens LL: Some difficulties in giving schizophrenic and borderline patients medication. *Psychiatry* 1968;31:44–50.
39. Van Putten T, Crumptom E, Yale C: Drug refusal in schizophrenia and the wish to be crazy. *Arch Gen Psychiatry* 1976;33:1443–1446.

3

The Psychiatric Laboratory

Mark S. Gold
A. Carter Pottash
Irl Extein

All psychiatrists utilize the laboratory and laboratory testing to a certain extent. Until recently, this utilization has been limited and predominantly focused on medical advances that occurred more than 25 years ago. The screening of new psychiatric patients and hospital admissions for syphilis, gross medical (SMA-22), and gross infectious or hematopoietic disease (urinalysis; CBC with differential) and pregnancy testing (females) is so commonplace that most psychiatrists instinctively order these tests in new outpatient referrals and all inpatients. This use of the laboratory continues in spite of changes that have occurred in the patterns and types of psychiatric referrals and frequency of disease entities having a psychiatric presentation. The yield for all laboratory tests changes over time. For example, nearly all new admissions have a test (RPR) for syphilis wherein the yield is closer to zero than it is to 1%. But no psychiatrist would want to miss syphilis even to prevent embarrassment and malpractice suits which are not defensible. This "admission profile" CBC, SMA, U/A, RPR, and pregnancy test is not a use of the laboratory or modern medicine; it is preventive malpractice. When the laboratory is used in this manner, it is not unusual to find that the busy practitioner has not reviewed even these "severely limited" data very carefully. Consultants, nurses, or even future admissions reveal that suspicious data existed which could have led to a correct diagnosis. Remembering that as many as one of three major depressive episodes

29

turn out to be secondary to a known medical or related illness, it is difficult to imagine that a psychiatrist can make a differential diagnosis and rule out of active consideration all competing illnesses with this admission panel and screening physical exam.

The usefulness of the laboratory is not limited to one type of test or procedure. It is not limited to new evaluations or admissions, but impacts in many areas of psychiatric practice. However, it is only recently that psychiatrists have begun to recognize the relatively wide scope of these applications. Many psychiatrists fail to see the laboratory and only see specific tests. Of those psychiatrists who utilize existing laboratory resources, many become familiar with only one application of the laboratory to inpatient practice, such as use of therapeutic drug monitoring, neurochemical testing of urine, applications of psychoneuroendocrinology to diagnosis, identification of biologically relevant state markers, etc. When we begin to review the area, we see that the clinical laboratory is a major component of the practice of medicine.

Laboratory tests in medicine vary with respect to sensitivity and specificity. The sensitivity of a test, as we will use the term here, describes the ability of the test to correctly identify a percentage of patients with a given syndrome (true positives) through an abnormal or positive result. The remaining unidentified patients are the false negatives. *Specificity* is a measure of the test's ability to exclude false positive patients. The *confidence level* describes the likelihood that an abnormal laboratory result in a given population will identify a true positive patient. Contrary to beliefs held by many psychiatrists, for a test to be useful in clinical practice or laboratory medicine, neither perfect (or 100%) sensitivity and specificity nor confidence level is necessary or even expected. What would be the sensitivity, specificity or diagnostic confidence for a chief complaint (eg, depression) or working descriptive syndromal diagnosis (eg, major depression)? It is the physician's responsibility to become familiar with the uses and limitations of each particular laboratory test in every specific psychiatric syndrome. For these and other reasons, laboratory tests can never replace physicians. Diagnosis in laboratory medicine is often based on the review of the results derived from a number of unrelated tests, each with a different sensitivity and specificity. The best example of this is the use of the laboratory in the diagnosis of various endocrinopathies or autoimmune diseases. Some of the most commonly used laboratory tests in these diseases have very low sensitivities or specificities, although the results of sequential, provocative or additive tests can make important contributions to the diagnostic process.

Many psychiatrists entered psychiatry with the hope of leaving the stethoscope, physical examination, and blood and urine tests to others. Diagnostic testing is important in modern psychiatric practice; which specific tests are useful or outdated will remain in flux.

DIAGNOSTIC TESTING

Drug Abuse Detection

The ability of clinicians to rapidly document the abuse of prescribed or illicit drugs is critical in accurate diagnosis and development of appropriate treatment plans for psychiatric patients. Given the fact that most psychiatric admissions have used drugs and/or alcohol, maximizing detection is the main issue. Failure to detect drugs of abuse results in failure to address the diagnostic issue of a drug-related, drug-contributed or drug-independent syndrome. A blood alcohol test and additional testing for particular drugs of abuse should be ordered on all new evaluations, patients, or admissions unless there is a good reason not to.

General medical laboratories performing routine "drug screens" frequently generate perplexing results that are difficult for clinicians to understand. For example, urine samples from known abusers and patients maintained on methadone frequently return with negative results. Patients rarely admit to drug use, but when they complain of taking or smoking something and becoming paranoid, manic, depressed, psychotic, etc, the drug screen may be negative. Important and commonly abused psychoactive compounds, such as methaqualone (Quaalude), marijuana, tetrahydrocannabinol (THC), phencyclidine (PCP or "angel dust") or heroin (morphine), are not tested for in most drug screens. Other important drugs of abuse, such as amphetamine and cocaine, cannot be detected in low doses in the typical drug screen. These problems are not a result of laboratory error or incompetency, but instead reflect limitations of the most commonly used method for drug abuse screening. The consumer beware: In this case the psychiatrist is the consumer. Psychiatrists are unaware of the sensitivity of the various drug abuse detection tests or whether the test they ordered can detect the drug they are trying to measure in order to decide on drug-induced, drug-related or naturally occurring etiologies. The failure to order the correct test(s) or to understand the limitations of those ordered frequently results in misdiagnosis, confirming or adding to a psychiatric stigma and to treating someone who has a drug or alcohol problem in the wrong treatment program, or with the wrong medication. This failure perpetuates itself as the physician never learns what X, Y or Z drug is or is not, and he is supported by self-fulfilling prophecies. The patient who is psychotic, with a history consistent with schizophrenia or mania, who has a negative drug screen *and* responds to haloperidol, is a schizophrenic or manic: wrong. Cocaine, amphetamine, other stimulants, and PCP behave the same way.

Drugs can be detected in human urine by any of several analytical techniques, including colorimetry, gas chromatography, fluorometry, and antibody-based assays. High pressure liquid chromatography, gas chromatography with mass spectroscopy, and other specific techniques can be used to quantify and detect most drugs of abuse in blood. Quantitative and specific blood testing for cocaine and amphetamine can add to the clarity of diagnosis of affective states. Blood PCP is used in the differential diagnosis of psychotic states, and plasma methadone is used on admission to document safe dose and level of tolerance. Quantitative assays in blood, while sensitive and specific, are costly. They are critical in certain clinical situations and irrelevant in others. The routine drug screen performed by most general laboratories uses the rapid, inexpensive, thin layer chromatographic (TLC) technique; being fast and inexpensive are the TLC tests main virtues. This traditional toxicology urine screen is less than ideal for psychiatrists' use as a rapid documentation of subtoxic levels of a known or unknown drug in a random sample of urine. TLC screens are technically cumbersome and involve crude and highly interpretive methods. When the physician is testing for drugs that TLC methods can identify, when the quantities ingested are large, and when the sample is obtained shortly after the drug abuse event, the TLC tests may be useful. This is the case while other more specific and reliable testing is pending. TLC is of little or no use in testing for admission, forensic psychiatry, differential diagnosis or establishing a drug level baseline. Since identification in urine of the low dose use and abuse (the most common type of abuse in the psychiatric patient) is desired, antibody-based, gas chromatography (GC) capillary, or GC/MS (mass spectroscopy) methods are preferable. We have found urine antibody screening methods useful in most clinical situations to give a sensitivity and specificity up to 50 times superior to TLC results for certain drugs of abuse. In addition, antibody-based assays can readily identify synthetic opiates, marijuana, methaqualone, THC and high concentrations of PCP.

The clinical applications are clear and relate to the questions being asked by the hospital or psychiatrist. For example, identifying the psychotic patient who has used cocaine, amphetamine or PCP is of critical importance in the clinical setting. Many of these patients are unwilling or unable to admit to drug use and, when they do, the exact drug taken is always a mystery. Every psychiatrist recognizes that these drugs are in the differential diagnosis, but only a few will vigorously rule it out of active consideration with a detailed history and specific laboratory tests. In many cases, especially first break cases, both urine (antibody) and plasma (GC or GC/MS) testing should be ordered. In one recent study, 145 consecutive patients seen in the psychiatric emergency service of an urban public hospital were tested specifically for PCP. A surprisingly high 43% of the patients showed positive plasma PCP levels. In other reports, cocaine or cannabis has been shown to produce a clinical picture very similar to that seen in euphoric or manic states and in schizophrenia. Both drugs are easy to identify in blood and urine. The major reason that these tests are not utilized is the psychiatrists' false belief that a drug screen will suffice.

The treatment plan for the depressed patient who by testing is found to be in a post-stimulant state, a low-dose barbiturate or alcohol abuse state, or a person on a self-styled Quaalude or marijuana maintenance program, is specific and markedly different from that of the atypical or pure endogenously depressed patient, especially if the depression clears once the patient is off drugs of abuse. Similarly, drug-related or induced euphoric or psychotic states require special attention and specific treatment to prevent their continuance or recurrence. Patients minimize and rationalize drug use and deny the association of alcohol and other drugs with their chief complaint. Patient answers such as people drink, smoke pot, use X, Y, Z, and I do a little, can be evaluated with quantitative testing. Quantitative testing and a medication and drug-free trial can make the diagnosis and provide for effective aftercare.

Inpatient treatment units in hospitals, especially adolescent units, often set limits on acceptable behavior, including prohibitions against bringing drugs or alcohol onto the unit by patients or visitors, or taking drugs while in the hospital or on a hospital pass. In many hospitals, a common consequence of proven drug use is discharge of the patient or transfer to a more restrictive facility. Considering the false positives and negatives of TLC techniques and given the staff response to such drug use by inpatients, antibody-based assays or blood levels are indicated in such cases to preserve the integrity of the inpatient program, insure accuracy, and enable hospital staff to remove patients who are pretending to be in treatment but wasting valuable resources and needed bed space.

All analytical methods have limitations. Sample integrity, time of day of the sample, time and dose of the last drug ingestion, as well as drug structure, half-life, affinity for the brain and their lipophilic profile, all affect the length of time the drug can be detected in a urine sample. In psychiatry, supervised first voided urines are necessary. In addition, the measurement of urinary specific gravity should be done in all urine drug testing samples to eliminate the possibility that the sample has been tampered with and diluted with tap water.

In freestanding specialty hospitals where patients are generally referred for evaluation and treatment after failing in outpatient treatment, a complete drug abuse evaluation is essential. A comprehensive drug abuse evaluation includes, at a minimum, antibody-based tests for opiates (morphine equivalents), barbiturates, alcohol, amphetamine, benzodiazepines, methadone, phencyclidine (PCP), cocaine, cannabinoid (marijuana and THC), and methaqualone. Simultaneously, urine specific gravity is measured. Although a comprehensive drug abuse evaluation, including all the common drugs of abuse, is indicated in many cases, in some patients with a clear presenting symptom limited testing may be more cost effective. For example, evaluation of a newly admitted patient with natural or drug-related euphoria should at least include specific testing for amphetamines, cocaine, methadone, opiates, PCP, methaqualone and alcohol. Psychotic patients should be tested for amphetamines, barbiturates, cocaine and PCP. A minimum depressant drug abuse evaluation should include antibody testing for benzodiazepines methaqualone, barbiturates, cocaine and alcohol. Newly admitted adolescent patients usually are tested for amphetamines, barbiturates, benzodiazepines, cocaine, methaqualone, marijuana/THC, PCP, and alcohol, if a comprehensive drug abuse evaluation is not ordered. Positives by any method should be confirmed in duplicate and confirmed by a second, independent method. Patients admitted after first voided urine, in a suspected drug withdrawal, drug-intoxicated or drug-related psychosis should have blood testing immediately for the suspected drug(s), while the urine can be taken as soon as possible for comprehensive evaluation. First voided urine is preferred for demonstrating drug use, abuse or drug-related states. Once a comprehensive admission screen is completed, a repeat test can be readily interpreted by conparison with the initial laboratory findings.

Diagnostic Neuroendocrine Testing

In a typical depressive disorder, patients display both affective and "hypothalamic" symptoms. Affective symptoms may include depressed mood with a loss of interest, motivation, enjoyment and a prevailing attitude of pessimism, worthlessness, helplessness and hopelessness. Ruminative thinking, anhedonia and suicidal thoughts may be present. In addition, somatic symptoms which may be described as hypothalamic may be present, including anorexia, anergia, decreased libido and aggressive drive, insomnia with a sleep continuity disturbance, psychomotor changes (retardation or agitation) and a diurnal variation in symptoms.

Depression is the most common of psychiatric symptoms and occurs in many psychiatric illnesses which have depressed mood in common. A major depressive disorder can be distinguished by sleep and appetite disturbance and other hypothalamic signs and symptoms.[1-4] Major depression now can be subdivided[1-4] into unipolar and bipolar depressive illness on the basis of a past history of mania in bipolar illness, and into primary and secondary depression. Secondary depression and minor depressive illness occur in medical illness and in nonaffective psychiatric illness such as obsessive-compulsive neurosis, personality disorders, schizophrenia, drug and alcohol dependence, and sexual dysfunction, respectively. These categories have been helpful in improving diagnostic reliability between psychiatrists and reducing heterogeneity in diagnostic groups. They improve understanding of pathophysiology, and facilitate prediction of treatment response and prognosis. Meeting RDC or DSM-III criteria does not help the psychiatrist determine whether the illness is psychiatric or medical (eg, vitamin deficiency) or endocrinological (eg, hypothyroid), etc. Biological tests have been developed that can support a clinical impression or diagnosis as well as a primary, psychiatric etiology. A number of important biochemical subgroups of unipolar major depression can be identified with these biochemical tests.[5-15]

After medical, endocrinological and other tests are ordered and are proven negative, psychiatric diagnostic tests are then ordered, which are now clinically useful as confirmatory tests for diagnosis of active major depression and are adjuncts to assess and confirm responses to treatment. Of these diagnostic/prognostic tests, the most extensively studied and consistently reported abnormality in major depression is hypersecretion of cortisol and failure to suppress cortisol secretion after dexamethasone administration.[5-9,14,15]

Diurnal Cortisol Test (DCT)

The most frequently reported endocrine abnormality in depression is hypersecretion of cortisol. The DCT is a test of the hypothalamic-pituitary-adrenal (HPA) axis which measures cortisol levels and endogenous diurnal rhythm. Normal levels at 8 AM range from 10–25 $\mu g/100$ mL. In normal patients, diurnality is present and cortisol falls below 14 $\mu g/100$ mL by 4 PM and is significantly lower by midnight (< 6 $\mu g/mL$). In the test, the patient goes to bed and rises at his or her regular time. Plasma samples for cortisol by radioimmunoassay (RIA) are taken as frequently as possible, but at least by 8 AM, noon, 4 PM, and midnight.

In patients with major depression, there is excessive secretion of cortisol, increase of cortisol production rates, and cortisol secretion is above normal in every sample, although sometimes this is seen only in the 4 PM or midnight samples. The hypersecretion is not due to anxiety, psychotic decompensation, stress, or to a change in cortisol metabolism. In most cases of major depressive disorder, although there is hypersecretion of cortisol, diurnality is preserved. Failure to demonstrate normal diurnality, or finding a reversal of diurnality in a patient with endogenous depression, may be associated with "jet lag" or a major depression that is relatively nonresponsive to antidepressants.

Adrenal insufficiency is suggested by persistently low plasma cortisols. High values in all samples may suggest Cushing's syndrome. Both of these diagnoses have been made "by accident" in patients with a chief complaint of depression who were tested with the DCT.

The DCT is an independent test which identifies a different patient group than the dexamethasone suppression test (DST). Because the endorphin antagonist naltrexone produces depression and DCT hypersecretion, but with normal dexamethasone suppression test abnormalities, DCT may be a test for the endorphin subtype of depression.

Dexamethasone Suppression Test (DST)

The DST is another test of the HPA axis that has been extensively studied in psychiatric patients. The abnormalities seen in patients with affective disorders have been reported and reproduced by researchers all over the world. The DST is not perfect, but it is better than two psychiatrists agreeing that the patient has the diagnosis they saw in the psychiatric dictionary (DSM-III).

The patient receives 1 mg of dexamethasone orally at midnight. The patient may eat regularly. No subjective effects are reported from the test. Blood is then taken over the next 24 hours (a minimum sampling of 8 AM, noon, 4 PM, and midnight) for RIA plasma cortisol determination. The failure of dexamethasone to cause a normal suppression indicates significant limbic-hypothalamic-pituitary system dysfunction, similar to that observed in Cushing's syndrome and certain other specific physical illnesses. Elimination of any of these sample points decreases sensitivity. These patients are biological treatment responsive (eg, ADS, ECT).

Using the six-point DST in major depression, patients frequently are found who are suppressors when using only the 4 PM and midnight points but nonsuppressors when using all six points. Using the time-point 8 AM, noon, 4 PM, and midnight, one of three patients with primary major depression fail to suppress. The sensitivity goes from one-third to one-half by adding an 8 PM and 10 PM sample and by using all six time-points. Increasing the number of postdexamethasone cortisol measurements increases the percentage of patients with primary major depression who are correctly identified as nonsuppressors on the DST. Therefore, if you value as positive the DST, it is wise to maximize the odds of finding it, if it is present. The finding is that four post-DST time-points are better than two, and six are better than two, and four are consistent with the pulsatile nature of cortisol secretion. More sampling increases the likelihood of measuring a nonsuppressed cortisol peak. By increasing the time-points from the two 4 PM and midnight points, proposed by Carroll et al[16,17] and now in common outpatient use, to six points, the sensitivity of nonsuppression on the DST for primary major depression increases to approximately 50%. This increase is not minor or insignificant as it is an increase of 42% in sensitivity. In our experience with 300 study patients, we have found that the extra time-points increase sensitivity by identifying more patients with a "late escape" pattern of nonsuppression.

As compared to other laboratory tests in medicine, the DST is a very reliable test. The specificity of an abnormal DST in the diagnosis of major depression is 90% to 96%, ie, the failure to suppress on the DST is extremely rare in other psychiatric disorders, with a false positive rate 5% to 10%. The sensitivity is approximately 50% to 67%, partially depending on the total number of time-points used in the protocol. In summary, a positive DST (lack of suppression) is of considerable practical usefulness in diagnosis and treatment. It is a test with unusual diagnostic power in that a positive test confirms the diagnosis and helps predict treatment outcome. The DST does not appear to be affected or interfered with by oral contraceptives or by the common psychotropic agents, except perhaps by high doses of benzodiazepines.

Normalization of the DST after successful treatment has been reported in many studies. Interestingly, depressed patients who show apparent clinical recovery, but whose DST remains abnormal, are at serious risk for early relapse. In such cases, continued DST abnormalities may indicate need for alternative antidepressant treatment or ECT, or, at the minimum, continued somatic treatment and observation. Some clinicians successfully use normalization of the DST as a guide to when to discontinue treatments in a course of electroconvulsive therapy. Other clinicians have suggested the DST returns to normal before clinical response to antidepressants in patients who are on their way to recovery.

In addition to its primary role in identifying patients with major depression, the DST also has been applied in a variety of other ways. It is possible that an abnormal DST will identify patients for whom treatment for depression may be indicated, although they carry other presumptive diagnoses such as schizoaffective depression, severe character disorder, dementia, or catatonia. In fact, a DST positive diagnosis may have more prognostic, medication prediction, and relapse power than any other diagnosis. In addition, nonsuppression in depression in children and adolescents may support use of somatic treatments in such cases where clinical presentations are varied and due to a multitude of factors. Results at the present time regarding the DST's ability to predict response to a particular antidepressant are conflicting, but the data support biological treatment responsiveness.

Thyrotropin Releasing Hormone (TRH) Test

Thyroid stimulating hormone (TSH) response to thyrotropin releasing hormone, the TRH test, is useful in confirming a major, unipolar depression diagnosis and relapse prognosis as demonstrated in our studies[12,13] and data reported in the literature.[18-20] Patients with unipolar depression, but not other depressed patient groups or controls, have reduced a maximal TSH response, or a ΔTSH of $\leq$ uIu/mL. The actual cut-off for ΔTSH varies according to TSH assay methodology.

Thyrotropin releasing hormone (TRH) is a tripeptide found in the hypothalamus. When released, it causes secretion of thyroid-stimulating hormone (TSH) from the anterior pituitary gland. TSH then acts directly on the thyroid gland. Endocrinologists have long used the TRH test as a test of thyroid axis functioning. Synthetic TRH, in a 500-μg dose, is administered intravenously to the patient at bedrest after an overnight fast. Samples for TSH are taken at baseline, and at 15, 30, 60, and 90 minutes after TRH administration via an indwelling venous catheter. TSH is measured in duplicate by radioimmunoassay (RIA). Delta TSH (ΔTSH) is the maximum TSH response, derived by subtracting the baseline TSH level from the peak. Subjective response to TRH infusion is limited to mild transient autonomic symptoms such as an urge to urinate.

In our studies, the mean ΔTSH for each major patient group is: unipolar depression, 7.0 ± 0.9; minor depression, 11.2 ± 1.2; bipolar depression, 14.7 ± 1.4; mania, 5.5 ± 0.9; schizophrenia, 9.5 ± 1.1; schizoaffective mania, 9.8 ± 1.5; schizoaffective depression, 8.0 ± 1.1. Unipolar patients have significantly lower ΔTSH values than bipolar depressed patients. In comparison to patients with minor depression, patients with unipolar depression had significantly lower ΔTSH values, whereas bipolar depressed patients had significantly higher ΔTSH values. Manic patients had significantly lower ΔTSH values than patients with schizophrenia, undifferentiated subtype, and patients with schizoaffective disorder, manic type. There were no significant differences in ΔTSH values between normal controls or patients with schizophrenia undifferentiated subtype, schizoaffective disorder manic type, or schizoaffective disorder depressed type or minor depressions.

Our results are consistent with the widely recognized and reported finding that the TRH-induced TSH elevation is blunted in patients with active, major depressive disorder, specifically in primary unipolar major depressive disorder, but not minor depressive disorder.[21-35] Our data also suggest that bipolar depressed patients have an increased response to TRH, consistent with other reports in the literature.[12,13,31,36] Our studies find a significant decrease in TSH response to TRH in mania, consistent with several reports of both nonsignificant trends to blunted response,[32,37] and significant decreases in response.[36,38] In addition, it appears that the TSH response to TRH switches with mood changes in manic depressive illness.[12,36] The results here are consistent with previous reports of normal TSH response to TRH in secondary and characterological depression, and in schizophrenia.[12,30,32,35] The differences in the TSH response to TRH between unipolar, bipolar, and minor depression, and between mania and schizophrenic psychosis do not seem to be artifacts of any of the factors known to influence the TRH test, and may reflect basic biological differences in these psychiatric disorders.[39]

In the differential diagnosis of depression either a blunting or augmenting of the TSH response to TRH may help distinguish patients with major depressive disorder from those with minor depressions. This distinction is important because patients with major depressions are more likely to require and benefit from antidepressant medications than patients with minor depressions.[40-42] Among patients with major depressions, the TSH response to TRH may help in the differential diagnosis of unipolar versus bipolar depression, and hence may have implication for prognosis and pharmacotherapy. A bipolar depressed patient would be more likely to have an antidepressant response to lithium,[42,43] or need lithium as an adjunct to a short course on tricyclic or monoamine oxidase inhibitors (MAOI), both of which produce manias[44] or rapid mood cycling[45] in a significant portion of bipolar, but not unipolar depressed patients. Investigation of the pharmacological response and course of patients whose TRH test "disagrees" with the clinical diagnosis, such as unipolar with an augmented TSH response, is particularly important. These patients may be "false unipolars"[42,46] who could perhaps be identified before they develop manic episodes. The "blunted" ΔTSH group may be biologically homogeneous, cut across syndromal diagnostic groupings, and relate more directly to biological treatment response (eg, lithium response). TRH testing has also been shown to predict high relapse potential in depressed patients when these patients are retested at the time of supposed clinical recovery.[47] Our data and the data in literature also suggest the potential utility of pre- and post-treatment TRH testing in psychiatric treatment decision-making. In the differential diagnosis of mania versus schizophrenic psychosis, a blunted TSH response to TRH may help identify the manic patient. The ability to differentiate mania from schizophrenic psychosis is crucial for several reasons, including the more optimistic prognosis of affective illness,[48,49] greater therapeutic efficacy of lithium in bipolar illness,[42,50-52] neuroleptics in schizophrenia,[48,53,54] and the risk of tardive dyskinesia in misdiagnosed bipolar patients treated with long-term neuroleptics.[54]

In conclusion, the TRH test is a neuroendocrine test that can be performed clinically and may be useful in psychiatric diagnosis and treatment planning.[12,13,38,55,56] The TRH test appears to be useful in differentiating similarly appearing unipolar, bipolar and minor depressive disorders,[12,13,57] and in differentiating mania from schizophrenic psychosis.[38] The TRH test,[12,13,21,36,38,57] dexamethasone suppression test,[8,9,58,59] and other biological tests[60-65] may at some time be added to the present standard diagnostic criteria[6,67] for affective disorders. Researchers need to explore the possibility that the TRH test may, by identifying biologically homogeneous subgroups of patients, help the clinician make treatment decisions, such as whether to use antidepressant medications, the choice of tricyclics versus lithium in depression, and the choice of lithium versus neuroleptics in acute pyschosis. Reviewing the TRH test as a diagnostic test for major unipolar depression in this and some other studies, sensitivity often ranges from 60% to 77% and specificity from 77% to 97%. Similar results, with slightly lower specificity, can be seen when the TRH test is used in the differential diagnosis of mania and schizophrenia.

Using both the DST and the TRH test, abnormalities in either can confirm the diagnosis of major depression (particularly unipolar depression) with high diagnostic confidence and with few false positives, especially when combined with a careful clinical interview. Any comprehensive evaluation program should use the DCT, DST and TRH test to increase identification of true unipolars 80% to 90%. When all testing is negative, a re-examination of other examinations and tests is in order to again rule out a secondary illness. As with the DST and DCT, use of the TRH test in inpatient psychiatry is becoming clearer. Its primary use is in the identification of hypothyroidism; its secondary use is in confirming a diagnosis of active major depression. In addition, changes in the TSH response to TRH in depressed patients have been used to predict response in a manner similar to the predictive utility of the DST. Nearly all depressed patients who failed to show a significant increase in ΔTSH after ECT relapsed within six months, while the majority of those who showed a change in ΔTSH after ECT remained cured during the same time period.

Thyroid Function Tests (TFTs) and Depression

Many of the symptoms of hypothyroidism are similar to the symptoms of depression. In hypothyroidism, depression and/or changes in cognition are common, both of which usually improve with replacement therapy. These observations have led to a great deal of interest in the incidence and coexistence of thyroid disease and depression. Often the covertly hypothyroid patient's first complaint is of depression or lethargy, sometimes leading to a visit to a pyschiatrist. Recently developed descriptive diagnostic criteria (DSM-III or RDC) are much improved over past diagnostic criteria, but meeting descriptive criteria does not rule out underlying thyroid disease. Actively ruling out the disorder is an essential prerequisite to assigning any psychiatric diagnosis. It is useful to note that if only "routine" thyroid testing had been done in either the inpatient or outpatient populations, only 10% of the hypothyroid patients would have been detected and the total incidence would be less than 1%. Since many psychiatrists merely take the patient's complaint and begin treatment, a number of these undiagnosed hypothyroid patients have been failures in psychiatric therapy and antidepressant treatment. Other physicians order routine thyroid function testing in all newly admitted psychiatric inpatients. Studies on such patients showed an incidence of thyroid dysfunction either equal to or greater than the general population. However, in most of these studies patients presenting with depression and/or anergia were not separated from patients with other diagnoses. In addition, the diagnostic evaluation included measurement only of peripheral thyroid hormone (TH) — usually thyroxine (T4) and triiodothyronine (T3) resin uptake, (T3) uptake, and occasionally, measurement of basal thyroid stimulating hormone (TSH). More recently, however, research has shown that the TRH test is the most useful test in identifying cases of incipient or evolving hypothyroidism.

Normally, as peripheral thyroid hormone levels fall, TRH receptor sensitivity increases, and TSH slowly increases in an attempt to boost thyroid gland output to maintain the individual's "normal" euthyroid state. Repeated compensatory pituitary changes in the face of frank thyroid failure eventually leads to the typical pattern in overt hypothyroidism of decreased T4 and markedly elevated TSH levels. Hypothyroidism may occur for a variety of reasons (eg, decreased dietary iodine, lithium administration, radioactive exposure, excessive ablation of thyroid tissue to treat hyperthyroidism, autoimmune thyroiditis with destruction of thyroid tissue and functions, or idiopathic hypothyroidism), but in each case, the thyroid gland fails to produce enough thyroxine and the pituitary compensation cannot retain "normal" circulating levels of thyroid hormone.

In hypothyroid patients, the ΔTSH is markedly increased and values of greater than 30 are common. This occurs at any time of reduced circulating thyroid hormone, because the pituitary is already producing extra TSH reserve to enable the individual to compensate for the decrease in thyroid hormones. Although resting TSH levels may be normal, the pituitary gland's TRH receptors are exceptionally responsive to TRH stimulation.[68-73]

Grades of hypothyroidism exist and can be identified using the TRH test. We have clearly demonstrated that a failing thyroid gland has a behavioral presentation and can be diagnosed only by waiting until the patient is overtly hypothyroid or doing a TRH test. Grade 1 (overt) rarely presents to the psychiatrist and is roughly equivalent to classical myxedema. All thyroid tests are abnormal, eg, thyroid hormones decreased, TSH increased, ΔTSH increased. Grade 2, or mild hypothyroidism, while also treatable with thyroid replacement, is more subtle than Grade 1. Patients with Grade 2 frequently present to psychiatrists complaining of depression, problems with concentration and memory, or lack of energy. Basal thyroid hormone testing is normal, TSH is borderline elevated, and ΔTSH is markedly increased. Of "depressed" patients, 3% to 4% are Grade 2 hypothyroid. Grade 3 patients have a predominantly psychiatric syndrome with the only evidence of thyroid change being pathologically elevated. Two to five percent of depressed patients are Grade 3 hypothyroid. In our experience, TRH/thyroid testing along with ΔTSH identifies those hypothyroid patients who are misdiagnosed by descriptive criteria and labelled as psychiatric. The TRH test also identifies thyroid hormone responders.

Given the high (1% to 7%) incidence of thyroid failure in "psychiatric" patients, one is interested to know something about the cause. The etiology of hypothyroidism is diverse. Autoimmune mechanisms, however, are frequently implicated and can be screened for with relative ease.[74-76] Endocrinologists have begun to focus on hypothyroidism as an evolving disease entity, rather than an "all or none" phenomenon. As hypothyroidism develops, all of the laboratory measures of thyroid function become abnormal over time.

Thyroid Autoantibodies

Screening for thyroid autoantibodies is one final test that is useful in assessing the status of the thyroid gland, although it is not a direct measure of thyroid function. The immune system is capable of making antibodies and destroying the thyroid gland. Serum can be tested for the presence of such antibodies. Two common antigens are thyroid microsomes and thyroglobulin, both of which are present in the thyroid gland. The presence of antibodies to either of these antigens is abnormal, and can be directly tested for by analyzing the patient's serum for anti-M or anti-T antibodies by available immunologic techniques.[77,78] In symptomatic patients, high antibody titers are considered as evidence of an autoimmune disease process involving the thyroid gland. Patients with an increased ΔTSH and positive antibodies are SAT or symptomless-autoimmune thyroiditis patients.

Measurement of MHPG

Many clinicians have found measurement of pretreatment urinary 3-methoxy-4-hydroxy phenylglycol (MHPG) to be of assistance in the prediction of a response to specific noradrenergic augmented antidepressant medications. MHPG is the major metabolite of brain norepinephrine. While there has been some disagreement about where the MHPG comes from and critical arguments about the misuse of urinary MHPG as a diagnostic test for depression, most studies (including the national collaborative study on depression) strongly support the use of the MHPG test to predict response to noradrenergic medication. As such, MHPG is the only well-validated pretreatment prognostic indicator.

Prior to a 24-hour urine collection, the patient should be on a low monoamine diet for at least two days and off psychoactive drugs for at least one week. Creatinine clearance and total urinary volume are measured at the same time as MHPG to rule out incomplete collection. In patients who are candidates for treatment with antidepressants, demonstration of low pretreatment MHPG levels ($< 1000 \ \mu g/24$ hours) predicts favorable response to antidepressants, such as imipramine, nortriptyline and maprotiline, which primarily affect noradrenergic systems.

B$_{12}$ and Folate

Most, if not all, psychiatrists order periodic CBCs and hematological studies on all new in- and out-patients. However, normal CBC and indices do not rule out vitamin deficiency states. Folic acid deficiency has been widely reported in psychiatric patients, alcoholics, drug addicts, epileptics maintained on anticonvulsant medications, women on oral contraceptives, eg, patients with malnutrition, malabsorption, or those who are pregnant, or even in the absence of anemia. A firm link between folic acid level and depressive mood only recently has been made, with research studies demonstrating an abnormally low folate level in 20% to 40% of nonanemic depressed patients. Other studies show that folate deficiency is more common in depressed patients and B_{12} deficiency more common in psychotic patients. Folate deficiency can impair monoamine (eg, norepinephrine) synthesis in the brain (folate is the co-enzyme for tyrosine hydroxylase). While folate deficiency is treated with replacement, it is unclear whether folate depression exists as a distinct entity, as a precipitant of an underlying vulnerability, or as a life-style side effect to depression. If patient-specific norms are unavailable, use age- and sex-controlled norms and, when decreased even marginally, folate replacement is indicated.

Investigators and biologically oriented clinicians have repeatedly found low B_{12} levels in psychiatric patients. Again, it has been reported that psychiatric symptoms may appear before the development of frank anemia in untreated pernicious anemia. B_{12} replacement is simple and indicated when absolute or relative deficiency is demonstrated. In one California survey, failure to diagnose just such a B_{12} deficiency without anemia led to the largest psychiatric malpractice settlement in five years. We suggest folate and B_{12} levels in the context of a comprehensive neuropsychiatric evaluation, especially in at-risk patients.

Tyrosine and Tryptophan

The two most widely held biochemical models of depression—the catecholamine (CA) and indolamine (IA) hypotheses—explain depression as a result of deficient transmission of the CA, norepinephrine (NE) or the IA, serotonin (5-HT). Vitaminologists have explained depression as a form of vitamin or amino acid deficiency. Both models may have contributions to make. Due to dietary and other factors (eg, hereditary) depressed patients and patients with anorexia may have absolute or relative deficiencies in these precursor amino acids. In these cases replacement is indicated. Another use for the measurements of tryptophan and/or tyrosine is as an antidepressant in which the goal is to titrate levels to increase brain levels of NE and 5-HT. For this purpose, the 5-HT precursors tryptophan and 5-hydroxytryptophan (5-HTP), and the NE precursors tyrosine and dihydroxyphenylalanine (DOPA), have been administered to depressed patients. In addition, tryptophan and tyrosine have been utilized as potentiators of response when added to trazodone or nortriptyline treatment.

The enzyme tryptophan hydroxylase is not normally saturated with its amino acid substrate in vivo and, therefore, the rate of brain serotonin synthesis can be influenced by changes in available tryptophan concentration.[79] Brain tryptophan concentration varies directly with its available plasma concentration. This relationship is complicated by the sum of the plasma concentration of the other large neutral amino acids (LNAA) — leucine, isoleucine, valine, phenylalanine, tyrosine — which compete with it for 5-HT uptake into the brain.[80] Thus, tryptophan administration, or the ingestion of a carbohydrate-containing meal (which elicits insulin secretion, thereby lowering the plasma level of competing LNAAs), results in increases in brain tryptophan and, hence, in brain 5-HT. Tryptophan levels and monitoring are essential as it is reported that the blood concentration of nonalbumin-bound tryptophan determines the rate of tryptophan uptake into the brain. A tryptophan therapeutic window may exist for the use of tryptophan as an antidepressant. Tryptophan has been well studied as an antidepressant with efficacy limited to an inverted "U" plasma level range.[81-91]

Just as the fact that tryptophan hydroxylase is not fully saturated allows for the use of a precursor to increase available neurotransmitters, only 75% of tyrosine hydroxylase is saturated.[92] This means that tyrosine administration can raise brain tyrosine concentrations and can cause parallel changes in CA synthesis.[93,94] Increases in brain tyrosine levels lead to increased NE release and turnover, as measured by the accumulation of MHPG.[95] This makes tyrosine a unique "vitamin" treatment for depression or, if not as effective as traditional antidepressants, a potentiator of NE antidepressant response. We have also found tyrosine (100 mg/kg) qid as an effective treatment for cocaine withdrawal states.

Unlike the biogenic amines DA, NE, and 5-HT, their precursors — DOPA, tyrosine, 5-HTP, and tryptophan — easily cross the blood-brain barrier. Tryptophan raises brain 5-HT levels, producing measurable increases in CSF 5-HIAA.[87,96] Orally administered tyrosine raises plasma tyrosine in man and increases urinary excretion of NE and MHPG.[97] Tryptophan alone or in combination with serotonergic antidepressants, or tyrosine alone or in combination with noradrenergic antidepressants, may help improve efficacy and allow for more "natural" treatments. To administer either amino acids will require pretreatment levels and therapeutic amino acid monitoring.

It is clear that dietary intake is essential, and tryptophan is frequently low in depressed, anorexic, drug abusing and alcoholic patients, on the basis of a dietary deficiency. This deficiency may explain sleep and mood changes, aggressiveness, and irritability in these patients. Tryptophan replacement can reverse this dietary deficiency. In addition, lithium may cause a tryptophan deficiency possibly by accelerating the enzymatic conversion of tryptophan to serotonin. We have theorized that this may explain postmania depression in some patients on lithium, and depressed mood in some long-term lithium patients. Tryptophan test levels, taken at 8 AM (fasting since midnight) on two consecutive days may be indicated in patients who are "pre-lithium" and those who could have a dietary deficiency (eg, depression, anorexia nervosa, drug abuse, alcoholism) with simple tryptophan replacement, if indicated. Cocaine abuse now appears to produce tyrosine deficiency which may respond to replacement.

Magnesium and Electrolyte Imbalance

Electrolyte imbalance may cause syndromes that could be mistaken as psychiatric problems, such as depression or dementia. On the other hand, patients' psychopathology may lead to behavior that causes electrolyte imbalance, eg, anorexia nervosa or water intoxication in schizophrenia. Both hypokalemia and hypercalcemia are well known to cause depression or organic brain syndrome. Hyponatremia, secondary to excessive water ingestion, may produce a clinical picture of lethargy and withdrawal, or decreased concentration. Both hypernatremic and hypocalcemic patients often display signs of irritability or impaired cognition. Decreases in magnesium levels may lead to organic brain syndrome or depression, especially in alcoholics. For these reasons, we advocate routine monitoring of serum electrolytes at the time of admission. Sodium, potassium, and calcium usually are included as part of a SMA-22 battery of admission tests. In addition, magnesium levels should be ordered in all patients presenting with impaired cognition, organic brain syndrome, alcoholism or drug abuse.

THERAPEUTIC DRUG MONITORING

Antidepressant Levels

The use of standard dose regimens unrelated to plasma levels has been identified as a major source of antidepressant nonresponse. The reasons for this fact are numerous, but include pharmacokinetic, pharmacodynamic, and other factors. For example, liver microsomal enzymes metabolizing antidepressants and converting tertiary tricyclics to secondary may show large intersubject variability (greater than 30-fold). Antidepressant absorption from the gastrointestinal tract is highly variable among patients and in the same patient over time. Absorption may be markedly affected by antacids, sodium bicarbonate and vitamin C, to name a few. Drug interactions may seriously affect blood levels of antidepressants. Antipsychotic medications often increase antidepressant levels, while smoking and prior or current drug abuse will often lower antidepressant levels. Physicians sometimes forget that poor compliance is a major factor in drug nonresponse even in the most motivated patient.

All these factors explain why measurement of antidepressant levels is indicated for patients on these medications, especially for inpatients, many of whom have just started intensive treatment.

There are other reasons that justify the use of such levels. Cardiotoxicity, including prolonged QRS duration and dysrrhythmias, has been correlated with high plasma levels. Geriatric patients often show unusual patterns of drug metabolism, and often can least tolerate the cardiotoxic effects. On the same dose, elderly patients have higher drug levels than younger patients. In addition, other subjective side effects of antidepressant use may be correlated with plasma concentration.

Another reason many clinicians have delayed use of the plasma levels is because of suggestions in the past that all nonresponders merely require a higher dose of the antidepressant. It was once said that no antidepressant trial in the face of nonresponse was complete without a period on high or very high doses. However, now it is clear that not only is that incorrect, but in fact the practice is dangerous, since some patients would end up with extremely toxic levels on high dosages. Two other factors that relate to clinicians' delay in full use of plasma levels have been questions of expense and superiority of clinical judgment. Some doctors feel that antidepressant levels add an unnecessary expense for the patient. However, given the much greater expense of a single hospital day, any test that decreases length of stay in an inpatient facility even by one day, and decreases side effects, is cost effective. It is clear that there is a risk to the patient of being on an antidepressant with substandard levels—the risks of not getting better, suicide, and suffering, as well as the medical risks.

One difficulty many clinicians encounter when they attempt to use antidepressant levels is that laboratories vary greatly in their methodology and accuracy in the performance of the tests. Some methods are affected by other psychoactive medications, have low recovery of known standard concentrations, and cannot differentiate between active and inactive metabolites. Measurement of antidepressant levels is a very difficult and sensitive procedure and is not done routinely in many laboratories. When a laboratory does not perform the test in-house, it must send the sample to a reference laboratory, which in many cases increases the length of time it takes for the clinician to receive the results. Clearly, for antidepressant levels to be clinically useful, the results must be returned to the clinician rapidly, to enable the test to be used when making clinical decisions about dosage. It should take a laboratory no more than 24 hours to perform the assay.

Why blood levels of antidepressants? For any given dose of an antidepressant medication, there are marked interindividual variations in resultant steady-state antidepressant concentrations. Some patients have 30 times the blood level of other patients given the identical dose. Increasing evidence, as recently reviewed by numerous authors, suggests that for many antidepressants there are critical ranges of steady-state plasma concentrations of parent antidepressants and psychoactive metabolites that must be achieved for optimal efficacy. These ranges may not be achieved in approximately 40% of patients given standard therapeutic dosages, ie, imipramine 200 mg/day or trazodone 150 mg/day. Furthermore, even when therapeutic plasma concentrations are attained, these antidepressant levels may be altered and clinical response reversed by exogenous factors such as weight change, dietary alterations, changes in smoking status, differences in bioequivalence among pharmaceutical preparations, and the addition or withdrawal of concurrent medications, and, subsequently, toxicity or clinical relapse may occur. When therapeutic ranges are wide or when there is a linear relationship between plasma antidepressant concentration and clinical response, plasma level determinations occasionally may be useful to minimize toxicity or reduce adverse side effects by adjusting dosage to maintain therapeutic levels, but at lower concentrations. Any antidepressant with a therapeutic window that has few, if any, relevant active metabolites is a clear medication whose efficacy can be increased when compared to standard dose antidepressants, which produce active metabolites.

Why blood levels in inpatients? Antidepressant plasma level monitoring is clinically useful in the pharmacological treatment of depressed inpatients. In general inpatient psychiatry, the relationship between plasma antidepressant concentrations and therapeutic response is exploited to maximize response and reduce side effects, noncompliance, and length of hospital stays in the pharmacotherapeutic management of endogenously depressed patients. This is of special importance for nortriptyline (Pamelor) in which use of dose prediction test, therapeutic window, and the defined trial (21 consecutive days at therapeutic levels) can bring the response rate from 50% to 80% or 90%. Routine monitoring of plasma antidepressant concentrations in all medicated subjects is helpful and warranted in inpatients on both intellectual and cost effectiveness grounds. Desipramine also appears to have a window which may be exploited to increase efficacy.

Reducing toxicity Individuals who are at increased risk for toxic effects of antidepressants benefit from frequent plasma level monitoring. While most antidepressants have adverse effects, knowing plasma level-response relationships and using plasma levels can reduce or eliminate side effects. In certain patients with cardiovascular disease, prolonged atrioventricular conduction times may lead to ventricular arrhythmias and potentially, death. Consequently, any patient particularly at risk for toxic effects of antidepressants (eg, those elderly with cardiovascular disease; those with drug and/or alcohol abuse history, with liver disease, or with a family or personal history of side effects to low doses of antidepressants) may be medicated with nortriptyline, using concurrent frequent plasma level monitoring to remain within the lower limits of the therapeutic range to minimize any potential toxicity.

Why blood levels in outpatients? Tricyclic and other antidepressants usually may be used effectively in outpatients without frequent monitoring of plasma concentrations. However, response rate may only be 50% to 60%. When plasma levels are not used, all available antidepressants are equal in efficacy.

More than 50% of outpatients may be efficiently and appropriately treated by the simple use of standard doses of antidepressant, with a single blood level after dosage stabilization and response beginning to appear within two to four weeks. In these patients, additional bi-weekly or weekly plasma level monitoring is not necessary or indicated. However, weekly levels ensure compliance. In a relapsing patient, regular levels may save the financial, familial and personal cost of a relapse. If outpatients have not begun to experience a marked therapeutic benefit within two to three weeks, or seem to be sustaining unusually severe side effects, frequent plasma level determinations will be necessary. Dose adjustments can be eliminated or reduced, antidepressant trial integrity preserved, efficacy increased, and side effects decreased, by the use of the nortriptyline dose prediction test and monitoring NT plasma levels to ensure that the patient has a trial of ≥ 21 consecutive days at therapeutic levels.

Plasma level determinations are appropriate for several reasons. It may be that the patient simply will not benefit from that particular pharmacological agent and, thus, may need a trial of another antidepressant, or a trial with monoamine oxidase inhibitors, or electroconvulsive therapy. However, the managing physician cannot know this without a plamsa level determination. We have placed antidepressant nonresponders, and even supposed nortriptyline nonresponders, in 21 consecutive day trials, using a therapeutic levels protocol, and found that true nonresponse is very unusual. Furthermore, not knowing if the patient has a therapeutic plasma concentration of tricyclic or other antidepressant, blind raising or lowering of the dosage may precipitate toxicity or simply prolong an unsuccessful pharmacotherapeutic approach. Plasma level determinations in these instances allow the clinician to immediately know if any alternate therapy is appropriate, or if an increase or decrease in dosage is indicated. (See toxicity and relapse prevention sections.)

Outpatients: Preventing Relapse

Some patients in clinical remission, on maintenance antidepressants, may benefit from plasma antidepressant concentration determinations. As noted above, a variety of exogenous factors may alter steady-state concentrations of antidepressant medications. For example, neuroleptics, methylphenidate, corticosteroids, disulfiram, dipropylacetamide, vitamins, and weight loss, may all markedly increase plasma levels of antidepressants and potentiate toxicity or cause relapse in those anti-depressant agents with therapeutic windows. Conversely, barbiturates and tobacco smoking may markedly lower plasma tricyclic concentration and allow relapse in patients treated with all classes of antidepressants. There are likely to be numerous other drug-drug interactions affecting tricyclic plasma concentrations and, when adding or deleting a concurrent medication to a patient's pharmacological regimen, a plasma level determination may be appropriate.

Finally, differences in bioequivalence among pharmaceutical preparations of the same tricyclic agent have resulted in changes in plasma tricyclic concentrations and caused clinical relapses or precipitated toxicity, and the clinician must be alert to this if a patient changes pharmacies.

Compliance

It is well known that the majority of patients do not take medications as prescribed. This is a fact in outpatient *and* inpatient psychopharmacology. Noncompliance or partial compliance causes wide fluctuations in plasma levels and reduces response to treatment. Frequent monitoring of antidepressant levels is the best way to insure compliance and guarantee the integrity of the medication trial. Prevention of compliance problems is recommended to avoid wasted hospital time and risk of untreated severe depressions. Remember that proper utilization of blood levels will ultimately depend on your ability to get clinical access to research quality levels. Rather than discovering that your laboratory cannot measure antidepressants, send known samples and split samples before sending patients.

Neuroleptic Drug Levels

There is a smaller body of research into clinical use of neuroleptic or antipsychotic levels. However, many of the basic principles of therapeutic drug monitoring discussed above also apply to neuroleptic levels. Direct neuroleptic levels or levels of functional activity Dopamine Radio Receptor Assay (DA-RRA) will become routine, or at least common within the next few years. These levels are already useful. For example, consistently low levels might indicate noncompliance. Patients with extremely high levels may be considered toxic, may have a high risk of developing tardive dyskinesia, and may require closer observation. Anticholinergic drugs appear to lower plasma concentrations of neuroleptics and may cause relapse. In one study, levels varied as much as 15-fold in children on the same daily dosage. More recently, research has shown a correlation between neuroleptic plasma level and clinical response and relapse. A number of studies have shown the presence of a therapeutic window for plasma levels of haloperidol. These levels by GC or on the basis of function by dopamine receptor binding levels are extremely useful in dose titration and side effect prevention. Relapse may also relate to blood levels.

Maintenance neuroleptic treatment has been clearly demonstrated to reduce the incidence of schizophrenic relapse. Nevertheless, relapse is common and occurs in over 25% of schizophrenic patients who are treated with neuroleptics.[56] Although some patients who have relapses have discontinued or reduced their doses of medication, compliance failure alone does not account for the high rate of relapse. Patients who take oral doses of fluphenazine hydrochloride and those given intramuscular doses of fluphenazine when followed for one year after hospital discharge are found to have a relapse rate approaching 40%.[98] In treating acute schizophrenia, medication can be adjusted to the patient's clinical response, but there is no similar end point to guide the use and maintenance of prophylactic medication in patients whose illness is in remission. Both of these are indications for use of blood levels. There are wide individual differences in the neuroleptic plasma levels of parent neuroleptic by GC or GC/MS or biological activity by DA-RRA with patients taking the same neuroleptic dose, clearly having widely divergent measurable neuroleptic activity.

Over the past three decades, neuroleptic medications have become the treatment of choice for schizophrenia, particularly for acute[55,99] and prophylactic[56] treatment of psychosis. However, a significant proportion of schizophrenic patients have an inadequate antipsychotic response to neuroleptics,[100] One source of failure to respond and intractability may be variability in plasma levels of medication. Several investigators have studied the relationship of neuroleptic levels and response to treatment.[101-105] Some of these investigators have suggested therapeutic windows for plasma levels of neuroleptics, including haloperidol.[101,103,105]

Haloperidol is a potent neuroleptic with a relatively low profile of sedation and cardiovascular effects that is extremely useful in the treatment of acute psychosis.[99] Steady-state plasma levels are achieved in about six days.[101] Because haloperidol has no significant active metabolites, it is an ideal medication to use for study of the relationship between clinical efficacy and parent neuroleptic levels. We have confirmed these haloperidol data with DA-RRA and recently expanded them to include thioridazine. Most other neuroleptics have active metabolites, and studies of plasma levels and clinical response to these medications must involve assays of multiple compounds or dopamine-receptor binding assays.[102] Magliozzi et al have recently reported a therapeutic window for haloperidol levels in schizophrenic outpatients.[105]

Our results suggest that a high proportion of acutely psychotic schizophrenic inpatients who respond to treatment with haloperidol do so at plasma levels in the range of 5–15 ng/mL. This is in basic agreement with a previous study showing outpatients who respond within this approximate range.[105] It is not certain that patients who respond within a given range of plasma levels would not respond at levels above or below this range, although it is likely that there would be no additional benefit and only risk would be involved. Our studies identify a range of plasma levels within which most acute schizophrenic patients who respond to haloperidol will fall. There is certainly no linear relationship between haloperidol levels and clinical response. The results here are consistent with either a therapeutic window or a threshold for effective plasma levels of haloperidol in acute schizophrenia. Individual patient data suggest that nonresponders will continue not to respond when haloperidol levels are increased above 15 ng/mL.

Our results, along with previous results from other investigations, suggest that measurement of plasma haloperidol levels may provide useful guidelines for adjusting medication dosage in schizophrenic patients. Single dose prediction tests may be developed if a window is confirmed. Most of the acutely psychotic schizophrenic patients reported here responded with plasma levels in the range of 5–15 ng/mL. Further research needs to be focused on better defining a possible therapeutic window or threshold for effective haloperidol levels in schizophrenic patients. There are certain practical advantages to measuring plasma haloperidol levels. First, because haloperidol has no known significant active metabolites,[105] assay of haloperidol alone measures the pharmacologically active compound. Second, the GC assay[106] is adaptable to a large volume of clinical samples.

For other neuroleptics, similar plasma level response relationships appear to exist but can only be seen with DA-RRA. Specific DA-RRA levels will be generated for each neuroleptic and for acute and chronic management. For patients with a schizophrenic syndrome responsive to neuroleptic treatment, the serum neuroleptic level during long-term treatment appears to be closely related to clinical course. Low neuroleptic levels that may result from nonadherence, low dosage, or individual differences in absorption and metabolism, appear to be predictive of relapse. This dose-response observation provides further evidence for the efficacy of neuroleptics in maintaining remission in some schizophrenic patients. As with many other therapeutic agents, the serum neuroleptic level appears to be critically related to its clinical effectiveness. Monitoring of neuroleptic levels has the potential to reduce both the incidence of untoward side effects related to high-dose neuroleptic treatment and the rate of schizophrenic relapse.

Platelet Monoamine Oxidase Measurements

Platelet MAO activity has been measured and reported decreased in schizophrenia, mania, alcoholism and other disease states.[107-108] While the use of platelet MAO as a confirmatory diagnostic test is controversial, the use of a quantitative measurement of platelet MAO activity before and during MAO inhibition treatment is routine in many modern medical centers. Efficacy with MAO inhibitors can be increased to approximately 80% by titrating dose to 80% to 90% inhibition of platelet MAO.

THE LABORATORY IN PSYCHIATRIC PRACTICE

What has limited the implementation of laboratory advances by psychiatrists has been the "training lag" and conflicts between psychiatrists who treat patients, psychiatrists who do not treat or evaluate patients, but nevertheless tell other psychiatrists what to do, and psychiatrists who are pervasively nonmedical. The failure to evaluate drug abusers and homosexuals for the various forms of hepatitis, the failure to adequately assess patients for nutritional state, etc, suggests psychiatrists have fallen so far behind that they cannot catch up. Many psychiatrists view the use of laboratory procedures as incompatible with their own theoretical approach to the patient, and others will not or cannot draw blood. Other physicians have unrealistic expectations of the infallibility of laboratory systems. Psychiatrists are well known in medicine as physicians who denounce their colleagues and argue about which mode of therapy or school of thought should be used in clinical practice. It is no surprise then that unanimity is elusive with regard to the laboratory or doing physical examinations on psychiatric patients. Physicians in other branches of medicine have always found ways to coexist with their peers. As part of their formal training and through the experience of trial and error they learn about laboratories and testing and have realistic expectations. They do not find a laboratory test useless or suspect if it fails to have accuracy of 99% or more. They learn that laboratory testing is one component in the diagnostic and treatment process. The discussions about utility yield a constant state of improvement and progress. Understanding the limitations of a particular test, they use the test results in the context of other signs and symptoms. They weighted the neurological exam before the spinal fluid exam was sufficiently improved, then in order, the EEG, the brain scan, the arteriogram and the CAT scan or PET scan. All this occurred because of an underlying bias that you cannot "smell syphilis" and the addition of an important third party to mediate clinical inconsistencies and disputes is necessary even when the mediator is imperfect. Recognition of imperfections led to the next diagnostic refinement and step, and not to a nihilistic return to nothingness. Some psychiatrists have never learned, or they fail to remember, these basic principles of laboratory medicine, and they express nihilistic views, suggesting a lack of sensitivity is proof of the uselessness of a test. In addition, as some types of specialized laboratory testing are a relatively new area, psychiatrists need to learn the concept of interim measures vis-à-vis these tests. NASA did not expect to land on the moon before orbiting the earth, and cardiologists would never have defined the uses and limitations of the cardiac enzymes unless they were widely used by clinicians. Psychiatrists need to have hands-on experience with the full spectrum of psychiatric laboratory tests to find out what syndromes they have been missing, and to improve their patient evaluation and treatment, as well as to impact upon the use and improvement of such procedures. Finally, psychiatrists need to remember that medicine has, as part of its tradition, new tools and techniques that have been developed since their residency which often necessitate additional postresidency training. Just imagine the consequences of a surgeon not learning the newer techniques of laparoscopy or arthroscopy. Some psychiatrists feel that they have learned enough and nothing "that" important has happened to force them to take an in-depth training program, or start to change the way they practice. These psychiatrists are being replaced by family physicians who have an interest in psychiatry. With clergy, social workers, nurses, psychologists, and other groups successfully competing with the psychiatrist, therapist, and family practitioner or internists, the psychiatrist is becoming "niche-less."

54

REFERENCES

1. Guze SB, Woodruff RA, Clayton PJ, et al: Secondary affective disorder: A study of 95 cases. *Psychol Med* 1971;1:426–428.
2. Feighner JP, Robins E, Guze SB, et al: Diagnostic criteria for use in psychiatric research. *Arch Gen Psychiatry* 1972;26:57–63.
3. Sweeney DR, Maas JW, Heninger GR: State anxiety, physical activity, and urinary 3-methoxy-4-hydroxyphenethylene glycol excretion. *Arch Gen Psychiatry* 1978;35:1418–1423.
4. Spitzer RL, Endicott J, Robins E: *Research Diagnostic Criteria*, ed 3. New York, Biometric Research, New York State Department of Mental Health, 1977.
5. Schlesser M, Winokur G, Sherman BM: Genetic subtypes of unipolar primary depressive illness distinguished by hypothalamic-pituitary adrenal axis activity. *Lancet* 1979;1:739–741.
6. Brown WA, Shuey I: Response to dexamethasone and subtype of depression. *Arch Gen Psychiatry* 1980;37:747–751.
7. Sacher EJ, Asnis G, Nathan RS, et al: Dextroamphetamine and cortisol in depression. *Arch Gen Psychiatry* 1980;37:755–757.
8. Carroll BJ, Curtis GC, Mendels J: Neuroendocrine regulation in depression: I. Limbic system-adrenocorticol dysfunction. *Arch Gen Psychiatry* 1976;33:1039–1044.
9. Carroll BJ, Curtis GC, Mendels J: Neuroendocrine regulation in depression: II. Discrimination of depressed from nondepressed patients. *Arch Gen Psychiatry* 1976;33:1051–1058.
10. Sweeney DR, Maas JW: Specificity of depressive disease. *Annu Rev Med* 1978;29:219–229.
11. Extein I, Pottash ALC, Gold MS: TRH test in depression. *N Engl J Med* 1980;302:923–924.
12. Gold MS, Pottash ALC, Ryan N, et al: TRH-induced TSH response in unipolar, bipolar, and secondary depressions: Possible utility in clinical assessment and differential diagnosis. *Psychoneuroendocrinology* 1980;5:147–155.
13. Gold MS, Pottash ALC, Davies RK, et al: Distinguishing unipolar and bipolar depression by thyrotropin release test. *Lancet* 1979;2:411–413.
14. Greden JF, Albala AA, Haskett RF, et al: Normalization of dexamethasone suppression test: A laboratory index of recovery from endogenous depression. *Biol Psychiatry* 1980;15:449–458.
15. Gold MS, Pottash ALC, Extein I, et al: Dexamethasone suppression tests in depression and response to treatment. *Lancet* 1980;1:1190.
16. Carroll BJ, Feinberg M, Greden JF, et al: A specific laboratory test for the diagnosis of melancholia. *Arch Gen Psychiatry* 1981;38:15–22.
17. Carroll BJ: Clinical applications of the dexamethasone suppression test for endogenous depression. *Pharmacopsychiatria* 1982;15(1):19–25.
18. Ettigi P, Brown GM: Psychoneuroendocrinology of affective disorders: An overview. *Am J Psychiatry* 1977;134:493–501.
19. Kirkegaard C, Norlem N, Lauridsen UB, et al: Prognostic value of thyrotropin-releasing hormone stimulation test in endogenous depression. *Acta Psychiatr Scand* 1975;52:170–177.
20. Sachar EJ, Asnis G, Halbreich U, et al: Recent studies in the neuroendocrinology of major depressive disorders. *Psychiatr Clin North Am* 1980;3:313–326.
21. Prange AJ, Jr, Wilson IC, Lara PP, et al: Effects of thyrotropin-releasing hormone in depression. *Lancet* 1972;2:999–1002.
22. Kastin AJ, Schalch DS, Ehrensing RH, et al: Improvement in mental depression with decreased thyrotropin response after administration of thyrotropin-releasing hormone. *Lancet* 1972;2:740–742.

23. Takahashi S, Kondo H, Yoshimura M, et al: Thyrotropin-releasing hormone in mental depression. *Folia Psychiatr Neurol Jpn* 1973;27:305–309.
24. Takahashi S, Kondo H, Yoshimura M, et al: Thyrotropin responses to TRH in depressive illness: Relation to clinical subtypes and prolonged duration of depressive episode. *Folia Psychiatr Neurol Jpn* 1974;28:335–365.
25. Coppen A, Peet M, Montgomery S, et al: Thyrotropin-releasing hormone in the treatment of depression. *Lancet* 1974;2:433–435.
26. Ehrensing RH, Kastin AJ, Schalch DS, et al: Affective state and thyrotropin and prolactin responses after repeated injections of thyrotropin-releasing hormone in depressed patients. *Am J Psychiatry* 1974;131:714–718.
27. Maeda K, Kato Y, Ohgo S, et al: Growth hormone and prolactin release after injection of thyrotropin-releasing hormone in patients with depression. *J Clin Endocrinol Metab* 1975;40:501–505.
28. Kirkegaard C, Norlem N, Lauridsen UB, et al: Protirelin stimulation test and thyroid function during treatment of depression. *Arch Gen Psychiatry* 1975;32:1115–1118.
29. Hollister LE, Kenneth LD, and Berger PA: Pituitary response to thyrotropin-releasing hormone in depression. *Arch Gen Psychiatry* 1976;33:1393–1396.
30. Lossen PT, Prange AJ, Jr, Wilson IC, et al: Thyroid stimulating hormone response after thyrotropin-releasing hormone in depressed, schizophrenic and normal women. *Psychoneuroendocrinology* 1977;2:137–148.
31. Gold PW, Goodwin FK, Wehr T, et al: Pituitary thyrotropin response to thyrotropin-releasing hormone in affective illness: Relationship to spinal fluid amine metabolites. *Am J Psychiatry* 1977;134:1028–1031.
32. Kirkegaard C, Bjorum N, Cohn D, et al: Thyrotropin-releasing hormone stimulation test in manic depressive illness. *Arch Gen Psychiatry* 1978; 35:1017–1021.
33. Brambilla F, Smeraldi E, Sacchetti E: Deranged anterior pituitary responsiveness to hypothalamic hormones in depressed patients. *Arch Gen Psychiatry* 1978;35:1231–1238.
34. Mandlewicz J, Linowski P, Brauman H: TSH responses to TRH in women with unipolar and bipolar depression. *Lancet* 1979;2:1079–1080.
35. Asnis GM, Nathan RS, Halbreich U, et al: TRH tests in depression. *Lancet* 1980;1:424–425.
36. Extein I, Pottash ALC, Gold MS, et al: The thyroid-stimulating hormone response to thyrotropin-releasing hormone in mania and bipolar depression. *Psychiatry Res* 1980;2:199–204.
37. Takahashi S, Kondo H, Yoshimura M, et al: Thyroid function levels and thyrotropin responses to TRH administration in manic patients receiving lithium carbonate. *Folia Psychiatr Neurol Jpn* 1975;29:231–237.
38. Extein I, Pottash ALC, Gold MS, et al: Differentiating mania from schizophrenia by the TRH test. *Am J Psychiatry* 1980;137:981–982.
39. Extein I, Pottash ALC, Gold MS, et al: Using the protirelin test to distinguish mania from schizophrenia. *Arch Gen Psychiatry* 1982;39:77–81.
40. Goodwin FK, Extein I: The biological basis of affective disorders, in Lipton MA, DiMascio A, Killam KF (eds): *Progress in the Functional Psychosis.* New York, Spectrum Publications, 1979, pp 129–152.
41. Klein DF: Endogenomorphic depression. *Arch Gen Psychiatry* 1974;31: 447–454.
42. Goodwin FK: Drug treatment of affective disorders: General principles, in Jarvik MS (ed): *Psychopharmacology in the Practice of Medicine.* New York, Appleton-Century-Crofts, 1977, pp 241–253.
43. Goodwin FK, Murphy DL, Dunner DL, et al: Lithium response in unipolar versus bipolar depression. *Am J Psychiatry* 1973;129:44–47.
44. Bunney WE, Jr: Psychopharmacology of the switch process in affective

illness, in Lipton MS, DiMascio A, Killam KF (eds): *Psychopharmacology: A Generation of Progress.* New York, Raven Press, 1978, pp 1249–1259.

45. Wehr TA, Goodwin FK: Rapid cycling in manic depressives induced by tricyclic antidepressants. *Arch Gen Psychiatry* 1979;36:555–559.

46. Winokur G, Clayton PJ, Reich T: *Manic-Depressive Illness.* St. Louis, CV Mosby Co, 1969.

47. Kirkegaard C, Bjorum N, Cohn D, et al: Studies on the influence of biogenic amines and psychoactive drugs on the prognostic value of the TRH stimulation test in endogenous depression. *Psychoneuroendocrinology* 1977;2:131–136.

48. Pope HG, Lipinski JF, Jr: Diagnosis in schizophrenia and manic-depressive illness. *Arch Gen Psychiatry* 1978;35:811–828.

49. Robins E, Guze SB: Establishment of diagnostic validity in psychiatric illness: Its application to schizophrenia. *Am J Psychiatry* 1970;126:983–987.

50. Schou M, Juel-Nielsen N, Stromgren E, et al: The treatment of manic psychosis by administration of lithium salts. *J Neurol Neurosurg Psychiatry* 1954;17:250–260.

51. Davis JM: Overview: Maintenance therapy in psychiatry: II. Affective disorders. *Am J Psychiatry* 1976;133:1–13.

52. Hershman JM, Pittman JA, Jr: Control of thyrotropin secretion in man. *N Engl J Med* 1971;285:997–1006.

53. Casey JF, Bennett IF, Lindley CJ, et al: Drug therapy in schizophrenia. *Arch Gen Psychiatry* 1960;2:100–110.

54. Davis JM: Overview: Maintenance therapy in psychiatry: I. Schizophrenia. *Am J Psychiatry* 1975;132:1237–1245.

55. Extein I, Pottash ALC, Gold MS, et al: The TRH test in the differential diagnosis of depression, mania, and schizophrenia. *Abstract Book, XI International Congress of the International Society of Psychoneuroendocrinology.* Florence, Italy, 1980, p 65.

56. Kirstein L, Gold MS, Pottash ALC, et al: Clinical correlates of the TRH infusion test. *Abstract Book, XI International Congress of the International Society of Psychoneuroendocrinology.* Florence, Italy, 1980, p 71.

57. Gold MS, Pottash ALC, Extein I, et al: The TRH test in the diagnosis of unipolar depression. *Psychoneuroendocrinology* 1981;6:159–169.

58. Sachar EJ: Evidence for neuroendocrine abnormalities in the major mental illnesses, in Freedman DX (ed): *Biology of the Major Psychoses.* New York, Raven Press, 1975, pp 347–358.

59. Carroll BJ: Neuroendocrine function in psychiatric disorders, in Lipton MA, DiMascio A, Killan KF (eds): *Psychopharmacology: A Generation of Progress.* New York, Raven Press, 1978, pp 487–497.

60. Sachar EJ, Hellman L, Roffwang H, et al: Disrupted 24-hour pattern of cortisol secretion in psychotic depression. *Arch Gen Psychiatry* 1968;28:19–24.

61. Sachar EJ, Finkelstein J, Hellman L: Growth hormone responses in depressive illness: Response to insulin tolerance test. *Arch Gen Psychiatry* 1971;24:263–269.

62. Maas JS, Fawcett J, Dekirmenjian H: 3-Methoxy-4-Hydroxyphenylglycol (MHPG) excretion in depressive states. *Arch Gen Psychiatry* 1968;19:129–134.

63. Extein I, Pottash ALC, Gold MS, et al: Deficient prolactin response to morphine in depression. *Am J Psychiatry* 1980;137:845–846.

64. Pickar D, Davis GC, Schulz C, et al: Behavioral and biological effects of acute beta-endorphin injection in schizophrenic and depressed patients. Submitted for publication.

65. Gold PW, Reus VI, Goodwin FK: Vasopressin in affective illness — Hypothesis. *Lancet* 1978.1:1233–1236.

66. Spitzer RL, Endicott J, Robins E: Research diagnostic criteria: Rationale and reliability. *Arch Gen Psychiatry* 1978;35:773–782.
67. *Diagnostic and Statistical Manual of Mental Disorders.* American Psychiatric Association Task Force on Nomenclature and Statistics, ed 3. Washington, DC, The American Psychiatric Association, 1980.
68. Snyder PJ, Utiger RD: Inhibition of thyrotropin response to thyrotropin-releasing hormone by small quantities of thyroid hormones. *J Clin Invest* 1972;51:2077.
69. Snyder PJ, Utiger RD: Response to thyrotropin-releasing hormone in normal man. *J Clin Endocrinol Metab* 1972;34:380–385.
70. Snyder PJ, Utiger RD: Repetitive administration of thyrotropin-releasing hormone results in small elevation of serum thyroid hormones and in marked inhibition of thyrotropin response. *J Clin Invest* 1973;52:2305.
71. Saberi M, Utiger RD: Augmentation of thyrotropin responses to thyrotropin-releasing hormone following small decreases in serum thyroid hormone concentrations. *J Clin Endocrinol Metab* 1975;40:435.
72. Ridgway EC, Weintraub BD, Cevallos JL, et al: Suppression of pituitary TSH secretion in the patient with a hyperfunctioning thyroid nodule. *J Clin Invest* 1973;52:2783.
73. Vagenakis A, Rapoport B, Axixi F, et al: Hyper-response to thyrotropin-releasing hormone accompanying small decreases in serum thyroid hormone concentrations. *J Clin Invest* 1974;54:913.
74. Ingbar SH, Woeber KA: The thyroid gland, in Williams RH (ed): *Textbook of Endocrinology,* ed 6. Philadelphia, WB Saunders, 1981, pp 208–247.
75. Hall RCW, Popkin MK, DeVaul R, et al: Psychiatric manifestations of Hashimoto's thyroiditis. *Psychosomatics* 1982;23(4):337–342.
76. Fowler EF: The changing incidence and treatment of thyroid disease. *Arch Surg* 1960;81:733–740.
77. Cayzer I, Chalmers SR, Doniach D, et al: An evaluation of two new hemagglutination test for the rapid diagnosis of autoimmune thyroid disease. *J Clin Pathol* 1978;21:1147.
78. Delespesse G, Hubert C, Gawset P, et al: Radioimmunoassay for human antihyroglobulin antibodies of different immunoglobulin classes. *Horm Metab Res* 1976;8:50.
79. Fernstrom JD, Wurtman RJ: Brain serotonin content: Physiological dependence of plasma tryptophan levels. *Science* 1971;173:149–152.
80. Fernstrom JD, Wurtman RJ: Brain serotonin content: Physiological regulation by plasma neutral amino acids. *Science* 1972;173:414–416.
81. Bunney WE, Brodies HKH, Murphy DL, et al: Studies of alpha-methyl-paratryosine, L-DOPA, and L-tryptophan in depression and mania. *Am J Psychiatry* 1971;127:872–881.
82. Carroll BJ: Monoamine precursors in the treatment of depression. *Clin Pharmacol Ther* 1972;12:743–761.
83. Chouinard G, Young SN, Annable L, et al: Tryptophan nicotinamide, imipramine, and their combination in depression. *Acta Psychiatr Scand* 1979;59:395–414.
84. Dunner DL, Fieve RR: Affective disorder: Studies with amine precursors. *Am J Psychiatry* 1975;132:180–183.
85. Mendels J, Stinnett JL, Burns D, et al: Amine precursors and depression. *Arch Gen Psychiatry* 1975;32:22–30.
86. van Praag HM: Significance of biochemical parameters in the diagnosis, treatment, and prevention of depressive disorders. *Biol Psychol* 1977;12:101–131.
87. van Praag HM: Central monoamine metabolism in depression. I & II. *Compr Psychiatry* 1980;21:30–54.

88. Cole JO, Hartmann E, Brigham P: L-tryptophan: Clinical studies. *McLean Hosp J* 1980;5:37–71.
89. Cooper AJ: Tryptophan antidepressant: Physiological sedative, fact or fancy? *Psychopharmacology (Berlin)* 1979;61:97–102.
90. Growdon JH: Neurotransmitter precursors in the diet: Their use in the treatment of brain disease, in Wurtmann RJ, Wurtmann JJ (eds): *Nutrition and the Brain: Disorders of Eating and Nutrients in Treatment of Brain Diseases.* New York, Raven Press, 1979, pp 117–181.
91. Wirz-Justice A: Theoretical and therapeutical potential of indoleamine precursors in affective disorders. *Neuropsychobiology* 1977;3:199–233.
92. Carlsson A, Lindqvist M: Dependence of 5-HT and catecholamine synthesis of concentrations of precursor amino acids in rat brain. *Naunyn Schmiedebergs Arch Pharmacol* 1978;303:157–164.
93. Gibson CJ, Wurtman RJ: Physiological control of brain catechol synthesis by brain tyrosine concentration. *Biochem Pharmacol* 1978;26:1137–1142.
94. Wurtman RJ, Larin F, Mostafapour S, et al: Brain catechol synthesis: Control by brain tyrosine concentration. *Science* 1974;185:183–184.
95. Gibson CJ, Wurtman RJ: Physiological control of brain norepinephrine synthesis by brain tyrosine concentration. *Life Sci* 1978;22;1399–1406.
96. Goodwin RK, Post RM, Dunner DL, et al: Cerebrospinal fluid amine metabolites in affective illness: The probenecid technique. *Am J Psychiatry* 1973;130:73–79.
97. Glaeser BS, Melamed E, Growdon JH, et al: Elevation of plasma tyrosine after a single oral dose of L-tyrosine. *Life Sci* 1979;25:265–272.
98. Hogarty GE, Schooler NR, Ulrich R, et al: Fluphenazine and social therapy in the aftercare of schizophrenic patients. *Arch Gen Psychiatry* 1979;36:1283–1294.
99. Extein I: Psychopharmacology in psychiatric emergencies. *Int J Psychiatry Med* 1980;10:189–204.
100. Ayd FJ, Jr: Treatment-resistant patients: A moral, legal and therapeutic challenge, in Ayd, FJ, Jr (ed): *Rational Psychopharmacotherapy and the Right to Treatment.* Baltimore, Ayd Medical Communication, 1975.
101. Forsman A, Ohmen R: Pharmacokinetic studies on haloperidol in man. *Curr Psychiatr Ther* 1976;20:319–336.
102. Calil HM, Avery DH, Hollister LE, et al: Serum levels of neuroleptics measured by dopamine radioreceptor assay and some clinical observations. *Psychiatry Res* 1979;1:38–44.
103. Tune LE, Creese I, De Paulo JR Jr, et al: Clinical state and serum neuroleptic levels measured by radioreceptor assay in schizophrenia. *Am J Psychiatry* 1980;137:187–190.
104. Smith RC, Crayton J, Dekirmenjian H, et al: Blood levels or neuroleptic drugs in nonresponding chronic schizophrenic patients. *Arch Gen Psychiatry* 1979;36:579–584.
105. Magliozzi JR, Hollister LE, Arnold KV, et al: Relationship of serum haloperidol levels to clinical response in schizophrenic patients. *Am J Psychiatry* 1981;138:365–367.
106. Bianchetti G, Morselli PL: Rapid and sensitive method for determination of haloperidol in human samples using nitrogen-phosphorus selective detection. *J Chromatogr* 1978;153:203.
107. Wise DC, Potkin SG, Bridge TP, et al: Sources of error in the determination of Platelet Monoamine Oxidase: A review of methods. *Schizophr Bull* 1980;6(2):245–253.
108. Rosen AJ, Wirtshafter D, Pandey GN, et al: Platelet monoamine oxidase activity and behavioral response to pharmacotherapy in psychiatric patients. *Psychiatry Res* 1982;6:49–59.

Neurotransmitters and Receptors in Pharmacopsychiatry

Jerrold G. Bernstein

NEUROTRANSMITTERS IN PHARMACOPSYCHIATRY

As psychiatry comes of age as a medical discipline, theories regarding etiology and treatment are coming full circle. Centuries ago, before the distinct specialty of psychiatry became established, medical thinkers including Hippocrates subscribed to humoral theories of mental disorders. They believed the etiology of these conditions was not distinctly separated from theories about the etiologies of other medical conditions. Over the centuries, thoughts about the causation of mental disorders fluctuated between behavioral, biological and supernatural mechanisms.

In the last century or so, psychological theories as explanations of behavioral disorders were initially on the ascendency. On the other hand, the English chemist, Thudicum, began to do serious research on potential chemical factors in the causation of mental illness.[1] Nevertheless, the activities of Sigmund Freud and his contemporaries rather clearly established psychodynamic and behavioral explanations for psychopathology. These various psychological schools of thought also established their own forms of treatment of neurosis and other psychiatric conditions, to the extent that psychiatry began to move away from the main body of medical science. The sway of these schools of thought was indeed so strong that attempts to conduct biochemical and pharmacological research into the etiology and treatment of mental disorders were held in lower esteem than the reigning non-medical theories. Reports on chemical testing of biological fluids from psychiatric patients and experiments with a variety of medications in mentally ill individuals were scattered through the medical literature during the first half of this century, but were mainly published in journals of biochemistry, pharmacology or medicine rather than in journals devoted to psychiatry and behavioral science. Just a few decades ago, most clinicians found it impossible to make a logical connection between disturbed thinking or behavior and abnormal brain chemistry. The possibility that a tablet or injection could improve these abnormalities seemed like science fiction. Today it is almost taken for granted by psychiatrists that abnormal biology underlies many of the problems we treat.[2] Antidepressants and antipsychotic drugs have become as much a part of the armamentarium of the sophisticated psychiatrist as digitalis has for the internist.

We are reaching a point where it becomes increasingly more difficult to understand and treat psychiatric illness without some consideration of neurochemistry and pharmacology. Thus this chapter will review concepts of the interaction of chemical substances with receptor sites present in the nervous system of living organisms. Rather than focus on the complexities of organic, physical, and biological chemistry, these matters will be discussed in a simplified though hopefully accurate fashion in order to be readily understood and applied to the practice of pharmacotherapy in the psychiatric patient. It is impossible to present a complete discussion of neurotransmitters since countless numbers of compounds have been proposed to have neurotransmitter function. The present discussion focuses on those compounds that are most widely accepted and understood as neurotransmitters. Since the focus of this volume is the treatment of the psychiatric patient, this chapter will deal with the interaction of neurotransmitters, drugs, and receptor sites and the impact of this interaction on human behavior and mood.

NEUROPHYSIOLOGY AND NEUROTRANSMISSION

The human brain is comprised of several billion neurons. Each neuron consists of a cell body of multiple short fibers, termed dendrites, that receive information from other neurons. Each neuron also has extending from the cell body a fiber known as an axon that may be either short or long. The axon transmits information from the cell body to other neurons. Electrical impulses arising in the cell body travel through the axon to a specialized terminal known as the synapse. At the synaptic ending neurotransmitter substances are released; they diffuse across the synaptic cleft and thereby transmit information to the dendrite of the next neuron. Since the fibers of the multitude of neurons within the brain do not make physical connection with each other, electrical impulses generated within one neuron cannot jump the gap to the next neuron. Communication between them is dependent upon the release of specialized chemical substances termed neurotransmitters. The ability of vast numbers of nerve fibers to transmit information between the billions of neurons within the brain involves a large number of neurotransmitter substances and their specialized sites of action, known as receptors. This complex neuronal circuitry and the specialized action of a variety of neurotransmitters regulate information handling, memory, mood and behavior.[3] Structural and functional areas of the brain appear to be at least partially differentiated by their relative concentrations of chemically distinct neurotransmitters. The complexity of the electrochemical processes necessary for normal brain function makes the possibility of dysfunction readily understandable. As the electrical impulse travels down the axon, it causes the release of transmitters at the axon terminal. The transmitter substance then alters permeability of the dendritic membrane of the next neuron, resulting either in depolarization or hyperpolarization of the dendrites of the next neuron.[3] Once the transmitter has performed its function, it must be removed to terminate its action. It is understandable that the failure to terminate the action of a released neurotransmitter would be likely to prolong, inhibit, or exaggerate its action.[4] Likewise, the production and release of excess neurotransmitter or excessive sensitivity of the receptor site to the action of the neurotransmitter would produce an exaggerated effect at the cellular level, which may be seen as a clinical abnormality. On the other hand, deficient synthesis or release of neurotransmitter molecules, or decreased sensitivity of the receptor site also would be likely to produce a physiological abnormality that again could be manifested clinically in abnormalities of thought processes, mood, or behavior.[2]

Electron microscopic examination of neuronal junctions reveals that the width of the synaptic cleft separating the presynaptic membrane of the axon terminal from the postsynaptic membrane of the dendrite is approximately 100 to 500 Ångström units.[4] Within the presynaptic terminal are numerous small synaptic vesicles. It is in these vesicles that neurotransmitter substances are stored prior to their release. Once the electrical impulse has triggered the release of the neurotransmitter from the vesicles, the transmitter diffuses across the synaptic cleft, stimulates the postsynaptic receptors, and is released from those receptors back into the synaptic cleft.[3,4] In the case of acetylcholine, one of the more ubiquitous neurotransmitters, there is rapid hydrolysis through the action of the enzyme acetylcholinesterase.[5] In the case of norepinephrine, another prominent central nervous system transmitter, a portion of the released substance is repackaged into synaptic vesicles within the presynaptic nerve terminal. The remainder of the norepinephrine is then metabolically degraded through the action of the enzyme monoamine oxidase (MAO).

That portion of the released norepinephrine which has been repackaged into synaptic vesicles is not vulnerable to MAO-catalyzed inactivation, and it may be released again in response to an electrical impulse traveling down the axon in the fashion previously described.[3,6]

CLINICAL ASPECTS OF NEUROTRANSMITTERS

Having discussed in a very simplified form some aspects of neurotransmitter function, and before considering receptor sites and the actions of transmitters and drugs upon them, some clinical aspects of the material should be considered.[7] Neurotransmitter substances are formed endogenously within the central nervous system as well as within the autonomic nervous system. These substances are synthesized by the action of enzymes upon simpler chemical molecules absorbed into the circulation as a result of the metabolism of food. Neurotransmitter chemicals are complex charged molecules. Although the brain receives voluminous blood flow, the passage of substances from the circulation into the brain is selective. This selectivity is the result of what has been termed the blood-brain barrier.[3] For a circulating chemical to reach neuronal elements within the brain, it must pass through not only the dense capillary wall but also through a fatty barrier called the glial sheath. This sheath is made up of glial feet that are extensions of nearby astrocyte cells.[3] The structure and function of the blood-brain barrier is potentially protective, preventing certain substances from entering the brain, and is potentially disadvantageous, limiting access to the brain of certain chemical substances that we might wish to administer for therapeutic purposes. A case in point is, that due to the nature of this barrier and the molecular structure of neurotransmitter substances, we are unable to increase brain concentration of these substances by administering them directly to the patient.[2,3]

Recent investigations have found that administering large doses of dietary precursors of neurotransmitters will allow these substances to reach the brain and give rise to synthesis of increased quantities of certain neurotransmitters.[8] For example, oral administration of choline, a dietary precursor of acetylcholine formation, can produce increased brain concentrations of this neurotransmitter which may eventually have some therapeutic value.[9] Likewise, oral administration of tyrosine,[10] a precursor for norepinephrine, and tryptophan,[11,12] the precursor of serotonin, may prove to have therapeutic value in the treatment of depressive disorders wherein there may be a relative deficit or decreased sensitivity to these neurotransmitters.[13] The best known application of the administration of a neurotransmitter precursor is the longstanding therapeutic use of levodopa, which has considerable efficacy in Parkinson's disease, as a result of increased dopamine synthesis.[14]

The termination of action of neurotransmitters through their metabolic breakdown has previously been mentioned. If the metabolic breakdown of certain neurotransmitters can be reduced or inhibited, it stands to reason that the concentration and most likely the physiologic action of a neurotransmitter would be enhanced. Physostigmine inhibits cholinesterase, the enzyme responsible for terminating the action of the transmitter, acetylcholine.[5] The action of acetylcholine (cholinergic action) can be enhanced by the administration of physostigmine since decreased breakdown of acetylcholine leads to increased cholinergic activity. Physostigmine has been used for a number of years in the evaluation and treatment of patients suffering from toxic deliria induced by the administration of excessive doses of anticholinergic drugs.[15,16] The MAO inhibitors were the first effective antidepressant drugs. They also provided neuropharmacologists with an opportunity to understand some of the connections between neurotransmitters and mood.[2] By inhibiting enzymatic breakdown of norepinephrine and other centrally occurring monoamine neurotransmitters, MAO inhibitor antidepressants, such as phenelzine, allow for increased brain concentration of neurotransmitters whose actions may indeed be deficient in patients suffering from depressive illness.[1] The subsequently developed tricyclic antidepressants inhibit nerve reuptake of norepinephrine and serotonin, thus slowing the inactivation of these transmitters and perhaps enhancing their action, which appears to be diminished in depressive illness.[2] Thus a variety of techniques aimed at either enhancing neurotransmitter synthesis or inhibiting inactivation have found their way into the practice of clinical psychiatry and have provided tools for understanding nervous system function.[2,8,15]

RECEPTORS, TRANSMITTERS AND DRUGS

Having considered the formation and release of neurotransmitter substances as a result of the propagation of electrical impulses down the axon into the axon terminal, and their diffusion across the synaptic cleft to their site of action at the postsynaptic membrane, it is important now to consider the receptor site. A variety of complex molecules, most prominently protein in nature, are present within the membrane structure of each of the multitude of specialized cells that make up the human body.[2,3,4] The variety of specialized receptor sites within the body is enormous and uncountable, yet on the surface of any individual cell there may be only a few thousand receptor sites.[3] Any given cell may have one specific type of receptor, or conceivably could have a variety of receptors. In recent years we have begun to learn more about the specific nature of receptors, although the theoretical concept originated about a century ago.[3,4]

Postsynaptic membranes contain specialized membrane-bound protein molecules that act as receptors. These specialized molecules respond selectively to endogenously released chemical transmitter substances including the neurotransmitters we are considering, as well as a wide variety of hormones.[2,3] The selectivity of receptor sites appears to be based upon their individual physicochemical properties that make them uniquely responsive to particular molecular configurations.[2] If all endogenously released chemical substances act through combination with selective receptor sites, then one may question the relevance of this to the actions of newly developed therapeutic agents. In general, exogenously administered drugs act within the body by affecting a receptor site whose presence is presumably for the purpose of responding to an endogenous substance of physicochemical properties resembling those of the drug.[5,6] Thus, we have synthetically produced pharmaceutical products whose structural similarity is close enough to endogenously occurring substances that the drug product may mimic the naturally occurring substance. For example, the amphetamines are spoken of as sympathomimetic drugs because their action mimics the response to sympathetic nervous system stimulation. Indeed, they are chemically similar to norepinephrine, the naturally occurring transmitter active within the sympathetic nervous system.[6] Arecoline, a potent cholinergic compound, is spoken of as parasympathomimetic or cholinomimetic because its action mimics stimulation of the parasympathetic nervous system, presumably as a result of its ability to combine with and stimulate acetylcholine-sensitive receptor sites.[5,17]

As said previously, our understanding of the exact nature of receptor sites is still quite limited. Perhaps the best studied and most understood is the cholinergic receptor. This receptor appears to be composed of three or more subunits, each with a molecular weight of 40,000, which carry binding sites for cholinergic agonists and antagonists.[4,5] The interaction of agonist compounds (those that stimulate the receptor) with the receptor results in changes in sodium flux through the membrane as a result of change in state of a specific ionophore or ion-conductance modulator. Evidence suggests that this ionophore is a protein distinct from the receptor, with a molecular weight of 43,000, and that the receptor and ionophore are strongly associated with the cell membrane.[18,19] Those chemical substances, which stimulate a receptor site and produce a physiological effect similar to that produced by the action of the naturally occurring transmitter upon that site, are spoken of as agonists.[5] Chemical compounds whose molecular structure allows them to combine with receptor sites without stimulating the site or producing an agonist effect are known as antagonists.[2] An antagonist may be thought of as a receptor-blocking drug. The action of such compounds at receptor sites occupies the receptor and makes it unavailable to respond to endogenously released transmitter substance or to exogenously administered agonist compounds.

Haloperidol, a widely used antipsychotic drug, exerts its clinical action as a result of its ability to combine with and block dopamine receptor sites, thus it is a dopamine receptor antagonist.[20] Chlorpromazine, another antipsychotic agent, is an alpha-adrenergic antagonist. The ability of this compound to block alpha-adrenergic receptor sites in the peripheral vasculature accounts for its considerable ability to lower blood pressure.[1] Propranolol is a beta-adrenergic antagonist, which will decrease myocardial work, heart rate, and blood pressure[1] by blocking these receptor sites. The previously mentioned cholinergic agonist, arecoline, which stimulates acetylcholine receptors, may eventually find therapeutic application in the treatment of certain neurological and psychiatric conditions associated with decreased central nervous system acetylcholine activity.[17] Some drugs exert mixed agonist–antagonist activity and thereby may initially stimulate a receptor site and then block its further stimulation by other compounds, whether they be endogenously released or exogenously administered.[1,4]

CHEMICAL TRANSMITTERS
IN BRAIN FUNCTION

Most psychiatrists have at least a passing acquaintance with the neurotransmitter role of acetylcholine, norepinephrine, dopamine, and serotonin, since the actions of many psychotropic drugs are linked to these transmitters.[1,2] It must be emphasized, however, that these transmitters which we have come to accept as the most important ones act at only a minority of the nerve terminals within the central nervous system.[2] There is mounting evidence that histamine, long recognized as a mediator of allergic reactions, also serves a neurotransmitter role within the hypothalamus and perhaps other areas of the brain.[21] Quantitatively, a variety of amino acid-derived substances appear to have an even larger role in central neurotransmission than the more widely known, previously mentioned substances.[2]

In some areas of the brain, gamma-aminobutyric acid (GABA) serves a neurotransmitter function.[22] This compound may account for transmission in 25% to 40% of brain synapses.[2] GABA has the ability to inhibit firing of some neurons, and appears to function as the major inhibitory neurotransmitter.[22] The amino acid, glycine, appears to serve a similar inhibitory transmitter function in a large number of spinal cord and brain stem synapses.[2] On the other hand, glutamic acid and aspartic acid, present in large concentration within the brain, appear to act as excitatory neurotransmitters.[2] The widespread distribution of these amino acids throughout the brain and other body tissues has made it more difficult to study their role in neural function than has been the case with the previously mentioned neurotransmitters whose distribution is somewhat more discrete.[2] A variety of peptide substances, derived from several amino acid molecules linked together, act as hormones and neurotransmitters in the brain and throughout the body.[2] Opiate-like peptides known as enkephalins bind to specific sites within the central nervous system and are known to mediate pain perception. Opiate receptors are sensitive not only to these endogenously produced compounds but also to exogenously administered narcotic analgesics. A larger molecule made up of methionine-enkephalin, linked to 26 other amino acids, is known as beta-endorphin. It is present in a high concentration within the pituitary and may serve a neurotransmitter function.[2,23] Another polypeptide, substance P, appears to have a role as a neurotransmitter mediating pain sensation.[24,25] This substance along with GABA may function as naturally occurring tranquilizers, although much investigative work is still needed to clarify this role. Since each specific neuron within the brain generally utilizes only a single type of neurotransmitter compound, we have come to classify neurons not only on the basis of their physical structure and location, but also on the basis of which neurotransmitter they release.

Since the goal of this discussion is not an indepth view of neuroanatomy or neurochemistry but rather an attempt to correlate certain neurotransmitter functions with mental disorders and their treatment, the focus will continue on available knowledge as it applies to these concerns. There are two major norepinephrine tracts within the brain. The ventral pathway has cell bodies in several locations of the brain stem and axons that extend into the medial forebrain bundle and terminate at synapses, mainly in the hypothalamus and limbic system. This tract has terminals within the pleasure centers of the lateral hypothalamus, and appears to have a functional role in affective behaviors, including euphoria and depression.[2] The other major norepinephrine tract, the dorsal pathway, has cell bodies that are discretely localized to the locus ceruleus within the brain stem. Its axons also ascend in the medial forebrain bundle dorsal to those of the ventral pathway.[2] Terminals of the dorsal pathway are primarily localized in the cerebral cortex and hippocampus. Some axons from the locus ceruleus descend to form synapses with purkinje cells within the cerebellum. Some cells of the locus ceruleus give off axons that branch ascending fibers to the cerebral cortex, as well as the cerebellum. Thus, a single neuron may influence widespread areas of the brain. There is evidence that the dorsal norepinephrine pathway to the cerebral cortex may be associated with the control of alertness.[2]

There are a number of discrete dopaminergic tracts. The most prominent one has cell bodies in the substantia nigra and axons that terminate in the caudate nucleus and putamen, two structures of the corpus striatum that function to coordinate motor activity.[2] In Parkinson's disease there is deterioration of this pathway, giving rise to tremor and motor disorders that characterize this condition. Administration of the dopamine precursor, levodopa, helps to restore the neurotransmitter that is depleted and thus alleviates some of the symptoms of Parkinson's disease.[26] Other dopamine pathways have cell bodies close to the substantia nigra just dorsal to the interpeduncular nucleus, with terminals in the nucleus accumbens and olfactory tubercle which are components of the limbic system.[2] Furthermore, dopaminergic neurons within the cerebral cortex appear to have a role in emotional behavior. The ability of antipsychotic drugs to control symptoms of psychosis is directly related to blockade of these dopamine receptor sites.[20] Dopaminergic cells in the arcuate nucleus of the hypothalamus, with terminals in the median eminence, probably regulate the release of hypothalamic hormones which then act on the pituitary gland to regulate the release of pituitary hormones.[27] Dopamine inhibits the release of prolactin from the pituitary gland. Dopamine-blocking antipsychotic drugs thus elevate plasma levels of the hormone prolactin, potentially giving rise to the side effects of abnormal milk secretion and amenorrhea when these therapeutic agents are administered to women.[2,27]

Current research suggests that for any given transmitter substance there may be more than one type of receptor. Recent studies indicate that there may well be three or more species of dopamine-sensitive receptors.[27,28] The dopamine receptor just described, the one thought to be most important to the action of neuroleptic drugs, is known as DA-2.[27,28] The DA-1 receptors are found on intrinsic striatal neurons; they are involved in parathormone release and stimulate adenylate cyclase. These receptors are less sensitive to neuroleptic drugs than are DA-2 receptors. DA-3 receptors are likewise relatively insensitive to neuroleptics; they are involved apparently in autoregulation of dopamine neurons and are found on intrinsic striatal neurons as well as nigrostriatal terminals. The DA-2 receptors are found on intrinsic striatal neurons and on corticostriate afferents, as well as in the pituitary gland. DA-2 sites are not associated with increased adenylate cyclase, but are highly sensitive to neuroleptics and are the receptors generally referred to in the action of psychoactive drugs on behavior.[28]

Cell bodies of the serotonin containing neurons are localized in a series of nuclei of the lower midbrain and upper pons known as the raphe nuclei. It appears that most cells within these nuclei are serotonergic.[2] Axons of these cells ascend primarily in the medial forebrain bundle and give off terminals in all regions of the brain, although mostly within the hypothalamus. Destruction of the raphe nuclei in experimental animals produces agitation and insomnia.[2] Administration of the serotonin precursors, L-tryptophan or 5-hydroxytryptophan, will correct the serotonin depletion and induce sleep in the experimental animals.[29] Similarly, the serotonin precursor, L-tryptophan, has been employed clinically in normal subjects and patients with insomnia to induce sleep.[30] Stimulation of the raphe nuclei in experimental animals likewise induces sleep.[29]

BIOCHEMICAL BASES OF MENTAL
DISORDERS AND PHARMACOPSYCHIATRY

Over the years a variety of attempts have been made to find chemical abnormalities within the blood and urine of individuals suffering from mental disorders. Unfortunately, many of the earlier attempts were discredited by the inability of different groups of scientists to repeat the experiments with comparable results.[1] Another limitation to studies of the biological correlates of mental disorders has been the fact that essentially all of the neurotransmitters present within the brain are also present at other sites within the body. Thus, measurements of the substances in body fluid may reflect not only what is happening within the central nervous system, but within other tissues as well.

Over the years a number of clues have whetted our appetites and suggested biochemical correlations to psychiatric illness. About 50 years ago, epidemiologic studies within the mental institutions revealed a low incidence of allergic disorders in schizophrenic patients. Subsequent studies revealed that administration of histamine, a mediator of allergic reactions to schizophrenic patients, produced only minimal stimulation of gastric acid secretion in contradistinction to the effects of the compound on normal controls.[1] A number of years ago in my laboratory we found that levels of the histamine-metabolizing enzyme, histaminase, were significantly elevated in the blood of schizophrenic patients.[31] This finding correlated well with the decreased incidence of allergic disorders and decreased sensitivity to administered histamine that had previously been reported. At the time of this work, the possible neurotransmitter role of histamine was highly questionable. There is now increasing evidence to suggest that histamine may have an important neurotransmitter role.[21] Certainly most antihistaminic drugs exert pronounced sedative action. Furthermore, among tricyclic antidepressants a rather close correlation has been noted between sedative effect and histamine receptor-blocking potency.[32] Earlier experiments attempting to unravel the biochemistry of psychosis revealed that the administration of the amino acid tryptophan or methionine could produce an exacerbation of psychotic symptoms in schizophrenic patients who are clinically in remission.[1] Earlier investigation revealed the ability of MAO inhibitor drugs to exacerbate symptoms in asymptomatic schizophrenic patients presumably as a result of inhibition of catecholamine neurotransmitter metabolism.[1] The interaction of hallucinogenic drugs with serotonergic neurons has already been mentioned and may explain the ability of these compounds to provoke psychotic symptoms in normal subjects.[2]

Since data from studies of body fluids taken from patients have not been fully reliable and since, unlike other organs, we cannot remove a sample of brain tissue for analysis, our attempts to correlate brain chemistry with disease states depends on indirect documentation. The strongest source of data comes from our clinical experience with the administration of neuroleptic drugs to psychotic individuals and the correlation of the clinical findings with in vitro experiments.[33]Although the currently available neuroleptics are rather widely divergent in their chemical structure, they have one unifying characteristic in common, namely, their ability to antagonize or block dopamine receptor sites. Their clinical potency closely parallels their affinity for these receptor sites.[20] Inhibition of dopamine receptors accelerates the firing rate of dopamine neurons, increasing dopamine metabolites. Chronic blockade of dopamine receptors by prolonged administration of antipsychotic drugs produces supersensitivity at receptor sites and increased numbers of dopamine receptors.[2] These changes appear to correlate with the primary adverse effects of antipsychotic drugs, namely the possibility of producing tardive dyskinesia. Dopamine receptors can be measured by monitoring the binding to neuronal membranes of radioactive derivatives of neuroleptic drugs. To determine whether a drug blocks dopamine receptors, one ascertains if it will reduce the amount of radioactive neuroleptic bound to these sites. The relative potency of neuroleptics in blocking dopamine receptors measured in this way parallels their clinical potency, as previously mentioned.[20] Only drugs with neuroleptic activity antagonize dopamine receptors within the dose range used clinically.

PSYCHOTIC ILLNESS

In contrast to this specificity of action, the potency of neuroleptics as antagonists of nondopamine neurotransmitter receptor sites does not correlate with antipsychotic potency.[34,35] The findings correlating dopamine receptor blockade with clinical potency of antipsychotic drugs suggests that an abnormality in dopamine release or action may underlie schizophrenic illness.[36] Amphetamines, when administered in large doses, produce a psychotic state that is clinically indistinguishable from paranoid schizophrenia.[36] Furthermore, when administered to schizophrenic patients, even low doses of amphetamines will exacerbate psychotic symptoms. The symptoms precipitated by amphetamine administration in schizophrenic patients vary from individual to individual and correlate well with the pattern of symptoms previously seen in the particular patients under study.[2] The structural similarity of the amphetamines to norepinephrine and dopamine suggests that these compounds may facilitate the action of the catecholamine neurotransmitters within the brain.[6,36] Amphetamines trigger the release of norepinephrine and dopamine from nerve endings into the synaptic cleft.[6] Although the final answer is not available on the mechanism of schizophrenic illness, the ability of agents that stimulate the dopamine action to exacerbate psychosis, and the salutary effects of dopamine blocking drugs upon psychotic symptoms, strongly suggests that dopamine has a pivotal etiologic role in this form of psychotic illness.

It must be borne in mind that schizophrenia runs in families and that strong evidence supports a genetic factor in the etiology of this psychotic illness. Although the risk of developing schizophrenia is about 1% in the general population, 10% of siblings of schizophrenics are likely to develop the illness and 14% of children of affected patients are likely to develop schizophrenia.[2] If both parents suffer from schizophrenia, it is likely that about one-half of their children will become schizophrenic.[2] Although one may argue that environmental factors play a role in this predisposition, the studies of identical twins reared apart from each other and from their biological parents have attempted to correct for environmental influence, thus focusing on factors of genetic predisposition. Studies by Kety of biological and adoptive relatives of adopted children who later developed schizophrenia or schizophrenia-like disorders were compared for the presence of psychiatric disturbance.[37] As a control, biological and adoptive relatives of nonschizophrenic adoptees were also evaluated. There was a much higher incidence of definite severe schizophrenia in the biological relatives in schizophrenic adoptees than among those of control adoptees.[37] In contrast, schizophrenic-like disorders, such as schizoid personality, had about the same frequency in the two groups of relatives. This suggests that definite schizophrenia has a genetic basis that is lacking in the other disorders.

When the initial Copenhagen study was extended to the entire country of Denmark, a total of 74 schizophrenic adoptees and more than 1000 relatives were evaluated. In addition to corroborating the results of the initial study, the second investigation identified subtypes in the relatives with greater certainty.[37] Biological relatives of adoptees with definite schizophrenia had a high incidence of chronic but not of acute schizophrenia. Strikingly, biological relatives of acute schizophrenics showed very little evidence of schizophrenia-related disorders. Thus, we have further evidence that chronic schizophrenia has a genetic determinant that is not shared by acute schizophrenic illness.[37] Although psychological and environmental factors cannot be excluded in the genesis of schizophrenic illness, the evidence overwhelmingly supports the occurrence of a genetic predisposition to the development of a biochemical, ie, transmitter defect in the etiology of this condition.[1,2]

AFFECTIVE ILLNESS

In affective illness there is strong evidence for a genetic predisposition. In a summary of twin studies of affective illness, the overall concordance rate for bipolar illness in monozygotic twins was 72%, while the corresponding figure for dizygotic twins was only 14%.[38] In unipolar affective illness the concordance rate for monozygotic twins was 40%, while for dizygotic twins there was a concordance of only 11%. Numerous studies have suggested that the incidence of bipolar illness is much higher among relatives of bipolar patients than among relatives of unipolar patients.[2,38] A high frequency of hypomanic personality traits, even in the absence of clear affective illness, has been noted in family members of patients suffering from bipolar affective illness. Depressive personality traits are common in family members of patients suffering from bipolar affective illness. Depressive personality traits are common in family members of patients suffering from unipolar depression.[39] Alcoholism, which also appears to have a genetic predisposition, tends to be more common in the families of patients with major affective illness than in the population as a whole.[2] Although the etiologic role of life stresses in the precipitation of affective illness may be important, the genetic contribution appears to be of greater significance in those patients who begin to experience depression earlier in their life and in those individuals who have multiple recurrent affective episodes, whether they be depressive or manic episodes.[2] As in the case of schizophrenic illness, a genetic predisposition appears to give rise to a biochemical, ie, neurotransmitter, defect that eventually, on one or more occasions, becomes manifested in the life of the individual by affective symptoms. As in the case of schizophrenic illness, direct measurements of abnormal chemical factors within the brain cannot be made. Likewise, data from studies of biological fluids have provided only limited etiologic information.

Clinical and biochemical responses to administered drugs have provided most of the useful information supporting a biochemical etiology in affective illness. Serotonin and norepinephrine have both been implicated in the etiology of affective illness; both are localized in the limbic system and hypothalamus, brain areas that are known to be involved in the regulation of emotions.[2] Two serendipitous observations made about 30 years ago have given rise to much of our current appreciation of neurochemical correlates in mood disorders. Reserpine was widely used in the treatment of hypertension and frequently produced severe depressive illness and suicidal behavior, even in individuals with no prior history of affective disease.[1] This drug weakens binding sites for both serotonin and norepinephrine within the synaptic vesicles, causing these transmitters to gradually leak out into the synapse and become metabolically degraded.[2] The other important finding was the observation of hypomanic and manic behavior in tuberculous patients being treated with a new drug, iproniazid. This compound was known to inhibit the enzyme monoamine oxidase, thus blocking the ability of the brain to metabolize monamine neurotransmitters such as norepinephrine and serotonin.[1] Reserpine depletion of these neurotransmitters was associated with the production of severe depressive states, while iproniazid-induced enhancement of the brain concentration of these neurotransmitters was able to invoke the opposite mood-state, mainly hypomania or mania.[1]

Another accidental finding that occurred much later was the observation that the antihypertensive drug, alpha-methyldopa, which is known to interfere with the synthesis and release of norepinephrine, was capable of inducing severe depression.[40] In the search for safer and more effective antipsychotic drugs, the chlorpromazine derivative, imipramine, was administered experimentally to patients. Although this compound unfortunately lacked antipsychotic efficacy, an incidental observation revealed its ability to improve mood in depressed individual.[1] Imipramine and related tricyclic antidepressants inhibit nerve reuptake mechanisms, the primary mode of inactivation of serotonin and norepinephrine.[1,2] Thus, we have additional evidence correlating a decrement or increment in neurotransmitter activity with changes in mood state.

It would appear from these observations that any intervention decreasing central monoamine transmitter function would induce depression and that interventions enhancing central monoamine neurotransmission would exert an antidepressant effect. Electrically induced seizures in rats increase turnover of brain norepinephrine and appear to produce a net increase in both brain level and synthesis of this neurotransmitter.[41] Numerous studies have revealed decreased urinary excretion of MHPG (3-methoxy, 4-hydroxy-phenyglycol) in some depressed patients.[42] Urinary levels of MHPG have been observed to increase following a series of electroconvulsive therapy (ECT) treatments, suggesting a correlation between increased norepinephrine turnover and improvement in mood.[2,41] Those individuals who have low pretreatment MHPG are thought to represent depressive disorders whose mechanism involves decreased norepinephrine activity. Another group of depressed patients whose urinary and MHPG excretion is normal may show abnormally low cerebrospinal fluid levels of the serotonin metabolite 5-hydroxy indolacetic acid (5-HIAA).[42] Cerebrospinal fluid levels of 5-HIAA increase toward normal following ECT in many patient studies.[41] Thus, the metabolic changes in both serotonin and norepinephrine that have been associated with ECT both help to explain the mechanism of action of this effective therapeutic agent, and also lend further evidence to a biochemical understanding of depression. Among the tricyclics, tetracyclic and newer chemically unrelated antidepressant drugs, various compounds appear to exert selective action with respect to enhancing central serotonergic or noradrenergic (norepinephrine) activity.[1,32,42] This selective biochemical action appears to correlate with some selectivity of the beneficial clinically observed antidepressant effect of these compounds.

In addition to the drug-induced and ECT-induced changes in mood and neurochemistry, enhanced central serotonergic activity can be produced by administration of large doses of the precursor L-tryptophan.[11] Administration of L-tyrosine, a norepinephrine precursor that crosses the blood brain barrier and enters the brain, will increase central levels of the noradrenergic transmitter.[10] Preliminary studies of these two neurotransmitter precursors have revealed that each may exert a therapeutically useful antidepressant effect, thus again correlating increased central monoamine transmitter activity with improved mood in depressed patients.[10,11,12]

Manic behavior appears to have both clinical and neurochemical abnormalities that are essentially opposite those seen in depression.[2] Those drugs that improve depressive symptoms may trigger or worsen mania.[1] Drugs that may provoke depression, such as reserpine and neuroleptics, have an antimanic action.[1] Since acetylcholine appears to act in opposition to the catecholamine neurotransmitters, it would seem that cholinergic stimulation should decrease manic symptoms. The administration of anticholinergic drugs may worsen manic symptoms. The experimental administration of physostigmine, a cholinesterase inhibitor; arecoline, a direct cholinergic stimulant; or choline, an acetylcholine precursor; have all been shown to exert antimanic activity. This activity correlates with the ability of each of these compounds to increase central cholinergic function.[1,8,43] The neurochemical action of lithium remains quite intriguing, because this compound is capable of controlling and preventing mania, but also has the ability to improve and protect against recurrent episodes of depression. Information now becoming available suggests that lithium interacts with serotonergic, catecholaminergic and cholinergic sites within the brain. Furthermore, lithium appears to have a regulatory function in effecting the passage of sodium and perhaps other ions across cell membranes.[44]

ANXIETY

The central biochemical correlates of anxiety are still less well understood than even our rudimentary awareness of the neurochemical correlates of schizophrenic and affective illness. Specific benzodiazepine receptor sites have been identified within brain tissue.[45] Indeed, the possible role of GABA and substance P have been mentioned earlier in the context of their possible function as naturally occurring tranquilizers. The benzodiazepine receptor is functionally and perhaps structurally coupled to a receptor for GABA, the major inhibitory neurotransmitter.[2,45] An investigational antianxiety compound, buspirone, which is structurally different from the benzodiazepines, appears to exert an antianxiety effect but does not interact with the benzodiazepine/GABA receptor axis.[46] Interestingly enough, this novel compound appears only to interact with the dopaminergic system that produces a mixed agonist-antagonist effect.[47] If preliminary investigations on this compound can be carried further, we may be on the verge of understanding the connection between the neurochemical mechanism of anxiety and central dopamine receptor activity.

74

SUMMARY

This brief review has attempted to pull together correlations of mood, behavior, neurotransmitters and receptors in a way that will allow the clinician an opportunity to understand these complex interactions. Furthermore, ways in which receptor sites may be stimulated, blocked, or acted upon by compounds that produce both stimulatory and inhibitory effects and the clinical correlation of these actions have been reviewed. As pharmacophsychiatry advances, we are clearly looking toward a goal of better understanding the currently known receptors, discovering new receptors, and learning ways to modify these critical areas of neurotransmitter activity so that optimal care can be given to psychiatric patients. Those individuals who achieve little or no benefit from currently available therapeutic agents may eventually have the opportunity to benefit from hopefully more effective and safer therapeutic agents whose mechanism of action may bear little or no resemblance to the compounds we currently employ therapeutically. The possibility that amino acid and other compounds derived from dietary sources may modify synthesis and release of neurotransmitters and thus exert useful therapeutic action remains a promise for the future of pharmacopsychiatry.

REFERENCES

1. Bernstein JG: *Handbook of Drug Therapy in Psychiatry.* Littleton, MA, John Wright•PSG, 1983.
2. Snyder SH: *Biological Aspects of Mental Disorder.* New York, Oxford University Press, 1980.
3. Bloom FE: Neurohumoral transmission and the central nervous system, in Gilman AG, Goodman LS, Gilman A (eds): *Goodman and Gilman's The Pharmacological Basis of Therapeutics.* New York, Macmillan, 1980, pp 235–257.
4. Mayer SE: Neurohumoral transmission and the autonomic nervous system, in Gilman AG, Goodman LS, Gilman A (eds): *Goodman and Gilman's The Pharmacological Basis of Therapeutics.* New York, Macmillan, 1980, pp 56–90.
5. Taylor P: Cholinergic agonists, in Gilman AG, Goodman LS, Gilman A (eds): *Goodman and Gilman's The Pharmacological Basis of Therapeutics.* New York, Macmillan, 1980, pp 91–99.
6. Weiner N: Norepinephrine, epinephrine, and the sympathomimetic amines, in Gilman AG, Goodman LS, Gilman A (eds): *Goodman and Gilman's The Pharmacological Basis of Therapeutics.* New York, Macmillan, 1980, pp 138–175.
7. Baldessarini RJ: Drugs and the treatment of psychiatric disorders, in Gilman AG, Goodman LS, Gilman A (eds): *Goodman and Gilman's The Pharmacological Basis of Therapeutics.* New York, Macmillan, 1980, pp 391–447.
8. Wurtman RJ: Nutrients that modify brain function. *Scientific American* 1982;246:50–59.
9. Wurtman RJ, Hefti F, Melamed E: Precursor control of neurotransmitter synthesis. *Pharmacol Rev* 1981;32:315–335.

10. Gelenberg AJ, Wojcik JD, Growdon JH, et al: Tyrosine for the treatment of depression. *Am J Psychiatry* 1980;137:622–623.
11. Cooper AJ: Tryptophan antidepressant, "physiological sedative": fact or fancy? *Psychopharmacology* 1979;61:97–102.
12. Beitman BD, Dunner DL: L-Tryptophan in the maintenance treatment of bipolar II manic depressive illness. *Am J Psychiatry* 1982;139:1498–1499.
13. Moller SE, Amdisen A: Plasma neutral amino acids in mania and depression: Variation during acute and prolonged treatment with L-tryptophan. *Biol Psychiatry* 1979;14:131–139.
14. Calne DB, Kelabian J, Silbergeld E, et al: Advances in the neuropharmacology of parkinsonism. *Ann Intern Med* 1979;90:219–229.
15. Granacher RP, Baldessarini RJ: Physostigmine in the acute anticholinergic syndrome associated with antidepressant and antiparkinsonism drugs. *Arch Gen Psychiatry* 1975;32:375–380.
16. Baldessarini RJ, Gelenberg AJ: Use of physostigmine in antidepressant-induced intoxication. *Am J Psychiatry* 1979;136:1608–1609.
17. Sitaran N, Weingartner H, Gillin JC: Human serial learning: Enhancement with arecoline and choline impairment with scopolamine. *Science* 1978;201:274–276.
18. Birdsall NJM, Hume EC: Biochemical studies on muscarinic acetylcholine receptors. *J Neurochem* 1976;27:7–16.
19. Birdsall NJM, Burgen ASV, Hume EC: The binding of agonists to brain muscarinic receptors. *Mol Pharmacol* 1978;14:737–738.
20. Creese I, Burt DR, Snyder SH: Dopamine receptor binding predicts clinical and pharmacological potencies of antischizophrenic drugs. *Science* 1976;192:481–483.
21. Schwartz JC: Histamine as a transmitter in brain. *Life Sci* 1975;17:503–513.
22. Inversen LI: Biochemical psychopharmacology of GABA, in Lipton MA, DiMascio A, Killam KF (eds): *Psychopharmacology — A Generation of Progress.* New York, Raven Press, 1978, pp 25–38.
23. Kosterlitz HW, Hughes J, Lord JAH, et al: Enkephalins, endorphins, and opiate receptors. *Soc Neuroscience* 1977;2:291–307.
24. Euler US, Von Pernow B (eds): *Substance P.* New York, Raven Press, 1977.
25. Bury RW, Mashford ML: Substance P: Its pharmacology and physiological roles. *Aust J Exp Biol Med Sci* 1977;55:671–735.
26. Joseph C, Chassan JB, Koch ML: Levodopa in parkinson's disease. *Ann Neurol* 1978;3:116–118.
27. Snyder SH: Dopamine receptors, neuroleptics and schizophrenia. *Am J Psychiatry* 1981;138:460–464.
28. Creese I: Dopamine receptors explained. *Trends Neuroscience* 1982;5:40–44.
29. Aghajanian GK, Wang RY: Physiology and pharmacology of central serotonergic neurons, in Lipton MA, Di Mascio A, Killam KF (eds): *Psychopharmacology — A Generation of Progress.* New York, Raven Press, 1978, pp 171–184.
30. Hartmann E, Cravens J, List S: Hypnotic effects of L-tryptophan. *Arch Gen Psychiatry* 1974;31:394–397.
31. Bernstein J, Mazur WP, Walaszek EJ: The hystaminolytic activity of serum from schizophrenic patients. *Med Exp* 1960;2:239–244.
32. Richelson E: Tricyclic antidepressants and neurotransmitter receptors. *Psych Ann* 1979;9:186–195.
33. Snyder SH, Banerjee SP, Yamamura HI, et al: Drugs, neurotransmitters and schizophrenia. *Science* 1974;184:1243–1253.
34. Snyder S, Greenberg D, Yamamura HI: Antischizophrenic drugs and brain cholinergic receptors. *Arch Gen Psychiatry* 1974;31:58–61.

35. Snyder SH: Receptors, neurotransmitters and drug responses. *N Engl J Med* 1979;300:465–472.
36. Snyder SH: The dopamine hypothesis of schizophrenia: Focus on the dopamine receptor. *Am J Psychiatry* 1976;133:197–202.
37. Kety SS, Rosenthal D, Wender PH, et al: The biologic and adoptive families of adopted individuals who became schizophrenic: Prevalence of mental illness and other characteristics, in Wynee LC, Cromwell RL, Matthysse S (eds): *The Nature of Schizophrenia.* New York, Wiley and Sons, 1978, pp 25–37.
38. Allen MG: Twin studies of affective illness. *Arch Gen Psychiatry* 1976;33: 1476–1478.
39. Cadoret RJ, Winokur G, Clayton P: Family history studies VII. Manic depressive disease vs. depressive disease. *Br J Psychiatry* 1970;116:625–635.
40. Whitlock FH, Evans LEJ: Drugs and depression. *Drugs* 1978;15:53–71.
41. Modigh K: Long term effects of electroconvulsive shock therapy on synthesis, turnover, and uptake of brain monoamines. *Psychopharmacology* 1976;49:179–183.
42. Maas JW: Biogenic amines and depression. *Arch Gen Psychiatry* 1975;32: 1357–1361.
43. Janowsky DS, El-Yousef MK, Davis JM, et al: Parasympathetic suppression of manic symptoms by physostigmine. *Arch Gen Psychiatry* 1973;28: 542–547.
44. Ortiz A, Dabbagh M, Gershon S: Lithium: clinical use, toxicology and mode of action, in Bernstein JG (ed): *Clinical Psychopharmacology*, ed 2. Littleton, MA, John Wright•PSG, 1983.
45. Paul SM, Marangos PJ, Goddwin FK, et al: Brain-specific benzodiazepine receptors and putative endogenous benzodiazepine-like compounds. *Biol Psychiatry* 1980;15:407–428.
46. Paul SM, Skolnick P: Comparative neuropharmacology of antianxiety drugs. *Pharmacol Biochem Behav* 1982;17(Suppl I):37–41.
47. Taylor DP, Riblet LA, Stanton HC, et al: Dopamine and antianxiety activity. *Pharmacol Biochem Behav* 1982;17(Suppl I):25–35.

5

Evaluation and Treatment
of the Refractory Depressed Patient

Alan F. Schatzberg

With the advent of new antidepressants has come increasing hope that an even larger percentage of depressed patients can now be helped with effective antidepressant medications than had been helped previously. Although some of these new "second generation" antidepressants may act via alternative biochemical or pharmacologic processes and may have advantages in their side effect profiles, their introduction does pose potential problems for clinicians who must integrate these new drugs into their clinical practice. This may be particularly difficult because many clinicians have only recently become familiar with the subtle nuances in using tricyclic antidepressants and monoamine oxidase (MAO) inhibitors.

In spite of great efforts in continuing education, problems do remain in the prescription and monitoring of trials of first generation antidepressants. Unfortunately, many of the problems with poor response to first generation antidepressants have often stemmed from prescription practices, difficulties in diagnosis, etc, and have led to many treatment failures. The new antidepressants are not likely to overcome this problem, indicating that one would still expect a substantial portion of depressed patients not to respond to somatic therapy, although those refractory patients who had failed to respond, because of intolerance to side effects or because of a need for an alternative biochemical effect, may fare better. Obviously, refractory patients represent complex problems whose solutions offer a unique opportunity for developing effective treatments for less refractory patients. In this chapter, we will review key aspects regarding the management of refractory patients. Emphasis is placed on reviewing the previous history (including specifics of prior medication trials) and outlining a strategy for maximizing responses to antidepressant treatments.

ASSESSMENT

The assessment of any depressed patient must include careful history-taking, both physical and psychiatric, and an accurate diagnosis. In interviewing a depressed patient, the clinician must first ascertain whether the patient has a major depressive disorder as defined by DSM-III. While such criteria have been criticized by clinicians as being perhaps too broad and including too many patients, they do bear some similarity to the criteria proposed by various researchers for the diagnosis of so-called endogenous depression.[1-3] These criteria include a set of vegetative symptoms and signs. Most notably included are: a sleep disturbance (early, middle or late insomnia, or hypersomnia), anergia, anhedonia, psychomotor retardation, diurnal variation, anorexia and weight loss, anxiety and agitation, and suicidal ideation. It should be noted that suicidal ideation, while common in patients with depression, also occurs in patients with other types of psychiatric and medical illnesses. The importance in diagnosing an endogenous-type depressive disorder has been underscored by previous studies that have indicated that endogenous depressions are more responsive to somatic therapies, including psychopharmacologic treatments as well as electroconvulsive therapy, than are their nonendogenous counterparts.[4,5]

Nonendogenous depressive illnesses have been variously defined by different groups of investigators.[6-8] Early studies emphasized a negative definition, ie, the absence of neuro-vegetative signs and the presence of depressed affect on a more or less chronic basis.[6] More recently, some groups have attempted to specifically define nonendogenous disorders. One type appears to be the dysthymic disorder or depressive neurosis of DSM-III that bears some similarity to other classifications of nonendogenous syndromes. The Europeans, as well as some American groups, have defined nonendogenous syndromes on the basis of relative absence of pronounced neuro-vegetative signs, but in the presence of other signs and symptoms such as pronounced anxiety, obsessionality, histrionic behavior, tendency for tearful or whining behavior, self-pity, and some degree of acting out (eg, alcohol usage, etc).[7,8] These syndromes, over the years, have been felt to be less responsive to antidepressant treatments,[4,5] and many earlier surveys on so-called refractory depression pointed out that refractory depressed patients were, in fact, primarily nonendogenously depressed.[9-11] Because these syndromes may respond to certain antidepressant treatments, such as MAO inhibitors or perhaps more so to psychotherapy, these patients can be helped with treatment, although their response to standard antidepressants, (particularly tricyclics) has generally been less clear-cut and less pronounced than those seen in the endogenously depressed patient.

Having made the distinction between an endogenous and nonendogenous disorder, the physician must now look at qualifiers regarding the type of endogenous syndrome. Of particular importance are two other dichotomies that have entered into classification systems and find expression in the DSM-III. One categorization has been to divide endogenous syndrome into unipolar and bipolar types on the basis of the presence or absence of a previous hypomanic or manic syndrome.[12,13] A manic or hypomanic syndrome is characterized by a history of elevated mood, increased energy or vitality, increased sense of well-being, decreased need for sleep, spending sprees, elation or euphoria, pressured speech, or flight of ideas. Another categorization that has often been important in the diagnosis of major or endogenous depression has been whether the patient is psychotic or nonpsychotic. Psychotic depressive illnesses are clearly less common than nonpsychotic major depressive disorders, but they may be more common in the elderly.[14,15] Traditionally, this psychosis has been felt to be mood congruent, that is, an extension of pronounced depressed affect. Thus, such patients will show delusions of guilt and nihilism, often professing the belief that they are bad or that they will be punished because they are bad. When the cognitive distortion extends to paranoia in the absence of a lowered self-esteem and its more congruent delusions, the diagnosis of psychotic depression is less clear-cut. It is probable that many of these patients with paranoid psychoses in the absence of lowered self-esteem may, in fact, have a psychotic depressive illness that may be responsive to somatic therapies, particularly electroconvulsive treatment (ECT). Not uncommonly, careful history-taking reveals that such patients early in their episode demonstrated classic endogenous symptoms that were perhaps missed or discounted by patient and family.

It has been generally believed that endogenous depressive episodes last approximately six to nine months, and that they eventually leave the patient as abruptly or insidiously as they had arrived, either in response to treatment or by natural course of events. However, recent experience by our group and others has shown that a considerable proportion of depressed patients may be chronically depressed, and that even an endogenous depression may persist for prolonged periods of time.[16] Thus, the clinician cannot merely tell patients that if they wait long enough, their conditions will improve, and that even if they do not respond to any given treatment, eventually they will feel considerably better. Recently, we reported on a group of 110 patients who had been referred to us because they had failed to respond to treatment.[16] Of these patients, 16% had been chronically depressed (ie, had not had a three-month symptom-free interval) for 10 or more years, and an additional 10% had been depressed for more than five years. Thus, 26% of our sample had shown unremitting depressions for more than five years. These data indicate that depressed patients may develop chronic syndromes, as can patients suffering from a variety of other illnesses (eg, rheumatoid arthritis), and thus, endogenous depressions are not merely episodic.

Having assessed whether the individual is depressed and for how long, the physician must determine whether a contributing medical or neurological disorder may be involved in the patient's depressive illness. For the psychiatrist who is seeing a patient referral by an internist, this important task has probably already been done. Yet, a review of the patient's history, both with the patient himself/herself, as well as with the treating internist, appears wise since there are a host of medical illnesses that can lead to depression, or a constellation of symptoms that may suggest some form of a chronic depressive disorder. Commonly implicated causes are summarized in Table 5-1. Of note are the various endocrine disorders (particularly hyperthyroidism, hypothyroidism, and Cushing's disease), chronic hepatitis, and antihypertensive drugs — eg, reserpine and α-methyldopa. Many antihypertensives (including those noted above) may cause the individual to present with an anergic and retarded syndrome, although at times these patients will not have the full constellation of lowered mood, agitation, etc. Cerebral vascular accidents may be associated with depressive symptomatology such that strokes may not only cause aphasia and other neurological deficits, but also cause a depressive syndrome with neuro-vegetative signs and an abnormal Dexamethasone Suppression Test.[17,18]

Of particular importance in the elderly is the differential diagnosis between the pseudodementia of depression and early Alzheimer's disease. While it was once hoped that various advanced neuropsychologic, neuroradiologic, and neuropsychiatric techniques might be used to make this differential diagnosis, the diagnosis is often rather difficult.[19,20] Wells has pointed out that the false positive and false negative rate of these various procedures (including CT scanning, electroencephalography,

Table 5-1
Medical Problems Associated with Depression

1. Viral infections, eg, chronic hepatitis
2. Hypo- or hyperthyroidism
3. Addison's disease or Cushing's disease
4. Diabetes mellitus
5. Cerebral vascular insults
6. Covert seizure disorders
7. Parkinsonism
8. Collagen disorders
9. Antihypertensive agents

lumbar puncture, and neuropsychologic testing, etc) is rather high, indicating that the clinician must often rely on his experience to elicit and evaluate certain signs and symptoms that may help to differentiate pseudodementia from dementia.[20] For example, the pseudodemented patient can clearly define when his deficit began. The family can pinpoint the beginning of his disturbance and will often relate it to some stress or following a lowering in mood. The patient is aware of his deficit, complains of it, and will often not attempt various tasks. Thus, near misses are relatively uncommon on various neuropsychologic tests, but rather, one sees a pattern of anergic avoidance of all tasks. Recent memory is impaired; remote memory is maintained. The patient often shows lowered mood or depressed affect, and both a previous history and a family history of depression are more common in these patients.

In contrast, the demented patient shows neuropsychological deficits across the board, of which he is often unaware. The family has a great deal of difficulty pinpointing the onset of the condition. The patient will attempt to perform various tasks, demonstrate near misses on testing, and will try to hide his deficits. He will show a shallow affect, not commensurate with his poor performance. Deficits in both recent and remote memory are seen. A previous history of depression is less common, as is a family history of affective disorder. It was hoped that the Dexamethasone Suppression Test would discriminate demented from pseudodemented patients; however, some recent studies have shown a substantial proportion of elderly pseudodemented patients may demonstrate nonsuppression.[21] In spite of careful history-taking, the clinician is faced with a rather difficut differential diagnosis, such that treatment often has been recommended as a way of making the discrimination between dementia and pseudodementia, with failure to respond to vigorous treatment perhaps being a sign of dementia rather than pseudodementia.

PREVIOUS TREATMENT

Having ruled out a neurological/medical illness as contributing to the patient's depression, and having made a diagnosis, the clinician must evaluate the type of previous treatment that the patient has received. This is particularly important, not only to avoid repeating previously ineffective treatments, but also to determine whether previous treatments have either been well tolerated, or have been prescribed in adequate dosages and for adequate periods of time. The failure to prescribe an antidepressant, or to prescribe antidepressants in adequate amounts and for adequate periods, often reflects a lack of information on the part of the treater.[22] There are, however, patients who cannot tolerate an adequate trial of an antidepressant because they develop side reactions that preclude prescribing dosages in adequate amounts. These patients pose a rather separate problem for the clinician which will be addressed later in this chapter.

A number of years ago, Kotin et al at the National Institute of Mental Health reported that 18% of the depressed patients who had been referred to their specialty program had only been prescribed nonantidepressant medication, and 37% had been prescribed no medication for their illnesses.[23] Subsequent to that report, which appeared a number of years ago, increasing gains have been made in the use of antidepressant medications for the treatment of patients with serious depression. Still, in our survey of 110 patients seen between 1974 and 1978, we found that 76 of 110 patients (69%) had, in fact, received at least one antidepressant drug trial during their current episode. Of the remaining 31%, 14% had received some other form of drug therapy and 17% had received no medication for the current episode, although they had received medication for previous episodes. Only 26 of 110 patients (24%) received antidepressant medications only; 14% received nonantidepressant treatments only, and 45% received both antidepressant and nonantidepressant treatments.

The 91 patients received a total of 331 treatments (170 antidepressant and 161 nonantidepressant trials). Approximately two-thirds of the nonantidepressant treatments were with antianxiety drugs (24%) and antipsychotic agents (41%). These were prescribed often to treat some degree of anxiety or agitation, even though the literature that has emerged in recent years has indicated that such treatments (particularly benzodiazepines) are not effective primary antidepressant treatments.[24,25] Thus, while our percentage of patients who had not received antidepressant treatments was lower than that previously reported by Kotin et al,[23] the failure to receive an antidepressant still remains a problem in some clinician's hands and that this can be associated with the development of chronicity.

Selection or prescription of an antidepressant treatment represents the key first step in the treatment of patients with depressive disorders, and this must be followed by prescription of adequate dosages for adequate periods of time. Defining adequacy of treatment is not always an easy task. In recent years, considerable attention has been paid to developing so-called therapeutic blood level determinants for assessing adequacy of treatment.[26,27] In short, these blood level measurements provide a barometer for the clinician to assess whether a given treatment, which may have resulted in nonresponse, has been prescribed in adequate amounts.

The relationship between dosage and the attainment of blood level is somewhat bell-shaped, with some patients falling at either end of the spectrum, indicating that the difference between patients attaining blood level on a given milligram per kilo dose may vary as much as 30-fold.[28] Obviously, some patients will not respond because they may fail to develop adequate plasma levels in spite of vigorous treatment, either because they are rapid drug metabolizers, or because they take other medications that may increase the rate of drug metabolism in the liver, eg, barbiturates, chloral hydrate, nicotine, phenytoin, and other anticonvulsant medications.[28] Some patients who are slow drug metabolizers, either by nature or because of drug-drug interactions with such drugs as antipsychotics and methylphenidate,[29,30] may experience considerable side effects.[31] Such patients require treatment with lower dosages of tricyclics or discontinuation of other medication.

Not all clinicians have available to them reliable blood level determinations, and so the clinician himself must often develop a framework for determining the adequacy of treatment. Previously, we applied an artificial criterion of two-thirds of the manufacturers' recommended maximum dose, given for at least three weeks, to assess whether trials of antidepressant treatments were adequate. An adequate course of electroconvulsive therapy was defined as seven treatments. We had derived these empirically to provide us with some form of objective barometer to assess patterns of drug or somatic therapy prescription. Applying these criteria to our so-called resistant group, we found that only 39% of the 170 antidepressant trials met criteria for adequate trials. Of those 76 patients who had received one or more trials on a standard antidepressant, only 15 had received two or more adequate trials and these 15 patients did not differ remarkably in terms of endogenous or nonendogenous classification or syndromes. Of the 15 patients, nine had received adequate trials of ECT and 12 had received adequate trials of tricyclics. Thus, adequacy of treatment does not always result in effective response to antidepressant treatments, although most patients with so-called refractory depressive syndromes have received inadequate trials of antidepressants. Since depression is a severe illness, the clinican must be aware of this phenomenon and must push dosage to limiting side effects, or to maximum allowed dosages, in order to insure adequacy of treatment. Failure to do so only provides the patient with an increased risk of failing to respond. One exception has to do with the fact that certain medications (most notably nortriptyline) may have therapeutic windows such that reduction in dosage may be important in certain circumstances, although the dosage range recommended for nortriptyline generally places most patients within the so-called therapeutic window.

A problem that we inferred from our experience was that a considerable proportion of depressed patients are intolerant to antidepressant medications and they frequently demonstrate autonomic side effects (eg, dry mouth or constipation), agitation, or unpleasant sedation or grogginess that make trials or antidepressants difficult to continue. Of 170 antidepressant trials that our patients had received, 30% resulted in intolerance (ie, unpleasant side effects that resulted in discontinuation of the trial). Approximately one-half of the inadequate trials were associated with intolerance and, interestingly, only 6% of adequate trials were discontinued because of intolerance, suggesting that physicians will often increase dosage to some extent if patients can tolerate their medications.

Our experience suggests that the highly intolerant group does not overlap with those patients who failed to respond to adequate trials. Fourteen patients experienced intolerance of at least two antidepressant trials at dosages that we considered inadequate. Only one of these patients had also received two adequate trials with no response.

Intolerance to antidepressant trials can often be managed successfully by clinicians. In certain instances, key facets of the physician/patient relationship may enter into the development of intolerance or in assisting the patient to tolerate certain side reactions. A skeptical attitude on the part of the physician towards medication only enhances the patient's anxiety and increases his resistance to engage in drug trials. An over-inquisitive attitude regarding the side effects of medication can be harmful. As with any treatment, the physician must provide the patient with information regarding both risks and benefits; however, the physician must become familiar and comfortable with both the disease being treated and the medication being prescribed. The physician must be willing to tolerate a reasonable level of side effects in the patient and hidden biases against medications that come up in remarks as, "This is a problem with some medications and we better work it out in therapy," or, "I see this all the time and I don't like this or most medications," only enhances the patient's resistance and anxiety. Rather, the physician must develop an approach in which he listens to the patient's complaints, evaluates the degree and type of side effects, attempts to reassure the patient, and develops a strategy for dealing with a variety of specific side effects.

A general rule of thumb is that the development of early side effects is best handled by reassurance combined with a slower increase in dosages, extended over longer periods of time. For example, a patient who rapidly is escalated to a dose of 150 mg per day of imipramine and who develops significant orthostatic hypotension, anticholinergic side effects or agitation, may require a reduction in dosage and smaller incremental increases. In our hands, this is often effective even with orthostatic hypotension. Since this side effect occurs at relatively low imipramine plasma levels,[32] a change to nortriptyline—which causes hypotension at plasma levels above the therapeutic window—can be helpful.[33]

The antidepressant drugs of the tricyclic or tetracyclic class vary in the degree to which they bind to various receptors, and these effects may be associated with different side effects.[34,35] Of particular importance are the receptor-binding capacities to three types of receptors: acetylcholine, histamine-1 (H-1) and histamine-2 (H-2). The ability of the tricyclics and tetracyclics to block the peripheral acetylcholine receptor (muscarinic) as well as the central acetylcholine receptor (nicotinic) are important in the development of a variety of side effects including dry mouth, constipation, blurred vision, and confusion. The degree to which they bind to muscarinic receptors can be demonstrated using animal tissue paradigms, although these paradigms do not always correlate in a one to one fashion with the degree of side effects.[34] Of particular importance is the fact that protriptyline and amitriptyline are extremely potent blockers of muscarinic receptors, whereas desipramine and maprotiline appear to bind less vigorously to them, and thus produce less in the way of anticholinergic side effects.[35,36] Still, some patients will develop these side effects when treated with any of these agents and if severe, bethanechol may be used to overcome them.[37]

The histamine receptors (H-1 and H-2) produce various side effects when they are blocked. H-1 blockade is probably associated with weight gain and sedation. H-2 receptor blockade may be associated with the decrease in gastric acidity, a positive biplay to the tricyclic antidepressant.[38] While originally it was thought that muscarinic-blocking activity may be involved in producing sedation, as seen with amitriptyline, more recent evidence suggests H-1 blockade may be particularly important in the sedative effect of these drugs, as well as in the potentiation of weight gain. Desipramine and some other antidepressants appear to be less vigorous in their blockade of H-1 receptors, and therefore, represent an opportunity for switching within drug class.

Recent data from our group regarding urinary 3-methoxy-4-hydroxyphenylglycol (MHPG) suggest that urinary MHPG may be helpful in determining which patients are likely to demonstrate untoward side effects when treated with tricyclic or tetracyclic antidepressants. More specifically, whereas patients with low MHPG levels respond well, patients with high MHPG levels tend to respond less well to maprotiline or imipramine.[39-42] A further elaboration of our data has suggested that patients might be divided into three groups based on MHPG levels: low, intermediate, and high. In our experience, the patients with high and low MHPG levels do better when treated with maprotiline or imipramine than do patients with intermediate MHPG levels. High MHPG patients appear to require higher doses of maprotiline to respond than do low MHPG patients. In contrast, patients with mid-range MHPG levels often demonstrate intolerance to these drugs and show inadequate responses. Our hypothesis has been that these intermediate MHPG patients may have a disorder that does not involve norepinephrine systems, and that when challenged by potent noradrenergic drugs, such patients may indeed develop untoward side effects without experiencing beneficial antidepressant effects.[43] Further studies along this line are needed to see whether intolerance can be further defined by biological characteristics.

While it has been felt that amitriptyline and protriptyline are more potent in their anticholinergic effects and therefore less easily tolerated by many patients, our experience has been that some 15% of "refractory" patients do not tolerate any tricyclics, including desipramine. Tables 5-2 and 5-3 summarize our experience regarding drug trials in patients who experience intolerance. All of the tricyclic antidepressants were associated with intolerance, and the percentages of trials on each drug that had resulted in intolerance were approximately equal across all drugs, although amitriptyline was more commonly prescribed (Table 5-2). Further, treatment with antipsychotic agents, which also are potent muscarinic blockers, also resulted in frequent intolerance (Table 5-3). In contrast, intolerance to antianxiety agents was of a much lower order, indicating that intolerance is not related to medication in general, but is more related to specific biologic effects. Thus, for certain patients a switch in medication from one tricyclic to another may not offer positive benefit, although in some less treated patients it may prove useful.

If an individual has not received an adequate trial, the physician should prescribe a tricyclic and push the tricyclic to adequate dosages to attain adequate plasma levels, if these are available to him. If the patient has shown intolerance and intolerance cannot be mitigated against by increased patient contact, slower titration of dosage, or the addition of drugs that may potentiate cholinergic systems (eg, bethanechol), the physician must then consider a change to another type of antidepressant.

Although considerable attention over the years has been paid to tricyclic antidepressants, recently, greater interest has been shown to the monamine oxidase inhibitors (MAOIs). The British have argued that MAOIs are particularly effective in treatment of patients with nonendogenous depression, ie, those with considerable anxiety agitation, or phobic anxiety.[44] Our experience has been that endogenously depressed patients can be successfully treated with MAOIs, and these experiences dovetail with those of others in recent years, indicating that an increased turning to the MAOIs has again occurred.[45,46] These were originally spurned by observations that higher dosages of MAOIs might be required to effect a sufficient reduction in platelet MAO activity.[47] More specifically, for patients to achieve 80% inhibition in platelet MAO activity, they may require dosages of at least 60 mg per day of phenelzine. In our earlier experience with "refractory" patients, we found that seven of the first nine patients with endogenous depression who were assigned to MAOI showed a dramatic response to the drug, wherease only one showed intolerance and one showed no response. Dramatic response on MAOIs were obtained in the same patients who had failed on tricyclic antidepressants. Further, MAOIs are often better tolerated than are tricyclics, particularly because they have little affect on muscarinic receptors, although they may obviously affect blood pressure. There has been considerable interest in recent years as to whether elderly depressed patients show more tardy responses to the tricyclic antidepressant, and it appears that MAOIs may be rather useful in elderly patients, particularly those who have failed on tricyclics.[48]

In recent years, a number of interesting regimens have been proposed to maximize or bring out responses to tricyclic antidepressants. Two

Table 5-2
Intolerance to Tricyclic Antidepressants*

	Trials	Intolerant Trials	Percent Intolerance
Amitriptyline	24	21	87.5
Imipramine	16	8	50
Doxepin	9	6	66.7
Desipramine	6	4	66.7
Protriptyline	3	3	100
Nortriptyline	1	1	100
Fluotracen	4	0	0

*Patient number intolerance to antidepressants = 30; TCA intolerance number = 23.

Table 5-3
Intolerance by Drug Class: Patients*

	TCA	MAOI	Li	ECT	AP	Anx	Camb	Stim	Other
Patient Number	30	11	13	5	18	18	3	4	8
Number with Intolerance	23	7	9	1	10	7	2	1	4
Percent with Intolerance	76.7	63.6	69.2	20	55.6	38.9	66.7	25	50

*Patient number = 37.

regimens appear to have particular potential for the clinician. One approach involves the addition of T_3 in dosages of 25 to 50 μg per day to the tricyclic, which may bring out a response within three to five days in a nonresponding patient.[49] Our experience has been positive in several difficult patients. Failure to respond within seven days generally means it will not work and thus there is no need to continue for prolonged periods.

Another regimen that has been proffered by deMontigny et al[50] has been the addition of lithium carbonate to tricyclic antidepressants. This group has argued that lithium was not acting as a primary antidepressant because patients often responded at rather low doses and serum levels. Rather, it appears that the lithium may be unmasking the responsivity of dopaminergic or serontonergic neuronal systems. The regimen involves the addition of low doses of lithium carbonate for a few days. Again, if the patient does not respond within seven to ten days, the trial can be considered a failure. In our experience this has worked in only a few patients, and we have been more favorably impressed with the addition of T_3 than with lithium carbonate.

One approach that has been used for many years is combining MAOIs and tricyclic antidepressants in patients with refractory depression. Unfortunately, studies have failed to demonstrate that the combination works more effectively. However, one problem has been that relatively low dosages of both treatments have been used, indicating that the patient may have received two inadequate trials.[51] More recently, a number of colleagues have reported to me that pushing dosages of both medications has resulted in dramatic clinical responses in previously refractory patients without hypertensive crisis. Indeed, there has been a sense emerging that tricyclics, when combined with an MAO inhibitor might protect against hypertensive crises, and that the combination could indeed be safer than one might infer.[46] One difficulty in reading the older literature on the use of TCA-MAOI combinations has been that the untoward effects have generally been associated with overdosages,[52] such that serious interactions and serious adverse effects would have perhaps occurred with an overdose of either regimen alone. This has been extrapolated to the belief that the combination itself is extremely dangerous, although the evidence that the combination is dangerous is actually lacking. There has been some suggestion that some combinations are safer than others. The addition of the MAOI to the TCA (rather than vice-versa), or simultaneously starting both, appears wisest to decrease the risk of hypertensive crisis.[52] Still, today it should be left to experienced hands. If it does prove effective and safe, rewording of package inserts might be necessary to diffuse a charged issue.

A number of other possible treatments are available to individuals who have failed to respond to tricyclics, MAOIs, or ECT. Notably, the second generation antidepressants do offer alternatives. Trazodone is a nontricyclic, nonMAOI antidepressant. This drug appears to be pro-serotonergic, and to have a positive effect on mood and anxiety in many patients. It produces sedation, but relatively little anticholinergic effect, with the result that it does not cause marked constipation. It can produce dry mouth because of its alpha-blocking effect, an effect that can be associated with decreased salivation.

A number of other drugs are being investigated today for use in depression and several of these are near approval as antidepressants. One notable example is alprazolam (Xanax), a drug that is currently on the market for anxiety and anxiety with depression, and which can be helpful in certain depressed patients who have failed to respond to treatment[53] as well as in patients with panic attacks (see Chapter 6). Further, bupropion (Wellbutrin) is apparently an effective antidepressant and is near release. This drug apparently has no affect on histaminic or acetylcholine receptors, nor does it exert much effect on norepinephrine systems. Rather, it may act through dopaminergic pathways.

NEW HORIZONS

Other recent work from our group has suggested that some patients with refractory depression may not be suffering from a chronic depressive syndrome, but from a heretofore undiagnosed neurological condition. We have seen a number of refractory depressed patients who have developed an increasingly pronounced picture involving odd symptoms, such as perceptual distortion, chronic depersonalization, or auditory hallucinosis. Several of these individuals have had normal neurological evaluations and routine EEGs.

The use of computerized electroencephalography (BEAM Studies[54]) has revealed that many of these patients do have abnormal electrical brain activity which may be associated with these symptoms. An example of this is a woman who had a chronic depression of over two year's duration. She had failed to respond to every known antidepressant regimen available to us, including several investigational drugs. Over time, she complained of a perceptual distortion involving the world appearing tinged. About a year previously, she had a seizure while on doxepin at a dose of 225 mg per day. EEGs and CAT scan then had been unremarkable. BEAM study revealed a left anterior temporal lobe focus of increased beta activity and an abnormal auditory-evoked response in the same area. Repeat CAT scan suggested a contusion of the anterior tip of the left temporal lobe. She has shown a moderate and sustained response to carbamazepine. Obviously, further studies with various brain imaging techniques are required to determine how common such abnormalities may be in various atypical or nonresponsive patients.

REFERENCES

1. Schatzberg AF: Classification of depressive disorders, in: Cole JO, Schatzberg AF, Frazier SH (eds): *Depression: Biology, Psychodynamics, and Treatment.* New York, Plenum Press, 1978.
2. Kiloh LG, Garside RF: The independence of neurotic depression and endogenous depression. *Br J Psychiatry* 1963;109:451–463.
3. Kendell RE: The classification of depressions: A review of contemporary confusion. *Br J Psychiatry* 1976;129:15–29.
4. Carney MWP, Roth M, Garside RF: The diagnosis of depressive syndromes and the prediction of ECT responses. *Br J Psychiatry* 1965;111:659–674.
5. Kiloh LG, Ball JRB, Garside RF: Prognostic factors in treatment of depressive states with imipramine. *Br Med J* 1962;1:1225–1227.
6. Lange J: Uber melancholie. *Z Neurol und Psychiat* 1926;101:293–319.
7. Rosenthal SH, Gudeman JE: The self-pitying constellation in depression. *Br J Psychiatry* 1967;113:485–489.
8. Schildkraut JJ, Klein DF: The classification and treatment of depressive disorders, in Shader RI (ed): *Manual of Psychiatric Therapeutics.* Boston, Little, Brown, 1975.
9. Sethna ER: A study of refractory cases of depressive illnesses and their response to combined antidepressant treatment. *Br J Psychiatry* 1974;124:265–272.
10. Helmchen H: Symptomatology of therapy-resistant depressions. *Pharmakopsychiat* 1974;7:145–155.
11. Lopez-Ibor Alino JJ: Therapeutic resistant depressions: Symptoms, resistance and therapy. *Pharmakopsychiat* 1974;7:189–187.
12. Leonhard K: *Aufteilung der Endogenen Psychosen.* Berlin, Akademie Verlag, 1959.
13. Perris C: A survey of bipolar and unipolar recurrent depressive psychoses. *Acta Psychiatr Scand* 1966;(suppl)194:7–188.
14. Himmelhoch JM, Anchenbach R, Fuchs CZ: The dilemma of depression in the elderly. *J Clin Psychiatry* 1982;43(suppl):26–32.
15. Detre P, Jarecki HG: *Modern Psychiatric Treatment.* Philadelphia, Lippincott, 1971.
16. Schatzberg AF, Cole JO, Cohen BM, et al: Survey of depressed patients who have failed to respond to treatment, in Davis JM, Maas J (eds): *Affective Disorders.* Washington, American Psychiatric Press, 1983.
17. Ross ED, Ross AJ: Diagnosis and neuroanatomical correlates of depression in brain-damaged patients. *Arch Gen Psychiatry* 1981;38:1344–1354.
18. Finkelstein S, Benowitz LI, Baldessarini RJ, et al: Mood, vegetative disturbance, and dexamethasone suppression test after stroke. *Ann Neurol* 1982;12:463–468.
19. Wells CE: Pseudodementia. *Am J Psychiatry* 1978;135:75–77.
20. Wells CE: The differential diagnosis of psychiatric disorders in the elderly, in Cole JO, Barrett JE (eds): *Psychopathology in the Aged.* New York, Raven Press, 1980.
21. Spar JE, Gerner R: Does the dexamethasone suppression test distinguish dementia from depression? *Am J Psychiatry* 1982;139:238–241.
22. Ketai R: Family practitioners' knowledge about treatment of depressive illness. *JAMA* 1976;235:2600–2603.
23. Kotin J, Post RM, Goodwin FK: Drug treatment of depressed patients referred for hospitalization. *Am J Psychiatry* 1973;130:1139–1141.
24. Schatzberg AF, Cole JO: Benzodiazepines in depressive disorders. *Arch Gen Psychiatry* 1978;35:1359–1365.

25. Schatzberg AF, Cole JO: Benzodiazepines in the treatment of depressive, borderline personality, and schizophrenic disorders. *Br J Clin Pharmacol* 1981;11:175-225.
26. Glassman A, Perel J, Shostak M, et al: Clinical implications of imipramine plasma levels for depressive illnesses. *Arch Gen Psychiatry* 1977;34:197-207.
27. Asberg M, Cronholm B, Sjoquist F, et al: Relationship between plasma level and therapeutic effect of nortriptyline. *Br Med J* 1971;3:331-334.
28. Glassman A, Perel J: The clinical pharmacology of imipramine. *Arch Gen Psychiatry* 1973;28:649-653.
29. Wharton RN, Perel JM, Dayton PG, et al: A potential clinical use for methylphenidate with tricyclic antidepressants. *Am J Psychiatry* 1971;127:1619-1625.
30. Siris SG, Cooper TB, Rifkin AE, et al: Plasma imipramine concentrations in patients receiving concomitant fluphenazine decanoate. *Am J Psychiatry* 1982;139:104-106.
31. Appelbaum PS, Vasile RG, Orsulak PJ, et al: Clinical utility of tricyclic antidepressant blood levels. *Am J Psychiatry* 1979;136:339-341.
32. Glassman AH, Bigger J, Giardina E: Clinical characteristics of imipramine-induced orthostatic hypotension. *Lancet* 1979;1:468-472.
33. Roose S, Glassman AH, Bruno R: Tricyclic antidepressant induced postural hypotension; comparative studies. *New Research Abstract, American Psychiatric Association, Annual Meeting.* May 1980, NR33.
34. Baldessarini RJ: Overview of recent advances in antidepressant pharmacology: Part II. *McLean Hosp J* 1982;7:1-27.
35. Blackwell B, Stefopoulos A, Enders P, et al: The anticholinergic activity of two tricyclic antidepressants. *Am J Psychiatry* 1978;135:722-724.
36. Richelson E: Pharmacology of antidepressants in use in the United States. *J Clin Psychiatry* 1982;43:4-11.
37. Everett HC: The use of bethanechol chloride with tricyclic antidepressants. *Am J Psychiatry* 1976;132:1202-1206.
38. Mangla JC, Pereira M: Tricyclic antidepressants in the treatment of peptic ulcer disease. *Arch Intern Med* 1982;142:273-275.
39. Maas JW, Fawcett JA, Dekirmenjian H: Catecholamine metabolism, depressive illness, and drug response. *Arch Gen Psychiatry* 1972;26:252-262.
40. Rosenbaum AH, Schatzberg AF, Maruta T, et al: MHPG as a predictor of antidepressant response to imipramine and maprotiline. *Am J Psychiatry* 1980;137:1090-1092.
41. Schatzberg AF, Rosenbaum AH, Orsulak PJ, et al: Toward a biochemical classification of depressive disorders III. Pretreatment urinary MHPG levels as predictors of response to treatment with maprotiline. *Psychopharmacology.* 1981;75:34-38.
42. Schatzberg AF, Orsulak PJ, Rosenbaum AH, et al: Toward a biochemical classification of depressive disorders IV. Pretreatment urinary MHPG levels as predictors of response to imipramine. *Commun Psychopharmacol* 1981;4:441-445.
43. Schatzberg AF, Orsulak PJ, Rosenbaum AH, et al: Toward a biochemical classification of depressive disorders V. Heterogeneity of unipolar depressions. *Am J Psychiatry* 1982;139:471-475.
44. Tyrer P: Towards rational therapy with monamine oxidase inhibitors. *Br J Psychiatry* 1976;128:354-360.
45. Quitkin F, Rifkin A, Klein DF: Monamine oxidase inhibitors. *Arch Gen Psychiatry* 1979;36:749-760.
46. Pare CMB: Monamine oxidase inhibitors; A British point of view. *McLean Hosp J* 1977;2:24-38.

47. Ravaris CL, Nies A, Robinson DS, et al: A multiple dose, controlled study of phenelzine in depression-anxiety states. *Arch Gen Psychiatry* 1976;33: 347–350.
48. Georgotas A, Ferris S, Gershon S, et al: *Resistant depressions in the elderly and response to MAOI's.* Presented at 13th CINP Congress, Jerusalem, Israel, June 1982.
49. Goodwin FK, Prange AJ, Post RM, et al: Potentiation of antidepressant effects by L-triiodothyronine in tricyclic nonresponders. *Am J Psychiatry* 1982;139:34–38.
50. deMontigny C, Grunberg F, Mayer A, et al: Lithium induces rapid relief on depression in tricyclic antidepressant drug nonresponders. *Br J Psychiatry* 1981;138:252–255.
51. White K, Simpson G: Combined MAOI tricyclic antidepressant treatment: A reevaluation. *J Clin Psychopharmacol* 1981;1:264–282.
52. Sethna ER: A study of refractory cases of depressive illnesses and their response to combined antidepressant treatment. *Br J Psychiatry* 1974;124: 265–275.
53. Schatzberg AF, Altesman RA, Cole JO: An update of the use of benzodiazepines in depressed patients in Usdine E, Skolnick P, Tallman JF, et al (eds): *Pharmacology of Benzodiazepines.* London, Macmillan, 1982 pp 45–51.
54. Duffy FH, Burchfield JL, Lombrosos CT: Brain electrical activity mapping (BEAM): A method for extending the clinical utility of EEG and evoked potential data. *Ann Neurol* 1979;5:309–321.

6

The Treatment of Panic and Phobic Disorders

David V. Sheehan

To treat anxiety and phobic disorders predictably well, a reliable diagnostic system is needed as a guide to the choice of treatment. Diagnostic confusion will inevitably lead to a poor choice of treatment for many patients. Unfortunately, the severe anxiety-phobic disorder characterized by spontaneous symptom attacks lends itself to diagnostic confusion. It is a multidimensional disorder that impacts at the metabolic, behavioral, and psychological levels, and expresses itself through symptoms in widely scattered areas of the body. It is easy for the physician to be distracted by one or another of its many symptoms. Taking that symptom out of context, he may fail to appreciate the disorder as a whole. Because these isolated symptoms mimic other illnesses, this invites costly medical workups and multiple consultations. Historically, this disorder has attracted a diverse array of diagnostic labels. These labels often reflect the specialty interest or theoretical orientation of the diagnostician. Examples include cardiac neurosis, hyperventilation syndrome, hypoglycemia, agoraphobia, hysteria and anxiety neurosis, panic disorder, generalized anxiety disorder, and hypochondriasis. The DSM-III, although it represents overall a positive step towards diagnostic precision, allowed the precision to be misplaced in sorting out the diagnostic confusion in anxiety and phobic disorders. We have discussed this at length elsewhere.[1-4] This has several consequences at the practical clinical level. For example, consider the following cases:

Case 1: A patient is seen with surges of unprovoked autonomic hyper-activity, just short of panic attacks. He is diagnosed as having a general-ized anxiety disorder. He is treated with a benzodiazepine and does poorly or only moderately. Trials of behavior therapy, relaxation train-ing, biofeedback and psychotherapy may then be tried with little addi-tional success. Tricyclics or MAO inhibitors would rarely be considered. After all, it is argued the patient does not have panic attacks or obvious depression, so why should they be indicated?

Case 2: A patient has agoraphobia and several other phobias. She fears going far from home and crowded social situations. She denies having spontaneous panic attacks. She has intense spells of lightheadedness and imbalance, sometimes for little or no apparent reason. With a diagnosis of agoraphobia without panic attacks, such a patient is considered a suitable candidate for behavioral treatments, specifically in vivo ex-posure. Medication would be considered inappropriate.

Case 3: A patient complains of a single phobia — claustrophobia, par-ticularly in elevators and cars. This fear is quite intense and disruptive. At other times the patient gets attacks of diarrhea, with little or no prov-ocation, that is diagnosed as irritable colon syndrome. She fears that in closed spaces she may lose control of her bowels, or get an unreality feeling, and that a quick escape is impeded. With a diagnosis of simple phobia in this case, conventional wisdom would recommend behavior therapy alone. Even if that failed to yield full recovery, tricyclics would rarely be considered.

These are only three of many commonly encountered examples where the existing classification would have you believe that these pa-tients suffer from quite different disorders and require different treatment approaches. In reality, none of the above patients made a really satisfac-tory improvement until their spontaneous symptom attacks were first controlled by medication (tricyclics or MAO inhibitors).

NATURAL HISTORY

A more parsimonious classification would view these patients as suffering from the same basic disorder. It would stage each patient at a different level in the natural history of the disorder and consider each as having the disorder to a different degree of severity or chronicity. Much of the diagnostic confusion of the past stemmed from this disorder being subjected to cross-sectional rather than longitudinal analysis. In the early stages in the natural evolution of the disorder, it was given one diagnostic label, at a later stage another, and again later another, as if the patient had several disorders that were distinct from each other.

The typical patient with endogenous anxiety will describe several stages in the natural course of their illness over several years (Table 6-1).

Having spontaneous symptom attacks (one or two symptoms surging in isolation with little or no provocation) without full panic attacks is often the first stage. These symptoms could include sudden surges of tachycardia, lightheadedness, or shortness of breath (Table 6-2). Eventually, several of these symptoms occur at the same time and with increased intensity. The result is a panic attack. Because the patient is often at a loss to identify a justifiable psychosocial stressor for the symptoms, and because of an increase in fear, the patient fears that some serious medical disease must be causing the disorder (hypochondriasis). A severe panic attack can bring about a phobia to the situation in which it occurs by association (classical conditioning). For example, a panic attack may occur at the movies. Subsequently, the patient may have anticipatory anxiety when going to the movies and may phobically avoid it altogether. On

Table 6-1
Stages in Natural History of Endogenous Anxiety

Stage 1	Subpanic Symptom Attacks
Stage 2	Polysymptomatic Panic Attacks
Stage 3	Hypochondriasis
Stage 4	Single Phobia
Stage 5	Social Phobia
Stage 6	Polyphobic and Agoraphobic Behavior
Stage 7	Depression

Table 6-2
Diagnostic Criteria

Endogenous Anxiety	Exogenous Anxiety
1. Spontaneous, autonomous, clonic, phasic (subjectively reported) episodes of the following symptoms (1–2 for a minor attack, 3 or more together for a major attack): a. Skipping or racing of heart b. Dizzy spells or faintness c. Air hunger, difficulty getting breath, or hyperventilation d. Smothering or choking sensation e. Tingling or numbness (paresthesias) in hands, arms, feet, or face f. Nausea, upset stomach, or vomiting g. Sudden unexpected panic or anxiety feelings occurring with little or no provocation	1. No spontaneous panic or anxiety attacks or history of the same.

Table 6-2 (Continued)
Diagnostic Criteria

Endogenous Anxiety	Exogenous Anxiety
h. Hot flushes or cold chills	
i. Jelly legs or imbalance	
j. Shaking or trembling of hands or legs	
k. Derealization or depersonalization	
l. Chest pain, pressure, or discomfort	
m. Hypochondriasis	
n. Feeling will lose control, scream or "go insane" or die	
o. Spontaneous clonic alteration in sensory perception, eg, increased or decreased clonic sensitivity to light, sound, touch, temperature, taste, proprioception, muscle power	
p. Diarrhea attacks	
q. Sweating episodes.	
2. Such symptom attacks have persistently recurred for at least one month. Within a 3-month period, at least 3 discrete major attacks must occur for a diagnosis of major endogenous anxiety, or at least 3 discrete minor attacks for a diagnosis of minor endogenous anxiety.	2. Tension and symptoms of anxiety occur *only* in response to immediate, clearcut, identifiable environmental stimuli. Onset of each attack not very sudden or unexpected but related to immediacy of triggering stimulus. In the case of conditioned changes in motor, sensory, symptoms or special senses, the symptom may occur alone without any overt anxiety.
3. Phobic symptoms, particularly fear of a spontaneous panic attack (phobophobia) and fear of crowded places. Phobias start only after onset of first spontaneous panic attack. Phobia may fluctuate in intensity over time.	3. Phobia restricted to one specific focus. Monophobic rather than polyphobic. Phobia rarely fluctuates in intensity over time.
4. Depression, neurasthenia (excessive tiredness and feeling everything is an effort), obsessive compulsive symptoms present to some degree in over two-thirds of cases.	4. Depression, neurasthenia, obsessive compulsive symptoms and other gross psychopathology absent.
5. Anxiety profile of spontaneous panic attack as in Figure 6-1 (although anticipatory type may also occur).	5. Profile of anxiety attack as in Figure 6-3.
6. Spontaneous fluctuations on GSR.	6. No spontaneous fluctuations on GSR.

Table 6-2 (Continued)
Diagnostic Criteria

Endogenous Anxiety	Exogenous Anxiety
7. Slow habituation rate on GSR.	7. Normal or rapid habituation on GSR.
8. Elevated resting pulse rate.	8. Resting pulse within normal range.
9. Brisk reflexes.	9. Reflexes not hypertonic.
10. Family history of anxiety attacks and phobic symptoms especially among female relatives.	10. ?Positive family history rare (insufficient data at this time).
11. Age of onset usually 12–40 years.	11. May occur at any age.
12. 80% of cases occur in women.	12. ?Equal sex distribution (66% women).
13. More likely to have visited medical doctor and emergency ward several times for treatment of symptoms. Spontaneous anxiety must occur: a. In absence of medical illness that could cause such symptoms b. In absence of life threatening situations.	13. Rarely seeks medical or emergency ward treatment
14. More likely to have seen several psychiatrists in treatment over many years.	14. Infrequent psychiatric consultations.
15. More likely to have had a hospital admission and surgical treatment for symptoms.	15. Infrequent medical consultations.
16. Response to MAO inhibitors and imipramine good.	16. Response to drugs poor.
17. Response of all symptoms to behavior therapy alone poor. Avoidance behavior alone may(?) improve with exposure treatment, but not spontaneous attacks.	17. Response to behavior therapy good.
18. Autonomy of clonic phasic course eg, does not immediately improve when environmental circumstances seem favorable.	18. More clearly responsive to psychosocial stimulus.
19. Anxiety attacks precipitated by sodium lactate IV and by marijuana administration.	19. Anxiety attacks not precipitated by either lactate or marijuana.

the second exposure to a movie theatre, the anticipatory anxiety may make it more likely that a surge of panic will occur on top of the anticipatory anxiety and further reinforce the phobia. If these spontaneous panic attacks occur in more situations over time, more phobias develop. The problem generalizes and the patient's multiple phobias over time (stage 6) may develop and be reinforced in a variety of ways (eg, see reference 4).

With progressive disability, generalization of anxiety and no relief, patients become progressively depressed. If the examining clinician evaluates the disorder cross-sectionally, he may assign different diagnostic labels to each stage and even to different symptoms within each stage. If the disease is viewed as a single evolving process, longitudinally, this confusing fragmentation can be avoided.

AN ALTERNATIVE DIAGNOSTIC SYSTEM

We found the current classifications of anxiety and phobic disorders too complex and clinically confusing to be useful. Furthermore, they were not the best guides to the most appropriate management strategy. In the search for a simple, clear and concise classification that would have heuristic merit in guiding both research efforts and in guiding the clinician to a logical treatment strategy, we have found the approach outlined in Figure 6-1 helpful.[1-4] This decision tree guides the clinician, through a logical sequence of diagnostic steps, to a diagnosis that better predicts each patient's response to a specific treatment strategy. This chapter outlines the treatment strategies for each of the diagnostic categories. There is a special emphasis on the treatment of endogenous anxiety with or without phobias, since it is this condition which is so disabling and presents clinicians with the greatest diagnostic and therapeutic challenges.

The central question in the diagnostic differentiation is whether spontaneous anxiety attacks occur or have ever occurred. In their most dramatic form, these may be full blown polysymptomatic panic attacks with a flight response. In more subtle forms, these attacks may be expressed as sudden unexpected spells of isolated symptoms (Table 6-2) that arise with little or no immediate identifiable stress. The patient has endogenous anxiety if these attacks now occur or have occurred at any point during the natural evolution of the disorder. If these attacks never occur and never have occurred and the anxiety is clearly always a response to an immediate environmental stress, then the patient has exogenous anxiety. These two major classes of anxiety may be subtyped on the basis of severity and chronicity. However, this subtyping is only a refinement of the central differentiation. The different diagnostic criteria for these two major types of anxiety are listed in Table 6-2. The exogenous anxiety is a tonic reactive response to stress. The exogenous phobia usually results from a traumatic event, eg, a car crash. Such patients usually are monophobic and never experience anxiety attacks in other situations. In contrast, the endogenous anxiety is a spiky, clonic, phasic disorder that appears to be autonomous.

The exogenous anxiety is similar to the anxiety of normal man. The accumulating evidence suggests that endogenous anxiety appears to be a biological disease[5] to which there is a genetic vulnerability.[6] The first responds well to psychological or behavioral treatments. The second requires drug treatment for optimal results.[5,8]

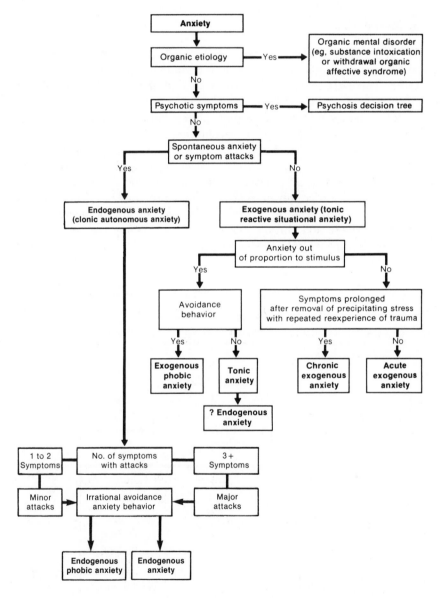

Figure 6-1 The decision tree approach to diagnosing anxiety. Reproduced from Sheehan DV: Current perspectives in the treatment of panic and phobic disorder. *Drug Therapy* 1982;12:49–63. Reprinted with permission.

TREATMENT

Endogenous and exogenous anxiety each require different treatment strategies. The treatment strategy for each is outlined in Figures 6-2 and 6-3, respectively.

Endogenous Anxiety

When a diagnosis of endogenous anxiety with or without complicating phobias is made, the first step is drug treatment for the core anxiety attacks. There are several classes of drugs that appear to be effective for this purpose: monoamine oxidase inhibitors;[8,9] tricyclic antidepressants;[8,10] the triazolobenzodiazepine, alprazolam;[11] the triazolopyridine, trazodone; and the tetracyclic, maprotiline.

Among the range of choices, the MAO inhibitor, phenelzine, is probably the single most effective drug overall. The differences in efficacy between these drugs may be small. In the milder and earlier stages of the disorder, any one of them would probably be effective if used correctly. Their differences and relative powers become more apparent in the more severe and chronic cases. Of these effective antipanic drugs, alprazolam appears to be the least toxic and the most rapidly effective.[11]

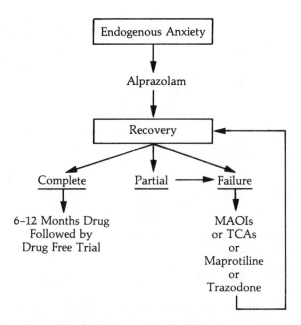

Figure 6-2   Management strategy for endogenous anxiety.

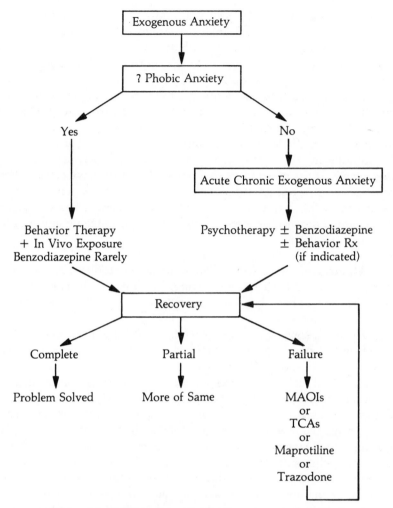

Figure 6-3 Management strategy for exogenous anxiety.

How it measures up against the MAO inhibitors and tricyclic antidepressants as an antipanic drug is now being studied under double-blind conditions. Its main advantage appears to be its superior safety and speed of action. For these reasons, I usually start the majority of patients on this drug first. For those who are very disabled and depressed in addition to their panic attacks, I generally favor either an MAO inhibitor or tricyclics first. Alprazolam appears to be a less potent antidepressant or mood elevator in these patients.[11]

Prescribing principles In general, most of the antipanic drugs are prescribed too casually and in doses that are too frequently subtherapeutic for the patient. In order to get good results, it is wise to approach this drug treatment as an endocrinologist would treat the diabetic patient who requires insulin. Time spent with the patient reviewing dose regulation and timing, and complication monitoring is all important. It is unusual to reach the final optimal dose in the first week or two of treatment. Patients tend to develop some tolerance to the side effects and benefits of lower doses. With most of these drugs, the dose at which the patient has some sensation of regular persistent side effects, is the dose at which they usually derive the best therapeutic effect. The physician's skill lies in adjusting the dose to strike the best balance between side effects and benefit. If the patient gets to a point where they have no side effects whatsoever, it is not unusual for this to be followed by some relapse of symptoms within a week or two. Correct adjustment of doses frequently makes the difference between a good treatment outcome and a failure with complications.

Alprazolam   This drug is unique among benzodiazepines in having a triazolo ring in its chemical structure. This may be the reason it is the only drug with a basic benzodiazepine structure that has significant antipanic properties.

The usual starting dose of alprazolam is 0.5 mg three times daily. It may help to have the patient take the drug at the end of each meal. This serves a dual purpose. This anchors the ingestion of drug to a set time every day and makes it less likely the patient will forget his medication. When taken following food, the drug is more slowly absorbed, the side effects (eg, drowsiness) are less acute, and its antipanic effect may be more protracted. Every two days the total daily dose can be increased by 0.5 mg/day. The escalation of the dose is stopped when the patient experiences either side effects (eg, drowsiness) or significant benefit. If a dose of 2 mg tid po is reached, further dose additions may be given at bedtime or the doses can be taken at four- to five-hour intervals. The drug's apparent duration of action against the panic is about four to six hours. If the doses are spaced too far apart (eg, eight to ten hours) some recurrence of symptoms may be experienced. Even when the dose is well adjusted, some patients may complain of anxiety feelings on first waking in the morning. This is the time when the blood level is lowest. It should be added that the half-life of benzodiazepines is not the best guide to their duration of therapeutic action. Clinicians should not be misled into thinking that because the half-life of alprazolam is 10 to 12 hours, this reflects its duration of therapeutic action.

Patients with panic may get a therapeutic effect at doses ranging from 3 to 9 mg/day. In three studies we have carried out on alprazolam, the average daily dose that delivers lasting therapeutic benefit was 6 mg/day. It often takes one to two weeks for patients to reach this level.

The most obvious side effects of alprazolam are drowsiness, ataxia, and slurring of speech if the dose is high. The drowsiness is much less apparent when the patient is active, and often quite marked when passive. At times, patients complain of memory lucunae (episodic forgetfulness), headaches, and irritability. These are most apparent in the early weeks of treatment. They generally subside with tolerance to the dose and/or dose adjustment. Sometimes a depressed, amotivational syndrome may be observed after a few weeks.

It is not unusual for patients to pass through two or three dose plateaus before they reach their final ideal dose. In other words, they reach a dose that gives benefit and side effects. Several days later the side effects clear, and a little later the patient loses the benefit. A small dose increase is called for. This may occur two or three times. However, there is a limit to the extent it occurs. It does not continue occurring endlessly. A similar phenomenon is not uncommon with all the effective antipanic drugs, if the dose is being regulated correctly. Under the circumstances, a small dose increase is called for if the patient loses all side effects and ceases to get benefit from a formerly effective dose.

If the dose has been properly regulated, after two to three weeks, the degree of recovery is reassessed (Figure 6-2). If recovery is complete, this regimen might be continued for six to 12 months. The spontaneous anxiety attacks should have stopped completely and the remaining anxiety syndrome should be under good control. After several months of recovery, the dose may be slowly lowered when the patient feels ready and confident. Because alprazolam is also an anticonvulsant, it should never be abruptly withdrawn, even when it is clearly ineffective. To do so could invite a withdrawal seizure at worst, or unpleasant withdrawal symptoms at best. An ideal withdrawal schedule would be to lower the dose at a rate of 0.5 to 1 mg every one to two weeks if the patient has done well for several months and is attempting a drug-free trial. If the drug is ineffective, it is not advisable to withdraw it at a rate faster than 1 mg every three days. A rate of 0.5 mg every three days would be preferable.

If the spontaneous panic attacks are not eliminated and the anxiety syndrome not really well controlled, or a satisfactory response is not achieved by 10 mg/day, then the alprazolam trial should be considered a therapeutic failure. The dose is then slowly lowered and one of the four remaining alternatives chosen. The heterocyclic antidepressant amoxapine (Asendin) and the investigational monocyclic antidepressant bupropion (Wellbutrin) do not appear to have comparable antipanic effects.[12]

Monoamine oxidase inhibitors There are two subtypes of MAO inhibitors currently available: the hydrazines, eg, phenelzine (Nardil), and isocarboxazid (Marplan); and the nonhydrazine, tranylcypromine (Parnate). Although both are effective for endogeous anxiety, the hydrazines have an edge in superior therapeutic potency at equivalent doses, especially in difficult cases. Among the MAO inhibitors, phenelzine has become the reference drug for endogenous anxiety. For a comprehensive overview on the use of MAO inhibitors in clinical practice, the reader is referred to references 13 and 14.

Dose Phenelzine may be started at 15 mg/day. The dose can then be increased by 15 mg every three or four days. After the 15 mg tid dose is reached, it can be increased further in weekly increments of 15 mg until some of the typical side effects appear. The doses are best taken with food. The reason is that the postural hypotension, which is often a troublesome side effect, is less, perhaps because there is a small amount of tyramine in the average diet that keeps the blood pressure up, while the drug is exerting its direct hypotensive effect. The food also delays the absorption of the drug. Probably the best single guide to the therapeutic dose is the presence of postural hypotension as measured by the sphygmomanometer. It is recommended that the blood pressure be taken sitting and standing at each visit. The blood pressure will be seen to drop and recover more slowly on standing, at doses close to the therapeutic level. At doses close to the therapeutic level, even small changes in the dose can make a considerable difference, both in bringing on side effects and in delivering benefit. Consequently, a patient may receive inadequate benefit at, for example, 15 mg tid po, yet when the dose is increased to 15 mg qid po, he may get excessive hypotension. If the dose is then adjusted to three and one-half tablets per day, an ideal balance may be reached. It is difficult to split the phenelzine tablets for this purpose. Because this situation is so frequent, it is quite regrettable that phenelzine is not manufactured in a form that is grooved to permit this easy division. Marplan is suitably manufactured for this purpose.

There are several other methods of minimizing the postural hypotension during the first month of treatment. Drinking coffee, tea, and colas (all caffeinated) tend to increase the blood pressure a little (but not too much) and counteract the tendency of the hydrazine MAO inhibitors to produce bradycardia which magnifies the hypotensive symptoms. Taking salt tablets, ensuring adequate hydration, and even adding 0.1 mg of fludrocortisone (Florinef) all have their advocates as temporary strategies to relieve the drug-induced hypotension.

Side effects The common side effects include some dry mouth and constipation, excessive sweating in the upper torso and head, and hot flashes, although these are less than at equipotent doses of tricyclics. Muscle twitching, delayed urination, orgasmic delay or retarded ejaculation, cold sensations, a craving for sweet foods, weight gain, edema and "electric shock sensations" are also quite common. Since the MAO inhibitors were derived from the hydrazine drugs, including isoniazid, well-known to produce Vitamin B_6 deficiency with long-term use, it is probably advisable to prescribe Vitamin B_6 200 to 400 mg/day, for patients on MAO inhibitors more than four to six months. This B_6 deficiency has been associated with an increased incidence of carpal tunnel syndrome. The "electric shock sensations" which occur on turning the head or eyes usually only occur after four to six months of treatment. Some patients have found Vitamin B_6 helpful in minimizing this side effect.

Another side effect sometimes seen with both MAO inhibitor and tricyclic use is cheilosis — a red, raw soreness in the angles of the mouth, sometimes associated with cracked lips. Two to four lysine tablets per day usually clears this problem up in four to seven days.

Food restrictions   The essential principle to remember regarding food restrictions when taking MAO inhibitors is that the prohibited foods are usually aged, fermented or decayed in some way. Cheese, aged or smoked meats, overripe fruit, are well-known examples. Theoretically a great many foods, particularly meats if they are spoiled, could cause reactions, since the tyramine content of foods increases with aging and spoiling. This is true even when the food in its normal state is quite safe to take with MAO inhibitors. Among the different restricted substances there is a hierarchy of danger. Some foods (eg, cheese and red wine) and over-the-counter cold medicines are always very dangerous. Other foods (eg, chocolate and coffee) usually cause only small rises in blood pressure, unless taken in great quantities. In our experience, almost 90% of such reactions have occurred on cheese, wine, or cold medicines (decongestants). These are the important items to stress to the patient to avoid. If a patient has a question about the safety of any food with MAO inhibitors and it is not on the written list, the degree of aging, fermentation, or spoiling is the best guide to its potential danger.

It is wise never to prescribe an MAO inhibitor without giving the patient a printed list of the restricted foods. These are easily available from the drug companies free of charge. Alternately, a list that the clinician has found helpful may be copied and given to the patient (eg, see references 13 and 14).

As a regular practice, it is best to have patients avoid all cheese. While it is true that aged cheese causes the most serious hypertensive reactions, most people are quite unable to tell by appearance, brand or type, the tyramine content of any cheese. If exceptions are made, some patients will take further liberties with the exceptions. Similarly among the wines, red wines are more dangerous, but it is prudent to avoid all wine for simplicity. This prohibition includes sherries, vermouth, and cognac, which are variants of wines and contain tyramine.

Hypertensive reactions to MAO inhibitors are very rare and the majority follow deliberate infractions by the patient. The best advice is to have the patient who experiences flushing, severe headache and throbbing to immediately go to the nearest emergency room for evaluation of blood pressure. Regitine, 5 mg intravenously, slowly, is the treatment of choice.

The practice of giving anxious patients on MAO inhibitors some hypotensive agent (eg, chlorpromazine) to treat a hypertensive reaction, cannot be recommended. Patients have often incorrectly decided they are having a hypertensive reaction when precisely the opposite is occurring — they are hypotensive. To take a large dose of a hypotensive in such circumstances could spell serious problems. Furthermore, hypotensive reactions on MAO inhibitors (particularly the hydrazines, phenelzine and isocarboxazid) greatly outnumber the hypertensive reactions.

Drug restrictions All drugs containing sympathomimetic amines should be avoided. For practical purposes, this includes over-the-counter medications, decongestants, inhalants, antiallergy or asthma medication, or diet pills. If patients are to have dental work, some local anesthetic without epinephrine (eg, Carbocaine) is preferable.

If patients insist on having some medicine for a cough or cold, plain guaifenesin (Robitussin) is safe. For patients in considerable pain that does not respond to routine analgesics, we have encountered no difficulties using codeine. Morphine and meperidine are to be avoided.

Drug blood levels Although drawing plasma tricyclic and platelet MAO levels have become more widespread, their value has probably been overestimated. They are sometimes useful guides, and they are particularly useful medicolegally. However, all too often the plasma tricyclic level would suggest that the patient has an adequate dose, yet the patient may have no significant benefit or side effects. In such cases the clinician should follow his clinical judgment to increase the dose and not let the blood level dictate his actions. Similarly, with platelet MAO, achieving 80% MAO inhibition may not be sufficient to derive optimal benefit from the drug. Such platelet MAO levels should be taken before the drug is started if the clinician wishes a baseline reading against which to measure percentage inhibition. Finally, platelet MAO requires special preparation of the samples within four hours of the blood drawing if they are to be accurate. Drawing a blood sample to send by mail to a distant laboratory may yield entirely unreliable results.

Ceiling doses Although doses of tricyclics higher than 300 mg/day or of phenelzine higher than 90 mg/day are not recommended, it is occasionally necessary to increase the dose beyond those levels. Clinicians who frequently are referred "treatment resistant" cases find themselves very often having to do this. If the patient has no significant side effects or benefit at the maximum recommended dose, further increases should be considered. Failure to do so may leave the patient with a crippling disability and expose him to the danger of suicide.

Duration of treatment If adequate therapeutic benefit has not been achieved after three weeks on a good individualized therapeutic dose of alprazolam, or after six to seven weeks on any of the remaining drugs in Figure 6-2, a transfer to another drug should be considered. Once the correct drug and dose has been found, a trial of six to 12 months is recommended. Some tolerance may develop to any of the drugs after a few months. In these cases the dose will need to be increased. When the drug is being discontinued, it should be done slowly, preferably over a few weeks. Slow withdrawal minimizes the possibility of withdrawal effects reactivating the disorder.

Recent Antipanic Drugs

There are no systematic double-blind studies documenting the efficacy of trazodone or maprotiline for panic attacks with phobias. However, we have found them both useful in many cases in our unit, even in patients without significant concomitant depression. In spite of the early publicity to the contrary, these drugs can have troublesome side effects at therapeutic doses. However, trazodone appears to have a lower anticholinergic side effect profile than tricyclics. Sedation and nausea are not uncommon.

In contrast, we have not found buproprion[12] or amoxapine (Asendin) particularly helpful in panic states, although they are reputed to be satisfactory antidepressants.

With the range of choices now available, there are very few patients who cannot be helped with one or another of the above-mentioned drugs. As a general prescribing principle, it is best to find the best single drug for each patient before resorting to polypharmacy.

Behavior Therapy

After the medications control the spontaneous panic or symptom attacks, some phobic avoidance behavior may remain. In general, the more recent and milder the disorder, the more likely that the drug alone will help the patient overcome his disorder completely. The more chronic and intense the panic attacks, the more engrained the phobic avoidance becomes. In such cases, the patient may feel much calmer and know he is better, yet be reluctant to reenter the phobic situations. In such cases, exposure treatments are necessary to reduce the phobic disability. The active ingredient of many of the behavior therapies for phobias appear to be the extent of the real life exposure to the phobic stimulus. To the extent that it is intense, lasts for a long time (two to three hours), is repeatedly practiced, and that the usual avoidance response is prevented, there will be good extinction of the phobic avoidance behavior. The clinician takes action in bringing the patient physically into the real phobic situation. He then enlists the help of family and friends to ensure this is repeatedly practiced. Too much discussion without action in treating phobias is not very fruitful. In contrast, active real life exposure is.

Psychotherapy

When the patient has overcome his panic attacks with medication, and his phobic avoidance with exposure treatment, any remaining psychosocial problems may now come into sharper focus. The patient may see the issues more clearly and now has more emotional energy to deal with them. However, the old notion that all patients with anxiety attacks and phobias must have psychosocial problems troubling them is without foundation. Some do, but many others do not. Psychotherapy is indicated for those who do, and it should not be imposed on those who feel they do not.

Exogenous Anxiety

Patients with exogenous anxiety respond to a different treatment strategy than those with endogenous anxiety. If the problem is an exogenous phobia, and no spontaneous panic or symptom attacks are or have been present, then behavior therapy, particularly exposure treatments, is the intervention of choice. The exposure to the phobia is less frightening if it is done slowly in a graduated fashion. The patients usual flight response is prevented. Long exposure sessions, (eg, one and one-half to three hours) are much more valuable than shorter ones. If, for example, a patient fears cats, there is no substitute for introducing real cats into the treatment. The use of a benzodiazepine is rarely indicated. If the patient fails to improve after three months or 12 sessions using this approach, a trial of one of the drugs for endogenous anxiety may be indicated. The in vivo exposure is then repeated. At this point, extinction of the phobia can occur with exposure rather quickly, where it had failed to do so before using the drug. What appeared to be a single exogenous phobia on first examination may, on closer examination, later turn out to be a low grade or early phase of endogenous anxiety.

If the problem is an exogenous anxiety (either acute or chronic), the first step is to identify the stresses that either precipitate or continue to reinforce the symptoms. Psychotherapy may then be indicated to clarify the stresses or conflicts and to support the patient in making any changes necessary to resolve or work through them. Although benzodiazepines are often used in such cases, they are not always indicated. Finally, if these measures fail to bring about a significant therapeutic benefit within a reasonable period of time, then the drugs used for endogenous anxiety may deserve a trial. This is necessary only in a minority of cases. It is more likely to be necessary in those with chronic exogeneous anxiety and in those in whom the anxiety is disproportionate to the reality of the blamed stress.

REFERENCES

1. Sheehan DV, Sheehan KE: The classification of anxiety and hysterical states, Part I. Historical review and empirical delineation. *J Clin Psychopharmacol* 1982;2(14):235-244.
2. Sheehan DV, Sheehan KE: The classification of anxiety and hysterical states, Part II. Towards a more heuristic classification. *J Clin Psychopharmacol* 1982;2(6):386-393.
3. Sheehan DV, Sheehan KE: Diagnostic classification of anxiety and phobic disorders. *Psychopharmacol Bull* 1982;18(4):35-44.
4. Sheehan DV, Sheehan KE: The classification of phobic disorders. *Int Psychiatry Med* 1982-1983;12(4):243-264.
5. Klein DF, Rabkin JG (eds): *Anxiety: New Research and Current Concepts.* New York, Raven Press, 1981.
6. Pauls DL, Bucher KD, Crowe RR, et al: A genetic study of panic disorder pedigrees. *Am J Hum Genet* 1980;32;639-644.
7. Casey G, Gottesman I: Twin and family studies of anxiety, phobic and obsessive disorders, in Klein DF, Rabkin JG (eds): *New Research and Current Concepts.* New York, Raven Press, 1981, pp 117-136.
8. Sheehan DV, Ballenger J, Jacobson G: The treatment of endogenous anxiety with phobic, hysterical and hypochondriacal symptoms. *Arch Gen Psychiatry* 1980;37:51-59.
9. Tyrer P, Candy J, Kelley DA: A study of the clinical effects of phenelzine and placebo in the treatment of phobic anxiety. *Psychopharmacology* 1973;32: 237-254.
10. Klein DF: Importance of psychiatric diagnosis on prediction of clinical drug effects. *Arch Gen Psychiatry* 1967;16:118-126.
11. Sheehan DV, Coleman JH, Greenblatt DJ, et al: Some biochemical correlates of agoraphobia with panic attacks and their response to a new treatment. *J Clin Psychopharmacol* (Manuscript submitted for publication).
12. Sheehan DV, Davidson J, Manschreck TC, et al: Lack of efficacy of a new antidepressant (bupropion) in the treatment of panic disorder with phobias. *J Clin Psychopharmacol* 1983;3(1):23-31.
13. Sheehan DV, Claycomb JB, Kouretas N: MAO inhibitors: Prescription and patient management. *Int J Psychiatry Med* 1980;10:99-121.
14. Sheehan DV, Claycomb JB: The use of MAO inhibitors in clinical practice. in Manschreck TC (ed): *Psychiatric Medicine Update, Mass General Hospital Review for Physicians.* New York, Elsevier, 1983.

7

Lithium: Clinical Use, Toxicology, and Mode of Action

Aurelio Ortiz
Mamoun Dabbagh
Samuel Gershon

INTRODUCTION AND BACKGROUND

Lithium has had a checkered, although unique, history since its discovery in 1818. Due to its solubility, lithium salts were used as a treatment of gout in the 19th century. The bromide of lithium was employed in that era as a sedative and anticonvulsant as well. Thereafter, lithium salts were little used in the United States until the late 1940s, when lithium chloride became a popular salt substitute for patients on sodium free diets. It was being taken by patients with heart and kidney disease and some fatalities and serious poisoning resulted.[1]

This background would not appear to be an auspicious one for any new therapeutic claims for lithium. However, Cade[2], in 1949, reported an improvement in all 10 manic patients after administration of lithium salts, but not in patients suffering from dementia praecox or chronic depressive psychosis.

The introduction of the lithium ion into psychiatry in 1949 initiated the beginning of modern psychopharmacology. It predated the use of chlorpromazine and reserpine, the compounds most widely known for creating this revolution in psychiatry. Lithium, like the others, was introduced by a clinician and no reliable predictions based on preclinical pharmacological studies were made about the profile of its clinical activity.

The acceptance of lithium in the United States was in 1970. This tardy approval was due, in part, to reluctance of American physicians to accept the safety of this treatment. In addition, lack of commercial interest in this inexpensive, unpatentable mineral rendered the research in establishing its efficacy without industrial support.

PHYSIOLOGY

Absorption

Ingested lithium is readily and almost completely absorbed from the gastrointestinal tract. Less than 1% is detected in the feces.[3] Blood levels peak after single oral doses of lithium between two and four hours. Accordingly, in clinical practice, blood lithium levels are measured at least eight hours and usually 12 hours after the last dose to avoid sampling during these peaks. It is possible that by avoiding extreme fluctuation of blood lithium levels, the incidence of peak-related side effects, eg, nausea, slight abdominal pain and diarrhea, would be reduced. Thus, the sustained-release preparation versus the conventional preparations have the advantage of helping these unwanted peak-related side effects, although these sustained-release preparations vary in their property to yield smooth serum-concentration absorption curves, and may even be correlated with poor absorption due to incomplete release of lithium ion. Accordingly, each preparation should be evaluated on the basis of published absorption curves.[4]

The sites of lithium absorption in the gastrointestinal tract have not been fully defined. There is no interaction between lithium absorption and meals. The negative correlation between blood levels of lithum and body weight was noted. The correlations suggested that patients who weigh less achieve a higher serum lithium level.

Distribution

Lithium — in contrast to all psychotropic medication — is not protein bound, and thus it is distributed throughout the entire body water. Many experiments indicate that lithium is actively transported across cell membranes rather than passively diffused.[5,6] Accordingly, tissue lithium concentration depends on several factors: serum lithium concentration, water content of the tissue, and lithium influx and efflux; or the rates at which lithium penetrates and is removed from intracellular fluids. The rate of lithium influx or uptake into tissue is not uniform. Lithium is rapidly taken up by the kidney, and penetrates more slowly into the liver, bone, and muscle. Brain lithium uptake is even slower, which suggests low lithium permeability of the brain blood barrier.[7,8]

Lithium distribution in man was also found to be varied. By measuring plasma and cerebrospinal fluid (CSF) in steady-state during chronic lithium administration, it has been found that the mean plasma–to–CSF ratio is 2:1 or 3:1. A similar distribution between plasma and red blood cells (RBC) concentration has been observed with plasma–to–RBC ratio of approximately 3:1. It was suggested that the RBC concentration and the RBC/plasma lithium ratio might be more useful in monitoring lithium therapy and toxicity than plasma level alone.

The relationship of this ratio to psychiatric diagnosis, to short- and long-term responses to lithium therapy, and to the side effects of lithium administration has been studied. There is some evidence that patients with bipolar illness have higher lithium ratios in vivo than normal controls.[9,10] The evidence that patients who respond to lithium therapy have higher lithium ratio than nonresponders [11-13] has not been confirmed by other investigators.[14-15] Side effects of lithium therapy may be more highly correlated with intracellular lithium concentrations or the lithium ratio than plasma concentration.[16-18]

Elimination

Lithium is eliminated almost entirely in the urine, although less than 1% may be lost in sweat and feces. In normal volunteers, the range of recovery is 90% to 106%.[19-21] The lithium passes easily through the renal glomerular membrane since it is not protein bound, but only 20% is excreted; the rest is reabsorbed in the distal tubule of the nephron.

Lithium renal clearance normally ranges from 7 to 41 mL/min.[19,21,22] Lithium clearance has been found to correlate highly with creatinine clearance and the ratio of lithium–to–creatinine clearance range from 0.20 to 0.30 in man. The renal clearance is found to be independent of lithium plasma concentration and is not significantly affected by water loading. Day–night cycle and patient age may both alter renal clearance. Some evidence shows that nighttime excretion may be as much as 2.48 times that during the daytime. Many studies show reduction in lithium renal clearance in the elderly. Further, lithium clearance was positively correlated with weight, height and surface area.

The phases of lithium elimination were described.[20] The first phase consisted of a peak of six to eight hours' duration; this is followed by a very slow second phase which may last two weeks. Any diuretic that leads to sodium depletion (eg, furosemide, ethacrynic acid and thiazides) can increase lithium retention. However, osmotic diuresis with urea, which decreases proximal sodium reabsorption, increases lithium excretion. In addition, sodium bicarbonate and the carbonic anhydrase inhibitor, acetazolamide, also increases lithium excretion perhaps by increasing proximal tubular cation loss to accompany the unreabsorbed carbonate anion.

The percent of lithium eliminated with 24 hours varies widely but averages about 50%; in other words, the half-life or the elimination half-life is 24 hours. More than 90% is eliminated within 48 hours. No difference is found between conventional and sustained-release preparations.[23]

The longer the lithium treatment history, the longer the elimination half-life. Numerous studies have shown that bipolar patients have reduction in the lithium elimination rate. In the state of mania, elimination time has been directly correlated with the improvement due to lithium therapy.

THE CLINICAL USES OF LITHIUM

Lithium in the Acute Treatment of Mania

The large number of open and controlled studies, as well as extensive clinical experience of lithium in mania, indicate a remarkable degree of consistency in concluding that this ion has definite therapeutic properties in the great majority of manic patients. However, there are some unresolved questions concerning the efficacy of lithium as a treatment of acute mania. What is the efficacy of lithium versus phenothiazines or haloperidol? What criteria might be used to define the potential lithium responder? All these questions have no definite answers as yet.

To date, 11 studies[24-34] have used control groups: four used placebo,[24-27] six used chlorpromazine,[28-33] and one used haloperidol.[34] An assessment of these studies does not permit any direct comparison inasmuch as the experimental designs and methodologies varied. In summarizing the studies, it can be said that lithium is clearly superior to placebo in treatment of acute mania. Between lithium and chlorpromazine, three[29-31] failed to show statistically significant differences, although all investigators felt lithium was superior in totally normalizing the manic state and/or permitting discharge. In another investigation,[32] results with these two drugs were different depending on the division of manic patients into "highly active" and "mildly active," and lithium appeared to be the "better" treatment in mildly active patients. To date, there has been only one double-blind controlled study[34] comparing the efficacy of the butyrophenone, haloperidol with that of lithium or chlorpromazine. This most recent double-blind controlled study with severely ill, hospitalized manic individuals showed that lithium and haloperidol produced a highly significant improvement of manic symptoms without sedation. Both drugs were more effective than chlorpromazine, which, although producing considerable sedation, did little to alter the underlying mania qualitatively. While haloperidol had a more rapid impact on behavior–motor activity, lithium acted more evenly on the entire manic picture with total normalization realized during the third week of active treatment. The majority of lithium treated patients met discharge criteria at study termination; this was not the case for patients receiving either of the neuroleptic drugs.

An overview of studies indicated that despite some differences, the bulk of the available evidence does, nevertheless, suggest the following:

1. Lithium has a more specific/unique effect against "pure" mania than neuroleptic drugs such as phenothiazines or butyrophenones; lithium exerts its antimanic effects without the nonspecific sedation and tranquilization seen with neuroleptics.
2. Lithium produces its antimanic effects more slowly than neuroleptic drugs, particularly when the level of manic excitement and hyperactivity is intense; the mania begins to dissolve on lithium therapy after a lag period of four to ten days.
3. As more schizoaffective features are included in the patient population studied, the advantages of lithium diminish and the advantages of neuroleptics increase.
4. Most of the evidence suggests that lithium alone is the treatment of choice for those manic patients whose hyperactive behavior can be managed during the lag period before lithium begins to exert its effects; for those manic patients whose hyperactivity requires immediate control, chlorpromazine or haloperidol plus or followed by lithium is generally the best approach.

Lithium in the Acute Treatment of Depression

The use of lithium in the treatment of depression is still controversial. The acceptance of this is somewhat impaired by the availability of the tricyclic compounds which have definite efficacy in a large number of depressed patients. Furthermore, the notion that lithium is a specific antimanic agent enhanced the resistance to accept a single compound as both antidepressant and antimanic.

To date, 11 studies[26,35-44] have used control groups. All of these studies were designed with either placebo substitution, placebo comparison, or comparison with a standard antidepressant. Three of these[35-37] concluded that lithium had no antidepressant property, while the other reported a significant antidepressant effect. In comparison to tricyclic antidepressants (TCA), one controlled trial has reported that lithium is as effective as desipramine.[39] The other has reported that lithium is as effective as imipramine.[44]

From an overview of the studies, in spite of many methodological short-comings, one can draw some tentative conclusions:

1. It is still premature to consider lithium as a standard therapeutic modality for depression, although some depressed
   patients do indeed benefit from it.
2. The more "endogenous" features in depression, the more
   favorable response to lithium.
3. The acute antidepressant responses to lithium were significantly more frequent in the depressed phase of bipolar patients compared to unipolar patients.

Lithium in Prophylactic Treatment of Recurrent Affective Disorder

The term prophylaxis is misleading. It is used in medicine to suggest complete prevention of illness. However, we will use it here to suggest a reduction in psychopathology, whether it be in frequency or severity.

Lithium carbonate has been the only drug proven to guard against or to minimize recurrences of the manic phase of bipolar illness. There are eight double-blind, placebo-controlled studies in which maintenance therapy for six months to several years has been continued.[45-52] The results have confirmed its efficacy. The same conclusion can be said about the efficacy of lithium in preventing a recurrence of depressed phase in bipolar illness. Further studies will have to be carried out in an effort to clarify the role of neuroleptics in preventing further manic episodes, including the use of haloperidol and chlorpromazine.

Six double-blind, placebo-controlled studies[45,47,49,51,53,54] suggest that lithium is an effective prophylactic therapy against recurrent depressive episodes in unipolar illness and is significantly superior to placebo. A recent double-blind controlled study[53] indicates that both lithium and imipramine were equally effective in staving off future relapses of acute depression, both were significantly better than placebo.

There is, in fact, strong evidence to suggest that TCA is significantly effective as a maintenance treatment for depression in unipolars. Thus, the problem confronting us is not whether lithium is effective against recurrent mania and/or depression but rather to determine if it is better than any other psychoactive drug and/or drug combination.

Lithium in the Treatment of Schizophrenia

There has been increasing interest in the use of lithium in schizo-phrenia and the so-called schizoaffective disorder. One of the most pa-tent difficulties in evaluating treatment outcome is the inconsistency in the diagnostic criteria used in both disorders. In addition, the issue of lithium specificity as an antimanic went too far; if the patient had re-sponded to lithium, his psychopathology became "atypical" mania, de novo.

The early studies about using lithium in treatment of schizophrenia found that it had no antipsychotic properties, was not effective in schizophrenia, and may actually be deleterious due to increased susceptibility of schizophrenics to lithium-induced neurotoxicity.[55,56] Some authors contend that clinicians overdiagnose schizophrenia and misdiagnose mania. Schizophrenic patients who responded to lithium are indeed "atypical" manic-depressives, and this favorable response indicates "re-arrangement" of the diagnosis.[57-59] In some studies, lithium has been found to be effective against pathologic excitement in schizoaffective disorder but not to be effective on schizophrenic behavior.[60] However, several studies have reported positive responses, at least in subgroups of "pure" schizophrenics.[61-64] Recently, several studies have been conducted to test the efficacy of combination lithium and neuroleptic medication.[65,66] Statistically, significant results were reported.

In summary, the use of lithium in schizophrenia (either alone or in combination with neuroleptics) is clearly a new and a significant issue, both clinically and theoretically. The data are not adequate as to size and control status to reach an unequivocal conclusion. Certainly, lithium appears to have a beneficial effect on the course of certain schizophrenics. However, no one has claimed that lithium is more effective than standard neuroleptics. Clearly, neuroleptic drugs remain the medication of choice for the treatment of schizophrenia. Moreover, with improvement noted in chronic patients when lithium was combined with neuroleptics, the need to search for "atypical manias" is less critical. More systematic studies with defined diagnostic criteria and diagnostic subtypes are needed to draw more clear conclusions.

Lithium in Other Psychiatric Disorders

Lithium has been evaluated in almost all psychiatric disorders. However, few placebo-controlled studies have shown promising results.

Placebo-controlled studies have failed to substantiate the claims of lithium effect in premenstrual tension, obsessive-compulsive disorder, and panic attacks. Some reports have suggested the usefulness of lithium in anorexia nervosa, affective psychosis in organic brain disorder, hypersexuality and transvestism.

Many reports have been published about the effects of lithium in the treatment of alcoholism. One double-blind, placebo-controlled trial[67] was able to show that those patients who were given lithium had significantly fewer drinking bouts than those given placebo. In another study no differences were reported between lithium and placebo in alcoholic patients without depression.[68]

Rifkin et al[69] have carried out a double-blind placebo-controlled crossover study of lithium in patients hospitalized with neurotic and personality disorder in whom a clear or presumptive affective component was present. Both lithium and chlorpromazine are effective in diminishing the mood fluctuation in emotionally unstable character disorder, but lithium appears to have fewer side effects and can more specifically control the short-lived mood swings.

A number of preclinical and clinical studies have dealt with lithium therapy for a variety of aggressive behaviors. A double-blind study was performed on prison inmates with a history of chronic assaultive behavior or chronic impulsive antisocial behavior. This study indicates a significant beneficial effect of lithium on aggressive behavior, probably with some specificity.[70] Studies of mentally retarded patients with disruptive behavior and temper outbursts indicate beneficial effects of lithium on both self-multilation and aggression toward others.

Lithium in Nonpsychiatric Disorders

The clinical utility of lithium in nonpsychiatric disorders has been suggested in a variety of diseases.

Lithium is well established to cause granulocytosis. Hence, lithium therapy has been tried for various granulocytopenic states. It was found to raise the leukocyte counts in a number, but not in all, cases of Felty's syndrome.[71] The clinical use of lithium for long-term treatment is unclear.

Lithium acts to inhibit adenylate cyclase in the kidney and hence to decrease cyclic AMP and antidiuretic hormone (ADH) response. This mechanism justified the use of lithium in inappropriate secretion of ADH. Treatment results have been mixed, some authors reported no effects,[72] others observed prompt water diuresis, normalization of urine osmolality, and correction of serum sodium.[73]

The clinical trials of lithium in hyperthyroidism demonstrate uniformly that lithium antagonized hyperthyroidism, but the practical value of this action is questionable. In addition, lithium has been combined with radioactive iodine in the treatment of metabolizing thyroid cancer.[74] Due to its inhibition of thyroid hormone release, lithium prolongs the presence of radioactivity in the gland and hence increases the ratio of gland irradiation to body irradiation. Lithium has been found no better than placebo in Meniere's disease in six month's double-blind crossover trial.

Lithium has been tried in various movement disorders. The positive results in using lithium in Huntington's chorea could not be validated in controlled studies. Anecdotal reports indicate positive treatment results in tardive dyskinesia, spasmodic torticollis, levodopa-induced hyperkinesia, and Tourette's syndrome.

The effectiveness of lithium in migraine and cluster headaches has been reported in several uncontrolled trials. The result is encouraging; however, more systematic investigations are needed to draw a clear conclusion.

PRACTICAL ASPECTS OF LITHIUM TREATMENT

The treatment procedure must take into account the two areas involved in the interaction, ie, the clinical aspect and the physiological and pharmacological properties of the drug. In the former, there are two considerations as to whether the treatment is for the control of the current manic episode, or for the prophylaxis during an interphase, and must also take into account, most importantly, the specificity of lithium as a mood stabilizer. The first issue, then, is proper selection of patients to whom lithium is to be prescribed, and second, the patient must be in reasonably good physical condition to adequately handle the lithium ion upon its introduction into the body. Besides doing a regular medical workup, the following investigations should be carried out: plasma creatinine, urea, electrolytes, fasting blood sugar, CBC, thyroid function test, pregnancy test and an EKG. A general guide to relative contraindication to co-existing medical conditions is given in Table 7-1.

Table 7-1
A General Guide to Contraindications to Lithium Therapy*

Condition or Drug	Strength of Contraindication
Renal failure	+ +
Renal tubular disease	+ + +
Acute myocardial infarction	+ + +
Cardiac conduction defects	+ +
Controlled cardiac failure	+ +
Epilepsy	+
Parkinson's disease	+ +
Tardive dyskinesia	+
Dementia	+
Cerebellar disorder	+
Myasthenia gravis	+ + +
Diabetes mellitus	+
Ulcerative colitis	+
Psoriasis	+
Senile cataracts	+
Pregnancy, 1st trimester	+ + +
Pregnancy, 2nd or 3rd trimester	+ +
Breast feeding	+ + +
Delivery	+ +
Diuretics, Na-losing	+ +
Indomethacin	+
Phenylbutazone	+
Digoxin	+ +
GABA agonist	+
Diphenylhydantoin	+

+ = caution + + = close expert psychiatric, medical, and laboratory monitoring
+ + + = contraindicated
*From Mann V, Gershon S: Absolute and relative contraindications to lithium treatment in, Johnson FN (ed): *Handbook of Lithium Therapy*, Baltimore, University Park Press, 1980, with permission.

Important conditions to keep in mind are enumerated below:

1. In cardiac diseases the lithium ion sensitizes the myo-cardium to the effects of low sodium and may cause arrhythmias, conduction defects, and aggravate heart failure. Patients with cardiac problems should be closely monitored when placed on lithium.
2. Toxicity to lithium dramatically increases with low salt and low fluid intake. Therefore, patients on diuretics or restricted salt or fluid regimen should receive lower doses of lithium and their intake of salt and fluid should be stable and regular. With lithium overdosage or toxicity, diuretics should be immediately stopped.
3. Renal diseases per se do not contraindicate lithium treatment. They demand careful monitoring of serum lithium level, regular determination of renal function, such as 24 hour urine volume and creatinine clearance determinations, and lower doses of lithium.[75]

Therefore, after selection of the patient for treatment, the therapeutic regimen may be considered in two phases. The initiation of lithium treatment in a manic patient may be considered similar to the institution of insulin in controlling a diabetic patient. The stabilization of a manic episode may take from five to ten days. Any of the lithium salts may be used, but the most readily available is lithium carbonate, which comes in tablets or capsules of 250 or 300 mg each, ie, equivalent to 6.75 or 8.0 mEq of elemental lithium. The range of daily dosage during this phase may vary considerably between 1 and 3 g in multiple divided doses over 24 hours. This initial higher level of dosage is given until the manic symptoms have abated. The size of the dose is determined by several factors such as the severity of the clinical condition, body weight, age, physical condition, and rate of renal clearance. Cooper et al[76,77] based on kinetic analysis, described a technique whereby the individual dosage requirement can be predicted from a single blood sample collected 24 hours after administration of a 600-mg dose of lithium carbonate.

The steady state between intake and elimination is reached in five to six days; thereafter the serum lithium concentration in blood samples drawn approximately 12 hours after the last intake of lithium should be within the range of 0.8 to 1.5 mEq/L. Plasma levels may be determined approximately every three or four days during the stabilization phase. In addition to such chemical surveillance, careful clinical observation is mandatory and may indicate the appearance of any toxic manifestations as well as the chemical assays. If toxic symptoms appear, or if the plasma lithium level approaches 2 mEq/L, the dose of lithium should be reduced; or if the toxicity is severe, the drug is temporarily withdrawn. In cases in which disruptive behavior becomes a significant management problem, a manic attack may also be treated with combination of lithium and a major antipsychotic such as chlorpromazine or haloperidol. The antipsychotic drug usually controls the more violent manifestation of the mania more rapidly, but when the effect of lithium becomes apparent, the former drug may be discontinued gradually.

After the manic episode remits, the initial high dosage of lithium may be reduced. The dosage should be lowered and plasma levels be continued until a stable plasma concentration is established. When the clinical condition is fully under control and a constant dose of lithium has been established, the patient can be safely managed at the level with continued ingestion and a regular check of plasma lithium levels and clinical surveillance. During maintenance treatment, the intake of lithium must equal the elimination, and since lithium is excreted almost exclusively through the kidneys, it is primarily the renal lithium clearance that determines the maintenance dosage. The renal lithium clearance is usually a fixed proportion, about one-fifth of the creatinine clearance. Like the latter, as mentioned above, it varies considerably between individuals and also falls with advancing years. Accordingly, the optimum maintenance dosage varies greatly from person to person. In general, this maintenance level of plasma lithium is between 0.6 and 1.2 mEq/L, although maintenance dosage should be adjusted to each individual case in accordance with the symptomatology and occurrence of side effects. Because of the usefulness of lithium medication as a prophylactic agent in manic depressive disease, this medication may need to be continued for many years. Although the addition of other psychotropic drugs to lithium in the treatment of either manic or depressive phase may be made without producing problems of drug interaction or increasing toxicity, some caution should be taken whenever lithium is combined with these medications.

TOXICOLOGY

Acute Effects of Excessive Dosage

The most common features associated with mild toxicity and slightly elevated serum lithium level (usually over 1 mEg/L) include anorexia, gastric discomfort, diarrhea, vomiting, polyuria, and hand tremor[26] (Table 7-2). These often coincide with serum lithium peaks and the effects may be related more to the steepness of the rise of the lithium levels than to the height of the peak. Often they disappear or diminish without reduction of dose. However, some may persist, such as polyuria and tremor.[78] The tremor induced by lithium does not respond to anti-Parkinson or anticholinergic medication, however, propranolol, the β-adrenergic blocking agent, may be useful in treating this occasionally disturbing effect.[79] The polyuria may continue and give rise to a diabetes insipidus-like syndrome that is resistant to ADH,[80] but responds to thiazide diuretics[81,82] and usually subsides on withdrawal of medication.[83]

Toxic effects seen at blood levels above 1.5 mEq/L are more serious and may include muscle fasciculation and twitching, hyperactive deep tendon reflexes, ataxia, somnolence, confusion, dysarthria, and, rarely, epileptiform seizures. These effects are often associated with reversible EEG alterations. A more reliable index of toxicity may be the intracellular lithium level rather than the serum level.[16-17,84]

There is no specific antidote for lithium intoxication. From the studies carried out to date, treatment should consist of general measures to correct the effects induced on water and electrolyte balance (Table 7-3). Schou et al[85] have suggested that forced diuresis should aid significantly in the elimination of lithium.

Table 7-2
Toxic Manifestations of Lithium Excessive Dosage*

Gastrointestinal Symptoms	Mental Symptoms
Anorexia	Mental retardation
Nausea	Somnolence
Vomiting	Confusion
Diarrhea	Restlessness and disturbed behavior
Thirst	Stupor
Dryness of the mouth	Coma
Weight loss	Cardiovascular System
Neuromuscular Symptoms and Signs	Pulse irregularities
General muscle weakness	Fall in blood pressure
Ataxia	ECG changes
Tremor	Peripheral circulatory failure
Muscle hyperirritability	Circulatory collapse
Fasciculation (increased by tapping muscle)	Miscellaneous
Twitching (especially of facial muscles)	Polyuria
Clonic movements of whole limbs	Glycosuria
Choreoathetoid movements	General fatigue
Hyperactive deep tendon reflexes	Lethargy and tendency to sleep
Central Nervous System	Dehydration
Anesthesia of skin	
Incontinence of urine and feces	
Slurred speech	
Blurring of vision	
Dizziness	
Vertigo	
Epileptiform seizures	

*From Gershon S: Lithium, in Usdin E, Forrest I (eds): *Psychotherapeutic Drugs*, vol 2. New York, Marcel Dekker, 1977, with permission.

Table 7-3*
Management of Severe Lithium Poisoning†

Clinical Procedures Recommended
1. Discontinue lithium.
2. Blood lithium level, stat; then daily or every two days as required.
3. Serum sodium and potassium estimations, stat; follow as required.
4. ECG, stat; periodically thereafter.
5. Temperature and blood pressure, every four hours.
6. Infection prophylaxis (eg, rotate patient).
7. Optional: spinal tap, EEG.
8. If question of infection exists, blood culture and viral studies of blood and CSF are indicated.

Treatment Methods Recommended
1. Replace water and electrolytes (sodium, potassium, calcium, magnesium) as needed. Total daily fluid intake should be at least 5 to 6 L per day. Do not oversalinize, and avoid abrupt changes in electrolyte intake. Monitor, if changes are made.
2. Forced lithium diuresis via urea, 30 g IV two to five times daily (urea contraindicated if severe renal impairment antedates toxicity), or mannitol, 50 to 100 g IV as total daily dose.
3. Increase lithium clearance with aminophylline (which also suppresses tubular reabsorption and increases blood flow), dosage 0.5 g by slow IV may cause sharp but transitory hypotension.
4. Alkalinization of urine with sodium lactate administered intravenously has been recommended as an adjunct.
5. If poisoning is severe, the patient should be dialyzed (peritoneal dialysis or artificial kidney).

*This table is a modification of one prepared by Dr. Gershon for the APA exhibit, San Francisco, 1970.
†Primarily via renal excretion: four-fifths of filtered lithium is reabsorbed in the proximal tubule (normal half-life of lithium is 24 hours).

Chronic Effects

These latter effects may be of considerable interest and have only recently been described. Lithium produces a generally benign diminution in the concentration of circulating thyroidal hormones. Several investigators have found decreases in the protein bound iodine and other thyroidal measures as early as 24 hours after the institution of lithium therapy.[85-88] Schou et al[89] found thyroid pathology consisting of euthyroid goiter in 12 of 330 patients (3.6%) treated with lithium for periods of from five months to two years. Shopsin et al[90] found mixed thyroid pathology (euthyroid goiter, three patients; goiter with hyperthyroidism, five patients; hyperthyroidism alone, one patient) in 11.7% of 77 patients treated from three weeks to three years with lithium alone. Significantly, both of these studies found an increase of lithium-related thyroid pathology after the first month of treatment. A related phenomenon, a benign, reversible exophthalmos, has also been observed during lithium therapy in 11% of the patients.[91] In most cases, the effects of lithium on thyroidal function are not of sufficient magnitude to require treatment. If necessary, thyroid supplementation may be administered. Underlying thyroid disorder is not a contraindication to lithium treatment if thyroid functioning can be properly assessed and if thyroid hormones can be maintained at acceptable levels, by exogenous supplement when necessary.[92]

The effects of lithium on blood glucose and on glucose tolerance are the complex product of numerous biochemical vectors. Reflecting this complexity are conflicting reports around these issues. Recently, Shopsin et al,[93] in heterogenous patient groups, found a significant increase in blood glucose level 30 minutes after acute ingestion and a decrease in glucose tolerance after two weeks of treatment. The implication of these studies are that decreased glucose tolerance accompanying lithium administration is due to physiological effects of this ion, and is not related to either psychiatric diagnosis, change in clinical state, or duration of treatment with a drug. This phenomenon is reversible upon withdrawal of medication.

Lithium produces a relative leukocytosis in most patients receiving treatment.[94-96] Shopsin et al[97] found elevations over baseline in 21 of 22 patients in whom lithium treatment was initiated. The leukocytosis was statistically significant and occurred irrespective of diagnosis. The mean leukocyte count in their patients increased from 9.116/cu mm before treatment to 14.716/cu mm after reaching therapeutic dosages. Following discontinuation of the treatment, values returned to a mean of 9.481/cu mm. The magnitude of leukocytosis has not correlated directly with the lithium blood level.[94-97] Analysis of the differential leukocyte response has revealed that the lithium induced leukocytosis is secondary to neutrophilia and is accompanied by a lymphocytopenia.[94-97] Since lithium-induced leukocytic changes have not been shown to have adverse effects in man and are reversible following discontinuation of lithium treatment, the issue of treatment for these effects does not arise.[98]

Many patients receiving therapeutic dosages of lithium manifest T wave flattening or inversion on the ECG. The T wave changes generally develop during the first few weeks of treatment, remain constant, and disappear in conjunction with the elimination of lithium from the body. Other cardiac effects of lithium occur infrequently.

Lithium has been noted to produce dermatologic lesions sporadically and infrequently. Most often, when they do occur, these lesions are maculopapular in type, appear in the first weeks of lithium treatment, disappear when lithium is discontinued, and do not necessarily return if lithium treatment is reinstated.[99,100]

Within this section, it is important to consider possible teratogenic effects of lithium that might arise in considering whether the patient should be maintained on this medication if a pregnancy intervenes. The

International Register of Lithium Babies[101-104] has been soliciting data on the offspring of mothers who received lithium treatment throughout their pregnancies. Of the 212 children on whom data was available, 22 had some form of malformation, and 17 of those had a cardiovascular malformation.[104] Lithium has been shown to pass freely across the placenta.[105] Its concentration in the fetus, therefore, closely reflects that in the maternal circulation. The data from animal studies has revealed definite teratogenic effects in animals.[106] Accordingly, we may conclude that, whenever possible, lithium treatment should be avoided during pregnancy, especially during the first trimester. However, there may be the occasion when the potential benefits of treatment outweigh the risks. In these instances, clinical judgment and certain precautions should be used.[98]

Finally, it should be noted that the lithium concentration in the mammary milk of lactating mothers is 30% to 100% of the serum. Furthermore, infants who are breast-fed attain serum lithium concentration closely approximating that found in the mother's milk.[107,108] Therefore, it would seem wise to counsel against breast-feeding in mothers who are receiving lithium treatment.

Nephrotoxicity

Lithium produces two distinct categories of renal effects. The most frequent and most benign effect is a nephrogenic diabetes insipidus syndrome. The other more serious effect is morphological damage, which is presumably irreversible due to chronic lithium intake. These two effects will be discussed below.

Polyuria and secondary polydipsia have long been known to occur with lithium treatment. These symptoms have been observed in more than half the patients starting lithium treatment, and approximately one quarter of all lithium-treated patients continue to exhibit these symptoms one to two years after initiation of treatment.[109] This diabetes insipidus-like syndrome is not related to the classic syndrome (ie, no posterior pituitary gland dysfunction). It is vasopressin-unresponsive and its renal mechanism has been established. It is recognized by low specific gravity, low osmolality, polyuria, inability to concentrate the urine, and no improvement from fluid restriction or administration of exogenous vasopressin.[110] The mechanism by which lithium reduces vasopressin responsiveness has been postulated. Vasopressin stimulates renal adenylate cyclase, which converts adenosine triphosphate (ATP) to cyclic adenosine monophosphate (AMP), which in turn mediates vasopressin response on a cellular level.[111] Lithium acts to inhibit adenylate cyclase and hence to decrease cyclic AMP and vasopressin response.[112] This syndrome is known to be fully reversible on discontinuation of the medication[113] and responsive to thiazide diuretics.[114,115]

The recent demonstration of lithium-induced histopathology in the kidney is the most pressing issue requiring proper evaluation.[116] In 1977 Hestbech et al[117] reported that patients receiving long-term lithium treatment with a history of lithium toxicity or lithium-induced nephrogenic diabetes insipidus showed changes characterized by chronic focal atrophy with interstitial fibrosis and numerous sclerotic glomeruli. These nonspecific changes were quantitatively different from those of a control group. Since lithium toxicity had occurred, the significance of the findings to uncomplicated lithium therapy was not clear.[118]

In a second study, the same group investigated the correlation between the histopathology and the functional impairment.[119,120] Morphologic alteration was correlated with duration of therapy, compromised urine concentrating capacity, and creatinine clearance. Bucht et al[121] reported the same finding and suggested that renal concentrating capacity might be impaired more by the combination of lithium and antipsychotic medications than by lithium alone. These reports, and others, have stimulated extensive studies and alerted the clinicians about the potential hazard of lithium therapy. However, Hullin et al[121] did not support the nephrotoxicity of long-term lithium therapy. Kincaid-Smith et al[123] failed to document histologic differences between renal biopsies in long-term lithium and non-lithium patients with affective disorder. Nonspecific nephropathies were observed in both groups. These findings raise doubts about whether such lesions are due to lithium alone.

In summary, the polyuric effects of lithium, despite their infrequent irreversibility, are not life threatening. The morphological changes do exist but the etiology is uncertain. The risk of renal insufficiency is remote. Better pre-lithium selection and renal workup, lower serum lithium levels and closer clinical and laboratory follow-up are advised.[110,124]

Neurotoxicity

The effects of lithium on the central nervous system (CNS) range from commonly observed mild effects to irreversible, life-threatening brain damage in rare instances of severe toxicity.

The most consistent anomalies found in neurotoxicity with lithium in ordinary therapeutic dosages are change in EEGs, including alteration in the alpha activity, diffuse slowing, accentuation of previous focal abnormalities, and appearance of previously absent focal changes.[98] Despite these consistent changes, the evidence suggested that these effects are benign. No evidence of impaired cortical function was found by using the Neuropsychological Battery to test for organic impairment in patients receiving 600 to 1500 mg of lithium daily for one year, two months to five years.[125]

Toxic neurologic side effects should be distinguished from the benign effects that are measurable in the majority of patients. This neurotoxic reaction is characterized by symptoms of organic brain syndrome such as disorientation, confusion, reduced comprehension, dysarthria, ataxia, somnolence, lethargy, and extrapyramidal signs.

This reversible reaction occurs at ordinary therapeutic lithium blood levels.[126] Schizophrenic patients in particular have been reported to be especially at risk for the development of neurotoxic, confusional states while receiving lithium treatment.[127,128] With increasing dosage and serum concentration, neurotoxic effects become more frequent and severe (see Table 7-2), although they are more closely correlated with preexisting EEG abnormalities and subsequent EEG alteration than with actual serum concentration.[127] Perhaps using a combination of lithium and neuroleptic medications may enhance a patient's vulnerability to neurotoxicity, since the neuroleptic may cause an increase in the intracellular lithium level.[129] One should remember that there are more cases of neurotoxicity reported with lithium alone than with the combination, and lithium is more often prescribed with other psychotropic medication than prescribed alone. Recently, a view has been put forward that lithium and neuroleptic combination can cause neuroleptic malignant syndrome.[130] Again, there is no convincing reason why the cause may not be the neuroleptic itself.

MODE OF ACTION

Ever since lithium was recognized to have a specific effect in mania, much interest was focused on understanding its mode of action. The fact that a simple substance, an alkali metal, could modify manic disorder and prevent recurrences of manic-depressive episodes has led to much research to clarify the mechanisms underlying bipolar affective disorders and the effects of lithium. Because of its physicochemical properties close to sodium, it was first thought that its effects were due to displacement of sodium from biological tissues, especially those in the central nervous system. Indeed, in some chemical and biological situations lithium behaves as a "weak" sodium[131] However, lithium also has comparable properties to those of the other three cations most abundant in cells: potassium, calcium, and magnesium, and may interact with ammonium groups including those of phospholipids in the cellular membrane and those of biogenic amines.[132] Furthermore lithium has specific properties on its own. It is the lightest of all solid elements, it has the smallest crystal radius of all the alkali metals, its electron affinity is higher than those of the other alkali metals, it has the largest energy of hydration, and upon hydration its radius is increased out of proportion to those of sodium, potassium, rubidium and cesium, indicating that in physiological situations lithium has the lowest diffusion coefficient. It is also the least lipid soluble of the alkali metals.[132,133] Since the therapeutic effects of lithium have been demonstrated when the intracellular concentration of sodium is 30-fold to 100-fold that of lithium, initially it was hypothesized that lithium could be correcting a defect unique to manic-depressive illness. The presence of either a specific "Li⁺-receptor" of the alteration of a central nervous system receptor or carrier which allows lithium to replace the normal substrate (Ca^{2+}, Mg^{2+}, Na^+, K^+) was then postulated.[134-136] In the second case, lithium would thus correct the defect and permit normal functioning.[136] Currently there are available data on the effects of lithium on: 1) electrolyte metabolism, 2) transport across biological membranes, 3) receptors and neurotransmitters, 4) endocrine functions, and 5) biological rhythms.

In man, lithium administration is accompanied by a rapid but transient diuresis of sodium and water,[137-139] which, in turn, produces increased aldosterone excretion that returns to previous levels after one week.[138,140] It is likely that lithium treatment first displaces sodium and potassium from intracellular (or extracellular) compartments.[141] Lithium can substitute for sodium, potassium, or both, under experimental conditions,[142] and can alter potassium, calcium, magnesium, and phosphate.[137,138,140,143-145] Lithium has been found to alter calcium and magnesium in the iris and visual cortex and potassium in the cerebellar cortex of the rat,[146,147] and calcium and magnesium in cerebrospinal fluid (CSF) and plasma in humans.[148-151] Thus, the interaction of the lithium ion with other cations with biological functions could explain some effects of lithium therapy.

Lithium was thought to enter and exit CSF and brain tissue via passive transfer kinetics, related to utilization of sodium–potassium (Na-K) pump.[152] However, more recent research seems to point out that lithium flow is by active transport, rather than passive diffusion. Thus, sodium and lithium appear to compete for a common binding site which exhibits greater affinity for lithium than sodium.[153-155] Lithium enhances blood-brain barrier (BBB) permeability at low cerebral blood flow,[156] stimulates the fast component of sodium entry,[157] reduces choline uptake,[158,159] increases CSF amino acid concentrations,[160] and lowers CSF cyclic AMP concentrations;[161,162] the last two effects mainly found in patients who have a previous history of lithium therapy. Lithium can activate sodium–potassium–magnesium ATPase in biological membranes[163] and has been described to interact with anionic membrane phospholipids which can modify these membranes, especially in nervous tissue.[164]

The uptake, storage, release, and metabolism of catecholamine and indolamine neurotransmitters can be affected by monovalent ions, such as lithium, as well as by divalent cations. These neurotransmitters have been implicated in affective disorders. Lithium has been found to decrease dopamine formation in striatum and limbic forebrain in the rat,[165] but experiments in humans have produced conflicting results on dopamine metabolism.[152,166] A great deal of research has been carried out on the development of dopamine receptor supersensitivity based on the idea that if the development of supersensitivity is important at the onset of mania, then lithium, which prevents such episodes, should also prevent the occurrence of supersensitivity.[152] In a series of experiments it was found that acute and chronic lithium administration can block pre-synaptic and postsynaptic dopamine receptor supersensitivity induced by nigrostriatal lesions or drugs that either block the dopamine receptor or decrease the availability of dopamine (denervation supersensitivity) at the receptor site.[132,167-176] These results may explain lithium ability to prevent recurrences of mania.[152]

Norepinephrine is the neurotransmitter thought to be the most influential in the causation of primary affective disorder.[152] It has been found in animal and human studies that lithium: 1) increases turnover of nor-epinephrine in the brain but not in the periphery,[166] 2) increases norepinephrine neuronal uptake,[166,177] 3) reduces the release of exogenously administered norepinephrine,[166,178,179] 4) inhibits the stimulus-induced norepinephrine release,[180,181] and 5) increases urinary excretion of norepinephrine metabolites, Vanillylmandelic acid (VMA), normetanephrine, and 3-Methoxy-4-hydroxyphenylglycol (MHPG)[166,182] and increases MHPG in CSF during initial lithium administration.[166] The effects of lithium on adrenergic receptors have also been studied. Decrease in β-receptor binding,[170,172,183] decreased density of β-receptors,[170,172] and increase or no effect in a α-receptor binding[183] have been found. These results have been related to prevention of supersensitivity of α- and β-receptors which develops after 6-hydroxydopamine lesions and lack of prevention of subsensitivity induced by imipramine.[152] It has been suggested that a reduction in synaptic norepinephrine in the brain may be associated with depression, so that a reduction of β-adrenergic receptor sensitivity is a better correlate of antidepressant treatment.[184] It also has been suggested that blockade by lithium of β-adrenergic supersensitivity in the brain may be associated with the therapeutic action of lithium in preventing recurrence of depressive states.[185]

More recent work has focused on the effects of lithium on serotonin (5-HT), due to the observation that lithium may induce improvement of previously nonresponsive depressions to various antidepressants.[186] Lithium can produce: 1) increase in brain concentrations of tryptophan, the precursor of 5-HT,[187,188] 2) stimulation of 5-HT synthesis,[165,189] 3) inhibition or lack of effect on 5-HT turnover,[190,191] 4) stimulation of 5-HT uptake in human platelets,[192] and 5) increase of 5-hydroxyindoleacetic acid (5-HIAA) in CSF.[193] Clinical reports have found a significant positive correlation between pretreatment levels of CSF 5-HIAA and lithium response, together with a nonsignificant increase of CSF 5-HIAA of 15% during treatment.[194] Chronic lithium administration may reduce 5-HT receptors in the brain.[195] It has been suggested that lithium treatment makes 5-HT and its receptors more flexible, rather than more stable.[152]

Because of evidence that increased cholinergic activity may induce depression, lithium has been thought to interact with the central cholinergic system.[152] Chronic lithium administration was found to produce acetylcholine (ACh) increase in cortex and midbrain in mice.[196] Lithium administration clearly affects the transport of choline by inhibition of transfer across the BBB and RBC membrane, and when given chronically, increases high affinity transport of choline in brain cells, increases ACh synthesis and release, and causes elevation of ACh and choline brain content.[152,197-201] It has been suggested that lithium may produce irreversible changes within the cell to release endogenously bound choline, stimulate cholinesterase activity within but not outside the neuron, and antagonize cholinergic neuronal transmission.[152] Although little work has been done on lithium and ACh receptors, it seems from the available data that lithium has an inhibitory effect on both affinity and number of ACh receptors.[152]

On other transmitters lithium has been found to have the following effects: 1) increase in met-enkephalin content in rat striatum, decreased binding affinity of opiate agonists and increased binding affinity of opiate antagonists, 2) decrease in number of binding sites of GABA receptors, due to activation of the GABA system to induce subsensitivity, and 3) increase of glycine in human RBC.[202-207]

Finally, lithium may affect the systems related to the activation by neurotransmitters and hormones of receptors and the biological response thus elicited. Induced increase of cyclic AMP, which is considered as the second messenger between receptor activation and the events that lead to the physiologic responses, is inhibited by the administration of lithium.[208-213] Adenylate cyclase, a magnesium-dependent enzyme that synthesizes cyclic AMP upon activation by a neurotransmitter or a hormone, can also be affected by lithium. Antidiuretic hormone (ADH)-sensitive adenylate cyclase is inhibited by lithium[214] as well as thyroid stimulating hormone (TSH)-sensitive adenylate cyclase,[154] therefore producing renal and thyroid effects. Lithium can also inhibit norepinephrine-sensitive adenylate cyclase and increase the activity of dopamine-sensitive adenylate cyclase.[214,215] In humans, plasma cyclic AMP was found to be respectively increased by lithium in the treatment of depression and decreased in the treatment of mania.[216] Long-term prophylaxis lithium treatment is found to be associated with decrease in plasma cyclic AMP.[217] Lithium treatment blocks chemically induced elevations in plasma cyclic AMP, as those induced by epinephrine and isoproterenol.[218] It has been suggested that, although lithium at toxic doses may act as a general inhibitor of cyclic AMP activity, its action at therapeutic doses to inhibit norepinephrine-induced increase of cyclic AMP may be important. Lithium at this dose would act to stabilize receptor changes important in reducing norepinephrine functional activity postsynaptically.[184,219] Cyclic GMP, which is thought to be important in the activation of adenylate cyclase, is also significantly reduced by lithium.[220] It has been proposed that the effect of lithium in mania may be due to inhibition, and its prophylactic effect to stabilizing cerebral adenylate cyclase.[221] Alternatively, as cyclic GMP is related to presynaptic α-adrenergic receptors, it has been suggested that cyclic AMP and cyclic GMP may be viewed as balancing systems, thus their interaction may provide a mechanism for the dual clinical effects of lithium in mania and depression.[184]

Lithium administration can affect the endocrine system. As stated earlier, enhanced aldosterone production after several days of lithium treatment is a result of renin stimulation which, itself, is secondary to the initial effects of lithium on water and electrolyte metabolism. In rats, subchronic and chronic lithium administration increases secretion of prolactin, possibly due to simultaneously enhanced 5-HT receptor sensitivity and decreased dopamine receptor sensitivity.[222] However, repeated human studies have found no effect on morning serum base levels and only minimal inhibitor effect on 24-hour secretion of prolactin.[159,223] Baseline growth hormone is not affected by lithium in humans, while drug-induced hormonal changes can be modified by lithium depending on the altered clinical state. For example, both men and premenopausal women have higher growth hormone levels after stimulation by insulin, thyrotropin-releasing hormone (TRH), and luteinizing hormone-releasing hormone (LHRH) in lithium-treated patients when compared to healthy controls.[224] Manic patients when given TRH show a more marked increase in plasma growth hormone after lithium treatment.[225] These actions may be related to effects of lithium on 5-HT and dopamine.[152] Although little work has been done on the effects of lithium on the secretion of TSH, follicle-stimulating hormone (FSH), and luteinizing hormone (LH), it seems that only TSH responses, but not those of FSH and LH, are altered after lithium treatment.[152,224,226]

Thyroid effects of chronic lithium treatment have been well documented. Lithium has been shown to produce hyperthyroidism and goiter. Lithium is concentrated in the thyroid gland and causes a reduction in triiodothyronine and thyroxine from euthyroid and hyperthyroid glands.[227] Thyroid effects of lithium may be related to the effects on the adenylate cyclase system or on the hypothalamic-pituitary regulation of the thyroid gland.[152,228] Lithium is known to induce mild hyperparathyroidism without clinical manifestations.[152,227] Chronic lithium treatment leads to increases in serum parathyroid hormone (PTH), calcium and magnesium with decreased bone mineral[229] and decreased serum phosphate. Serum calcium concentrations correlate significantly with serum lithium concentrations.[230] Laboratory and clinical work have demonstrated that lithium increases adrenal cortical activity. Plasma cortisol was increased in humans[231] and the zona glomerulosa and fasciculata of rat adrenals showed hyperactivity after lithium administration.[232] Another well-known effect of lithium is weight gain, which has been associated with changes in carbohydrate metabolism. Initially, there is a significant reduction of pancreatic islet insulin release[233] followed by high plasma glucose and glucagon that lead to compensatory stimulation of insulin.[152] Recent animal studies have shown that lithium decreases the levels of glucose-1,6-diphosphatase accompanied by reduction in the activities of phosphofructokinase and phosphoglucomutase.[234,235]

Most recently, attention has been focused on the effects of lithium on biological rhythms as changes in circadian rhythms of sleep, temperature, and hormones have been associated with bipolar disorders.[236] Laboratory studies done in animals have found that lithium can slow or delay circadian rhythms. It was observed in those studies that lithium administration affects circadian cycles in activity,[237,238] food and water intake, urinary activity, and body weight in rats.[239] It was also found that lithium delays the biochemical circadian rhythms of plasma prolactin, PTH, corticosterone, aldosterone, serum calcium and magnesium, and cerebellar calcium and magnesium.[240] Furthermore, chronic administration can modify the circadian rhythms in the rat brain of the α- and β-adrenergic, muscarinic, dopaminergic, opiate, benzodiazepine and α-melanocyte-stimulating hormone receptors,[241] and that of rat pineal N-acetyltransferase activity.[242] Another study has pointed out the capacity of lithium to promote resynchronization when an internal rhythm is faster than that of the environment.[238] As exciting as these findings can be, there are, however, few studies done in humans with the same results.[243–245] From the little available data, it has been hypothesized that lithium resynchronizes internal and external rhythms by lengthening circadian rhythms, the degree of this effect depending upon the amount of asynchrony.[152] This may explain the therapeutic and prophylactic effects of lithium.

Thus, lithium has many diverse and complex effects on biological tissues, especially in the central nervous system. Much work has been done on the mechanisms of action of lithium since its introduction in the treatment of affective disorders. It remains, however, far from clear how the mechanisms of lithium exert their therapeutic and prophylactic effects on bipolar affective disorders.

REFERENCES

1. Corcoran AC, Taylor RD, Tage IH: Lithium poisoning from the use of salt substitutes. *JAMA* 1949;139:685–688.
2. Cade JFJ: Lithium salts in the treatment of psychotic excitement. *Med J Aust* 1949;36:349–352.
3. Hullin RP, McDonald R, Dransfield GA: Metabolic balance studies of the effect of lithium salts in manic-depressive psychosis. *Proceedings of Fourth World Congress of Psychiatry* 1966;150:1900.
4. Caldwell HC, Westlake WJ, Conner SM, et al: A pharmacokinetic analysis of lithium carbonate absorption in man. *J Clin Pharmacol* 1971;11:349–356.
5. Pandey, GN, Dorus E, Davis JM, et al: Lithium transport in human red blood cells. *Arch Gen Psychiatry* 1979;36:902–908.
6. Duhm J, Becker BF: Studies on the lithium transport across the red cell membrane. II. Characterization of ouabain-sensitive and ouabain-insensitive Li^+ transport. Effects of bicarbonate and dipyridamole. *Pfluegers Arch* 1977;367:211–219.
7. Shou M: Lithium studies. 3. Distribution between serum and tissues. *Acta Pharmacol Toxicol* 1958;15:115–124.
8. Herrington RN, Ladir MH: Lithium, in Van Praag HM (ed): *Handbook of Biological Psychiatry*, Part 5. New York, Marcel Dekker, 1981, pp 61–72.
9. Lyttkens L, Soderberg R, Wetterberg L: Relation between erythrocyte and plasma lithium concentrations as an index in psychiatric disease. *Ups J Med Sci* 1976;81:123–128.
10. Lyttkens L. Soderberg R, Wetterberg L: Increased lithium erythrocyte-plasma ratio in manic-depressive psychosis. *Lancet* 1973;1:40–46.
11. Mendels J, Frazer A: Intracellular lithium concentration and clinical response: Towards a membrane theory of depression. *J Psychiatr Res* 1973;10:9–18.
12. Ramsey TA, Frazer A, Dyson WL, et al: Letter: Intracellular lithium and clinical response. *Br J Psychiatry* 1976;128:103–104.
13. Casper RC, Pandey G, Gosenfeld L, et al: Intracellular lithium clinical response. *Lancet* 1976;2:418.
14. Cazzullo CL, Smeraldi E, Sacchetti E: Letter: Intracellular lithium concentration and clinical response. *Br J Psychiatry* 1975;126:298–300.
15. Rybakowski W, Strzyzewski W: Red blood cell lithium index and long-term maintenance treatment. *Lancet* 1976;1:1408–1409.
16. Elizur A, Graff E, Steiner M, et al: Intra/extra red blood cell lithium and electrolyte distributions as correlates of neurotoxic reaction during lithium therapy, in, Gershon ES, Belmaker RH, Kety SS, et al (eds): *The Impact of Biology on Modern Psychiatry*. New York, Plenum Press, 1977, pp 55–64.
17. Hewick DS, Murray N: Red blood cell level and lithium toxicity. *Lancet* 1976;2:673.
18. Zakowska-Dabroska T, Rybakowski J: Lithium-induced EEG changes: Relation to lithium levels in serum and red blood cells. *Acta Psychiatr Scand* 1973;49:457–465.
19. Consbruch U, Degwitz R, Koufen H: Untersuchungen zur Lithium bilanzbei gesunden Probanden. *Pharmakopsychiatria* 1978;11:228–234.
20. Trautner EM, Morris R, Noack CH, et al: Excretion and retention of ingested lithium and its effect on ionic balance of man. *Med J Aust* 1955;2:280–291.
21. Amdisen A: Monitoring of lithium treatment through determination of lithium concentration. *Dan Med Bull* 1975;22:277–291.

22. Davis JM, Chang SS, Pandey NG, et al: Clinical pharmacology in psychiatry, in Usdin E (ed): *Lithium*. New York, Elsevier, 1981, p 183.

23. Thornhill DP: Pharmacokinetics of ordinary and substained-release lithium carbonate in manic patients after acute dosage. *Eur J Clin Pharmacol* 1978;14:267–271.

24. Schou M, Nuel-Nielson N, Stromgren E, et al: The treatment of manic psychoses by the administration of lithium salts. *J Neurol Neurosurg Psychiatry* 1954;17:250–260.

25. Maggs R: Treatment of manic illness with lithium carbonate. *Br J Psychiatry* 1963;109:59–65.

26. Goodwin FK, Murphy DL, Bunney WE Jr: Lithium-carbonate treatment in depression and mania: A longitudinal double-blind study. *Arch Gen Psychiatry* 1969;21:486–496.

27. Stokes PE, Stoll PM, Shamorian CA, et al: Efficacy of lithium as acute treatment of manic-depressive illness. *Lancet* 1971;1:1319–1325.

28. Johnson G, Gershon S, Hekimian LS: Controlled evaluation of lithium and chlorpromazine in the treatment of manic state: An interim report. *Compr Psychiatry* 1968;9:563–573.

29. Johnson G, Gershon S, Burdock EI, et al: Comparative effects of lithium and chlorpromazine in the the treatment of manic state. *Br J Psychiatry* 1971;119:267–276.

30. Spring G, Schrweid D, Gray G, et al: Double-blind comparison of lithium and chlorpromazine in the treatment of manic state. *Am J Psychiatry* 1970;126:1306–1310.

31. Platman SR: A comparison of lithium carbonate and chlorpromazine in mania. *Am J Psychiatry* 1970;127:351–353.

32. Prien SR, Caffey EM, Klett CJ: Comparison of lithium carbonate and chlorpromazine in the treatment of mania. *Arch Gen Psychiatry* 1972;26:146–153.

33. Takahaski R, Sakuma A, Itoh K, et al: Comparison of efficacy of lithium carbonate and chlorpromazine in mania. *Arch Gen Psychiatry* 1975;32: 1310–1318.

34. Shopsin B, Gershon S, Thompson H, et al: Psychoactive drug in mania: A controlled comparison of lithium carbonate, chlorpromazine, and haloperidol. *Arch Gen Psychiatry* 1975;32:32–42.

35. Hansen GJ, Retboll K, Schou M: Lithium in psychiatry: A review. *J Psychiatr Res* 1968;6:67–95.

36. Fieve RR, Platman SR, Plutchik RR: The use of lithium in affective disorder. I. Acute endogenous depression. *Am J Psychiatry* 1968;125:487–498.

37. Stokes PE, Shamoian CA, Stoll PM, et al: Efficacy of lithium as acute treatment of manic-depressive illness. *Lancet* 1971;1:1319–1325.

38. Goodwin FK, Murphy DL, Dunner DL, et al: Lithium response in unipolar versus bipolar depression. *Am J Psychiatry* 1972;129:44–47.

39. Mendels J, Secunda SK, Dyson WL: A controlled study of the antidepressant effects of lithium carbonate. *Arch Gen Psychiatry* 1972;26:154–157.

40. Noyes R Jr, Dempsey GM, Blum A, et al: Lithium treatment of depression. *Compr Psychiatry* 1974;15:187–193.

41. Johnson G: Antidepressant effect of lithium. *Compr Psychiatry* 1974;15: 43–47.

42. Baron M, Gershon ES, Rudy V, et al: Lithium carbonate response in depression: Prediction by unipolar/bipolar illness, average evoked response, catechol-O-methyl transferase, and family history. *Arch Gen Psychiatry* 1975;32:1107–1111.

43. Mendels J: Lithium in the treatment of depression states, in Johnson FM

(ed): *Lithium Research and Therapy*. New York, Academic Press, 1975, pp 43–62.

44. Watanbe S, Ishino H, Otsuki S: Double-blind comparison of lithium carbonate and imipramine in treatment of depression. *Arch Gen Psychiatry* 1975;32:659–668.

45. Baastrup PC, Poulsen JC, Schou M, et al: Prophylactic lithium: Double-blind discontinuation in manic-depressive and recurrent depressive disorders. *Lancet* 1970;1:326–330.

46. Melia PI: Prophylactic lithium: A double-blind trial in recurrent affective disorder. *Br J Psychiatry* 1970;116:621–624.

47. Copper A, Noguera R, Bailey J: Prophylactic lithium in affective disorder. *Lancet* 1971;2:275–279.

48. Hullin RP, McDonald R, Allsopp MN: Prophylactic lithium in recurrent affective disorder. *Lancet* 1972;1:1044.

49. Cundall RL, Brooks PW, Murray LG: A controlled evaluation of lithium prophylaxis in affective disorders. *Psychol Med* 1972;3:308–311.

50. Prien RF, Caffey EM, Klett CJ: Prophylactic efficacy of lithium carbonate in manic-depressive illness. Report of the Veteran's Administration and National Institute of Mental Health collaborative study group. *Arch Gen Psychiatry* 1973;28:337–341.

51. Prien RF, Klett CJ, Caffey EM: Lithium carbonate and imipramine in prevention of affective episodes: A comparison in recurrent affective illness. *Arch Gen Psychiatry* 1973;29:420–425.

52. Stallone F, Shelly E, Mendleweicz J, et al: The use of lithium in affective disorder. 3. A double-blind study of prophylaxis in bipolar illness. *Am J Psychiatry* 1973;130:1006–1010.

53. Fieve RR, Dunner DL, Kumbarachi T, et al: Lithium carbonate in affective disorders. IV. A double blind study of prophylaxis in unipolar recurrent depression. *Arch Gen Psychiatry* 1975;32:1541–1544.

54. Quitkin F, Rifkin A, Kane J, et al: Prophylactic effect of lithium and imipramine in unipolar and bipolar II patients; A preliminary report. *Am J Psychiatry* 1978;135:570–572.

55. Schou M, Juel-Nielsen N, Stromgren E, et al: The treatment of manic psychoses by the administration of lithium salts. *J Neurol Neurosurg Psychiatry* 1954;17:250–260.

56. Shopsin B, Kim SS, Gershon S: A controlled study of lithium vs. chlorpromazine in acute schizophrenics. *Br J Psychiatry* 1971;119:435–440.

57. Abram R, Taylor MA, Gaztanaya P: Manic-depressive illness and paranoid schizophrenia. *Arch Gen Psychiatry* 1974;31:640–642.

58. Carpenter WT, Strauss JS, Mulch S: Are there pathognomic symptoms in schizophrenia. V. An empiric investigation of Schneider's first rank symptoms. *Arch Gen Psychiatry* 1973;28:847–852.

59. Rapp MS, Edwards P: A high prevalence of affective disorder discovered in a "schizophrenia clinic." *Can Psychiatr Assoc J* 1977;22:181–183.

60. Perris S: Morbidity suppressive effect of lithium carbonate in cycloid psychosis. *Arch Gen Psychiatry* 1978;35:328–431.

61. Glesinger B: Evaluation of lithium treatment of psychotic excitement. *Med J Aust* 1954;41:277–283.

62. Taheri A: Letter: Lithium in schizophrenia. *Am J Psychiatry* 1976;133:1208.

63. Alexander PE, Van Kammen DP, Bunney WE Jr: Antipsychotic effects of lithium in schizophrenia. *Am J Psychiatry* 1979;136:283–287.

64. Hirschowitz J, Casper R, Garver DL: Lithium response in good prognosis schizophrenia. *Am J Psychiatry* 1980;137:916–920.

65. Small JG, Kellams JJ, Milstein V, et al: A placebo-controlled study of

lithium combined with neuroleptics in chronic schizophrenic patients. *Am J Psychiatry* 1975;132;1315–1317.

66. Van Putten T, Sanders DG: Lithium in treatment failures. *J Nerv Ment Dis* 1975;161:255–264.
67. Wren JC, Kline NS, Cooper TB, et al: Evaluation of lithium therapy in chronic alcoholism. *Clin Med* 1974;81:33–36.
68. Merry J, Reynolds CM, Bailey J, et al: Prophylactic treatment of alcoholism by lithium carbonate. *Lancet* 1976;2:481–482.
69. Rifkin A, Quitkin F, Carillo C: Lithium carbonate in emotionally unstable character disorder. *Arch Gen Psychiatry* 1973;27:519–523.
70. Sheard MH, Marini JL, Bridges CI, et al: The effect of lithium on impulsive aggressive behavior in man. *Am J Psychiatry* 1976;133:1409–1413.
71. Gupta RC, Robinson WA, Smyth CJ: Efficacy of lithium in rheumatoid arthritis with granulocytopenia (Felty's syndrome). A preliminary report. *Arthritis Rheum* 1975;18:179–184.
72. Forrest JN, Cox M, Hong C, et al: Superiority of demococycline over lithium in the treatment of chronic syndrome of inappropriate secretion of antidiuretic hormone. *N Engl J Med* 1978;298:173–177.
73. White MG, Fetner CD: Treatment of the syndrome of inappropriate secretion of antidiuretic hormone with lithium carbonate. *N Engl J Med* 1975;292:390–392.
74. Gershengorn MC, Izumi M, Robbins J: Use of lithium as an adjunct to radioiodine therapy of thyroid carcinoma. *J Clin Endocrinol Metab* 1976;42:105–111.
75. Kelwala S, Gershon S: Lithium, in Shader RI (ed): *Manual of Psychiatric Therapeutics.* Boston, Little, Brown, 1983 (In press).
76. Cooper TB, Bergner PEE, Simpson GM: The 24 hour serum lithium levels as a prognosticator of dosage requirements. *Am J Psychiatry* 1973;130:601–603.
77. Cooper TB, Simpson GM: The 24 hour lithium levels as a prognosticator of dosage requirements: A 2-year follow-up study. *Am J Psychiatry* 1976;133:440–443.
78. Schou M, Baastrup PC, Gross P, et al: Pharmacological and clinical problems of lithium prophylaxis. *Br J Psychiatry* 1970;116:615–619.
79. Kirk L, Baastrup PC, Schou M: Propranolol and lithium-induced tremor. *Lancet* 1972;1:839.
80. Brightwell DR, Halmi KA, Finn R: Lithium-induced polydipsia and polyuria: Mechanism of action. *Biol Psychiatry* 1973;7:167–171.
81. Levy ST, Forrest JN, Heninger GR: Lithium-induced diabetes insipidus: manic symptoms, brain and electrolyte correlates, and chlorothiazide treatment. *Am J Psychiatry* 1973;130:1014–1018.
82. Forrest J, Cohen A, Toretti J, et al: On the mechanism of lithium-induced diabetes insipidus in man and in the rat. *J Clin Invest* 1974;53:1115–1123.
83. Angrist BM, Gershon S, Levitan SJ, et al: Lithium-induced diabetes insipidus-like syndrome. *Compr Psychiatry* 1970;11:141–146.
84. Elizur A, Shopsin B, Gershon S, et al: Intra and extracellular lithium ratios and clinical course in affective states. *J Clin Pharmacol Ther* 1972;13:947–952.
85. Schou M, Baastrup P, Grof P: Pharmacological and clinical problems of lithium prophylaxis. *Br J Psychiatry* 1970;116:615–619.
86. Sedvall G, Jonsson B, Petterson U, et al: Effects of lithium salts on plasma protein bound iodine and uptake of 131I in the thyroid gland of man and rat. *Life Sci* 1968;7:1257–1264.

87. Cooper TB, Simpson GM: Effects of lithium on thyroid function. *Am J Psychiatry* 1969;125:1132.
88. Halmi KA, Noyes R: Occurrence of goiter during lithium treatment. *Biol Psychiatry* 1972;5:211.
89. Schou M, Amdisen A, Eskayaer-Jensen S, et al: Effects of lithium on thyroid function: A review. *Br Med J* 1968;3:710–713.
90. Shopsin B: Endocrine exophthalmus during lithium therapy of manic-depressive disease. *Dis Nerv Syst* 1970;31:237–244.
91. Segal RL, Rosenblatt S, Eliasoph I: Endocrine exophthalmos during lithium therapy of manic depressive disease. *N Engl J Med* 1973;289:136–138.
92. Shopsin B, Gershon S: Pharmacology–Toxicology of the lithium ion; in Gershon S, Shopsin B (eds): *Lithium: Its Roles in Psychiatric Research and Treatment.* London, Plenum Press, 1973, pp 107–146.
93. Shopsin B, Stern S, Gershon S: Altered carbohydrate metabolism during treatment with lithium carbonate. *Arch Gen Psychiatry* 1972;26:566–571.
94. O'Connell RA: Leukocytosis during lithium carbonate treatment. *Int Pharmacopsychiatry* 1970;4:30–34.
95. Freyhan FA, O'Connell RA, Mayo JA: Treatment of mood disorder with lithium carbonate. *Int Pharmacopsychiatry* 1970;5:137–148.
96. Murphy DL, Goodwin FK, Bunney WE Jr: Leukocytosis during lithium treatment. *Am J Psychiatry* 1971;127:1559–1561.
97. Shopsin B, Friedman R, Gershon S: Lithium and leukocytosis. *Clin Pharmacol Ther* 1971;12:923–928.
98. Reisberg B, Gershon S: Side effects associated with lithium therapy. *Arch Gen Psychiatry* 1979;36:879–887.
99. Callaway CL, Hendrie HC, Luby ED: Cutaneous conditions observed in patients during treatment of lithium. *Am J Psychiatry* 1968;124:1124–1125.
100. Kusumi Y: Cutaneous side effects of lithium: Report of two cases. *Dis Nerv Syst* 1971;32:853–854.
101. Schou M, Goldfield MD, Weinstein MR, et al: Lithium and pregnancy: I. Report from the Register of Lithium Babies. *Br Med J* 1973;2:135–136.
102. Weinstein MR, Goldfield MD: Cardiovascular malformation with lithium use during pregnancy. *Am J Psychiatry* 1975;132:529–531.
103. Schou M: What happened to the lithium babies? A follow-up study of children born with malformation. *Acta Psychiatr Scand* 1976;54:193–197.
104. Weinstein MR: Lithium treatment of women during pregnancy and in post-delivery period, in Johnson FN (ed): *Handbook of Lithium Therapy.* Baltimore, University Park Press, 1980, pp 421–429.
105. Schou M, Amdisen A: Lithium and the placenta. *Am J Obstets Gynecol* 1975;122:541.
106. Weinstein MR, Goldfield MD: Administration of lithium during pregnancy, in Johnson FN (ed): *Lithium, Research and Therapy.* London, Academic Press, 1975, pp 237–264.
107. Schou M, Amdisen A, Steenstrup OR: Lithium and pregnancy. II. Hazards to women given lithium during pregnancy and delivery. *Br Med J* 1973;2:137–264.
108. Catz CS, Giacora GP: Drugs and breast milk. *Pediatr Clin North Am* 1972;19:151–166.
109. Brown WT: The pattern of lithium side-effects and toxic reaction in the course of lithium therapy, in Johnson FN (ed): *Handbook of Lithium Therapy.* Baltimore, University Park Press, 1980, pp 279–288.
110. Lippmann S: Is lithium bad for the kidneys? *J Clin Psychiatry* 1982;43:220–224.

111. Dousa T, Hehter O: The effect of NaCl and LiCl on vasopressin sensitive adenylate cyclase. *Life Sci* 1970;9:765–770.
112. Schou M: Lithium prophylaxis: Is the honeymoon over? *Aust NZ J Psychiatry* 1979;13:109–114.
113. Anonymous. Lithium and the kidney: Around for cautious optimism. *Lancet* 1979;2:1056–1057.
114. Arof P: Renal toxicity of lithium may be exaggerated. *Clinical Psychiatry News* 1979;1:30–31.
115. Brante G, Franzen G, Lindholm T, et al: Lithium treatment: Exaggerated fear of irreversible kidney lesion? *Lakartidningen* 1978;75:1487–1488.
116. Jenner F: Lithium and the question of kidney damage. *Arch Gen Psychiatry* 1979;36:888–890.
117. Hestbech J, Hansen HE, Amdisen A, et al: Chronic renal lesions following long-term treatment with lithium. *Kidney Int* 1977;12:205–213.
118. Ayd FJ: A hazard of long-term lithium treatment. *International Drug Therapy Newsletter* 1978;13:25–30.
119. Hansen HE: Change in kidney function during long-term treatment with lithium. *Paper read at a meeting of the Scandinavian Society for Psychopharmacology.* Copenhagen, March 30–31, 1978.
120. Hestbech J: Renal lesions in patients given long-term treatment. *Paper read at a meeting of the Scandinavian Society for Psychopharmacology.* Copenhagen, March 30–31, 1978.
121. Bucht G, Wahlin A, Wentzel T, et al: Histological studies in kidney biopsies from patients on lithium and on neuroleptic treatment. Presented at Symposium: *"Lithium Treatment and Kidney Damage."* Copenhagen, October 1979.
122. Hullin RP, Coley VP, Birch NJ, et al: Renal function after long-term treatment with lithium. *Br Med J* 1979;1:1457–1459.
123. Kincaid-Smith P, Burrows GD, Davies DM, et al: Renal-biopsy findings in lithium and pre-lithium patients. *Lancet* 1979;2:700–701.
124. Lippmann S: Lithium: Status as a nephropathic agent, in Schwab, JJ (ed): *Psychiatry, Psychopharmacology, and Alternative Therapies: Trends for the 80s.* New York, Marcel Dekker, 1981, pp 53–61.
125. Friedman MJ, Culver CM, Ferrell RB: On the safety of long-term treatment with lithium. *Am J Psychiatry* 1977;134(10):1123–1126.
126. Schou M: Lithium in psychiatric therapy (stock taking after 10 years). *Psychopharmacologia* 1959;1:65–78.
127. Shopsin B, Johnson G, Gershon S: A controlled study of lithium vs. chlorpromazine in acute schizophrenia. *Int. Pharmacopsychiatry* 1970;5:170.
128. Prien RJ: Lithium in the treatment of schizophrenia and schizoaffective disorder. *Arch Gen Psychiatry* 1979;36:852–853.
129. Ostrow DG, Southam AS, Davis JM: Lithium–Drug interactions altering the intracellular lithium level: An in vitro study. *Biol Psychiatry* 1980;15:723–739.
130. Cohen WJ, Cohen NH: Lithium carbonate, haloperidol, and irreversible brain damage. *JAMA* 1974;230:1283–1287.
131. Williams RJP: The chemistry and biochemistry of lithium, in Gershon S, Shopsin B, (eds): *Lithium. Its Role in Psychiatric Research and Treatment.* New York, Plenum Press 1973, pp 15–31.
132. Bunney WE, Pert A, Rosenblatt J, et al: Mode of action of lithium: Some biological considerations. *Arch Gen Psychiatry* 1979;36:898–901.
133. Bunney WE, Murphy DL: The neurobiology of lithium. Introduction. *Neurosci Res Program Bull* 1976;4:115–116.
134. Bunney WE, Goodwin F, Murphy D: The "switch process" in manic-

depressive illness. III. Theoretical implications. *Arch Gen Psychiatry* 1972;27:312–317.

135. Lehn JM: Design of synthetic receptor and carrier molecules for the Li$^+$ cation. *Neurosci Res Program Bull* 1976;14:133–137.

136. Eigen M: Possible mechanism of action of lithium from the perspective of "receptor"-Li$^+$ interaction. *Neurosci Res Program Bull* 1976;14:142–144.

137. Baer L, Platman R, Kassir S: Mechanisms of renal lithium handling and their relationship to mineral corticoids: A dissociation between sodium and lithium ions. *J Psychiatry Res* 1971;8:91–105.

138. Murphy DL, Goodwin FK, Bunney WE: Aldosterone and sodium response to lithium administration in man. *Lancet* 1969;2:458–461.

139. Trautner EM, Morris R, Noack CH, et al: The excretion and retention of ingested lithium and its effect on the ionic balance of man. *Med J Aust* 1955;2:280–291.

140. Aronoff MS, Evens RG, Durrell J: Effect of lithium salts on electrolyte metabolism. *J Psychiatry Res* 1979;8:139–159.

141. Gershon S: Lithium, in Usdin E, Forrest I (eds): *Psychotherapeutic Drugs*, Vol 2. New York, Marcel Dekker, 1977, pp 1377–1411.

142. Schou M: Biology and pharmacology of the lithium ion. *Pharmacol Rev* 1957;9:17–58.

143. Rafaelsen OJ, Vendsborg PB, paper presented at the CINP meeting, Copenhagen, (1972). Quoted in Gershon S, Lithium, in Usdin E, Forrest I (eds): *Psychotherapeutic Drugs*, Vol 2, New York, Marcel Dekker, 1977, pp 1377–1411.

144. Mellerup ET, Plenge P, Ziegler R: Lithium effects on calcium metabolism in rats. *Int Pharmacopsychiatry* 1970;5:258–264.

145. Friezel D, Coppen A, Marks V: Plasma magnesium and calcium in depression. *Br J Psychiatry* 1969;115:1375–1377.

146. Reading HW, Isbir T: Action of lithium on ATPases in the rat iris and visual cortex. *Biochem Pharmacol* 1979;28:3471–3474.

147. Ulrich A, Baierl P: Extracellular potassium in rat cerebella cortex during acute and chronic lithium application. *Brain Res* 1980;192:287–290.

148. Rey AC, Jimerson DC, Post RM: Lithium and electrolytes in cerebrospinal fluid of affectively ill patients during acute and chronic lithium treatment. *Commun Psychopharmacol* 1979;3:267–278.

149. Jimerson OC, Post RM, Carman JS, et al: CSF calcium: Clinical correlates in affective illness and schizophrenia. *Biol Psychiatry* 1979;14:37–51.

150. Carman JS, Post RM, Teplitz TA, et al: Divalent cations in predicting antidepressant response to lithium. *Lancet* 1974;2:1454.

151. Pedersen EB, Amdisen A, Darling S: Plasma aldosterone and magnesium in serum and urine during lithium treatment. *Int Pharmacopsychiatry* 1977;12:80–85.

152. Goodnick PJ, Gershon S: Lithium, in Lajtha A (ed): *Handbood of Biochemistry, Vol 19. Alterations of Metabolism in the Nervous System*. New York, Plenum Press, 1983, Vol 19 (in press).

153. Pandey GN, Dorus E, Davis JM, et al: Lithium transport in human red blood cells: Genetic and clinical aspects. *Arch Gen Psychiatry* 1979;36:902–908.

154. Duhm J, Becker BF: Studies on the lithium transport across the red cell membrane. II. Characterization of ouabaine-sensitive and ouabaine-insensitive Li$^+$ transport. Effects of bicarbonate and dipyridamole. *Pfluegers Arch* 1977;370:211–219.

155. Meltzer HL, Rosoff CJ, Kassir S, et al: Active efflux of lithium from erythrocytes of manic-depressive subjects. *Life Sci* 1976;19:371–379.

156. Preskorn SH, Irwin GH, Simpson S, et al: Medical therapies for mood disorders alter the blood-brain barrier. *Science* 1981;213:469–471.

157. Hesketh JE: Effects of potassium and lithium on sodium transport from blood to cerebrospinal fluid. *J Neurochem* 1977;28:597–603.

158. Erlich BE, Diamond JM, Braun LD, et al: Effect of lithium on blood-brain barrier transport of the neurotransmitter precursors choline, tyrosine and tryptophan. *Brain Research* 1980;193:604–607.

159. Cornford EM, Braun LD, Oldendorf WH: Carrier mediated blood-brain barrier transport of choline and certain choline analogs. *J Neurochem* 1978;30:299–308.

160. Goodnick PJ, Fieve RR, Dunner DL: Factors in time-course of lithium response: Pharmacokinetics and CSF parameter changes. Abstract, *Third World Congress of Biological Psychiatry*, Stockholm, 1981.

161. Schulz HH: Lithium and adrenergic function in man: The changed cyclic AMP levels in cerebrospinal fluid during lithium treatment. *Prog Med* 1973;101:272.

162. Goodnick PJ, Fieve RR, Meltzer HL, et al: Lithium pharmacokinetics, duration of therapy, and the adenylate cyclase system. *Int Pharmacopsychiatry* 1982;17:65–72.

163. Dick DAT, Naylor GJ, Dick EG: Effects of lithium in sodium transport across membranes, in Johnson FN, Johnson S, (eds): *Lithium in Medical Practice*. Baltimore, University Park Press, 1978, pp 173–182.

164. Hauser H, Shipley GG: Crystalization of phosphatidylserine bilayers induced by lithium. *J Biochem* 1981;256:11377–11380.

165. Engel J, Berggren V: Effects of lithium on behavior and central monamines. *Acta Psychiatr Scand (Suppl)* 1980;280(61):133–143.

166. Schildkraut JJ: Pharmacology - the effects of lithium on biogenic amines, in Gershon S, Shopsin B (eds): *Lithium: It's Role in Psychiatric Research and Treatment*. New York, Plenum Press, 1973, pp 51–73.

167. Gallager DW, Pert A, Bunney WE: Haloperidol-induced presynaptic dopamine supersensitivity is blocked by chronic lithium. *Nature* 1978;273:309–312.

168. Flemenbaum A: Lithium inhibition of norepinephrine and dopamine receptors. *Biol Psychiatry* 1977;12:563–572.

169. Pert A, Rosenblatt JE, Sivit C, et al: Long-term treatment with lithium prevents the development of dopamine receptor supersensitivity. *Science* 1978;201:171–173.

170. Rosenblatt JE, Pert CV, Tallman JR, et al: The effect of imipramine and lithium on alpha- and beta-receptor binding in rat brain. *Brain Res* 1979;160:186–191.

171. Verimer T, Goodale DB, Long JP, et al: Lithium effects on haloperidol-induced pre- and postsynaptic dopamine receptor supersensitivity. *J Pharm Pharmacol* 1980;32:665–666.

172. Rosenblatt JE: Neurobiologic mechanisms of lithium action. *Scientific Proceedings of the American Psychiatric Association*. 1981; p 160.

173. Allikmets LKH, Nurk AM, Vliianie khronicheskogo vvdeniia khlorida liita na razuitie giperchuvst vite l-nosti dofaminovykh retseptorov pri otmene morfina u krys. *Biull Eksp Biol Med* 1981;925:571–572.

174. Tanimoto K, Maeda K, Chihara K: Inhibition by lithium of dopamine receptors in rat prolactin release. *Brain Res* 1981;223:335–342.

175. Meller E, Friedman E: Lithium dissociates haloperidol-induced behavioral supersensitivity from reduced DOPAC increase in rat striatum. *Eur J Pharmacol* 1981;76:25–29.

176. Wajda IJ, Banay-Schwartz M, Manigault I, et al: Effect of lithium and sodium ions on opiate- and dopamine-receptor binding. *Neurochem Res* 1981;6:321–331.

177. Patel PD, Shah DS, Patel SR, et al: Investigation of the mechanism of decreased sensitivity of the rat seminal vesicle to norepinephrine by lithium. *Pharmacology* 1979;18:64–71.

178. Katz RI, Chase TN, Kopin IJ: Evoked release of norepinephrine and serotonin from brain slices: Inhibition by lithium. *Science* 1968;162:466–467.

179. Katz RI, Kopin IJ: Release of norepinephrine-³H and serotonin-³H evoked from brain slices by electrical-field stimulation – calcium dependency and the effects of lithium, ouabain and tetrodotoxin. *Biochem Pharmacol* 1969;18:1935–1939.

180. Bindler EH, Wallach MB, Gershon S: Effect of lithium on the release of 14C-norepinephrine by nerve stimulation from the perfused cat spleen. *Arch Int Pharmacodyn Ther* 1971;190:150–154.

181. Chase TN, Katz RI, Kopin IJ: Release of [3H] serotonin from brain slices. *J Neurochem* 1969;16:607–615.

182. Greenspan K, Schildkraut JJ, Gordon EK, et al: Catecholamine metabolism in affective disorders. 3. MHPG and other catecholamine metabolites in patients treated with lithium carbonate. *Psychiatry Res* 1970;7:171–183.

183. Treiser S, Kellar KJ: Lithium effects on adrenergic receptor supersensitivity in rat brain. *Eur J Pharmacol* 1979;58:85–86.

184. Belmaker RH: Receptors, adenylate cyclase, depression, and lithium. *Biol Psychiatry* 1981;16:333–350.

185. Frances H, Maurin Y, Puech AJ, et al: Effect of chronic lithium treatment on isolation-induced behavioral and biochemical effects in mice. *Eur J Pharmacol* 1981;72:337–341.

186. DeMontigny C, Grunberg F, Mayer A, et al: Lithium induces rapid relief of depression in tricyclic antidepressant drug nonresponders. *Br J Psychiatry* 1981;138:252–256.

187. Laakso ML, Oja SS: Transport of tryptophan and tyrosine in rat brain slices in the presence of lithium. *Neurochem Res* 1979;4:411–423.

188. Tagliamonte A, Tagliamonte P, Perez-Cruet J, et al: Effect of psychotropic drugs on tryptophan concentration in the rat brain. *J Pharmacol Exp Ther* 1979;177:475–480.

189. Perez-Cruet J, Tagliamonte A, Tagliamonte P: Stimulation of serotonin synthesis by lithium. *J Pharmacol Exp Ther* 1971;178:325–330.

190. Corrodi H, Fuxe K, Schou M: The effect of prolonged lithium administration on cerebral monoamine neurons in the rat. *Life Sci* 1969;8:643–651.

191. Marini JL, Sheard MH, Kosten T: Study of the role of serotonin in lithium action using shock-elicited fighting. *Commun Psychopharmacol* 1979;3:225–233.

192. Martin K: Irreversible effects of lithium administration on transport processes in erythrocytes and platelets, in Johnson FN, Johnson S (eds): *Lithium in Medical Practice.* Baltimore, University Park Press, 1978, pp 167–171.

193. Ho AK, Loh HH, Craves F: The effect of prolonged lithium treatment on the synthesis rate and turnover of monoamines in brain regions of rats. *Eur J Pharmacol* 1970;10:72–78.

194. Bowers MB, Study RE: Cerebrospinal fluid cyclic AMP and acid monoamine metabolites following probenecid: Studies in psychiatric patients. *Psychopharmacology* 1979;62:17–22.

195. Treiser S, Kellar KJ: Lithium: Effects on serotonin receptors in rat brain. *Eur J Pharmacol* 1980;64:183–185.

196. Miyauchi T, Oikawa S, Kitada Y: Effects of lithium chloride on the cholinergic system in different brain regions in mice. *Biochem Pharmacol* 1980;29:654–657.

197. Hanin I, Mallinger AG, Kopp U, et al: Mechanism of lithium-induced elevation in red blood cell choline content: An in vitro analysis. *Commun Psychopharmacol* 1980;4:345–355.

198. Jope R: Effects of lithium treatment in vitro and in vivo on acetylcholine metabolism in rat brain. *J Neurochem* 1979;33:487–495.

199. Pestronk A, Drachman DB: Lithium reduces the number of acetylcholine receptors in skeletal muscle. *Science* 1980;210:342–343.

200. Jenden DJ, Jope RS, Fraser SL: A mechanism for the accumulation of choline in erythrocytes during treatment with lithium. *Commun Psychopharmacol* 1980;4:339–344.

201. Jope RS, Jenden DJ, Ehrlich BE, et al: Choline accumulates in erythrocytes during lithium therapy. *N Engl J Med* 1978;299:833–834.

202. Maggi A, Enna SJ: Regional alterations in rat brain neurotransmitter systems following chronic lithium treatment. *J Neuochem* 1980;34:888–892.

203. Shea PA, Small JG, Hendrie HC: Elevation of choline and glycine in red blood cells of psychiatric patients due to lithium treatment. *Biol Psychiatry* 1981;16:825–830.

204. Gillin JC, Houg JS, Yaug HY, et al: [MET 5] Enkephalin content in brain regions of rats treated with lithium. *Proc Natl Acad Sci USA* 1978;75:2991–2993.

205. Pert CB, Snyder SH: Opiate receptor binding of agonists and antagonists affected differentially by sodium. *Mol Pharmacol* 1974;10:868–879.

206. Amir S, Simantov R: Chronic lithium administration alters the interaction between opiate antagonists and opiate receptors in vivo. *Neuropharmacology* 1981;20:587–591.

207. Deutsch SI, Peselow ED, Banay-Schwartz M, et al: Effect of lithium on glycine levels in patients with affective disorders. *Am J Psychiatry* 1981;138:683–684.

208. Geisler A, Klysner R: Combined effect of lithium and fluopenthixol on striatal adenylate cyclase. *Lancet* 1977;1:430–437.

209. Schorderet M: Lithium inhibition of cyclic AMP accumulation induced by dopamine in solated rentinae of the rabbit. *Biochem Pharmacol* 1977;26:167–170.

210. Ebstein RP, Reches A, Belmaker RH: Lithium inhibition of the adenosin-induced increase of adenylate cyclase activity. *J Pharm Pharmacol* 1978;30:122–123.

211. Reches A, Ebstein RP, Belmaker RH: The differential effect of lithium on noradrenaline- and dopamine-sensitive accumulation of cyclic AMP in guinea pig brain. *Psychopharmacology* 1978;58:213–216.

212. Ebstein RP, Hermoni M, Belmaker RH: The effect of lithium on noradrenaline-induced cyclic AMP accumulation in rat brain: Inhibition after chronic treatment and absence of supersensitivity. *J Pharmacol Exp Ther* 1980;213:161–167.

213. Hermoni M, Lerer B, Ebstein RP, et al: Chronic lithium prevents reserpine-induced supersensitivity of adenylate cyclase. *J Pharm Pharmacol* 1980;32:510–511.

214. Ebstein RP, Belmaker RH: Lithium and brain adenylate cyclase, in Cooper TB, Gershon S, Kline NS, et al (eds): *Lithium: Controversies and Unresolved Issues*, Amsterdam, Excerpta Medica, 1979, pp 703–729.

215. Zatz M: Low concentrations of lithium inhibit the synthesis of cyclic AMP and cyclic GMP in the rat pineal gland. *J Neurochem* 1979;32:1315–1321.

216. Lykouras E, Varsou E, Gavelis E, et al: Plasma cyclic AMP in manic-depressive illness. *Acta Psychiat Scand* 1978;57:477–453.
217. Arato M, Rihmer Z, Felszeghy K: Reduced plasma cyclic AMP level during prophylactic lithium treatment in patients with affective disorders. *Biol Psychiatry* 1980;15:319–322.
218. Friedman E, Oleshansky MA, Moy P, et al: Lithium and catecholamine-induced plasma cyclic AMP elevation, in Cooper TB, Gershon S, Kline NS, et al (eds): *Lithium: Controversies and Unresolved Issues.* Amsterdam, Excerpta Medica, 1979, pp 730–735.
219. Geisler A: Reduced plasma cyclic AMP levels during prophylactic lithium treatment in patients with affective disorders. Address, World Congress of Biological Psychiatry, Stockholm, 1981, quoted in Goodnick PJ, Gershon S: Lithium, in Lajtha A (eds): *Handbook of Biochemistry, Alterations of Metabolism in the Nervous System.* New York, Plenum Press, 1983, vol 19 (in press).
220. Belmaker RH, Kon M, Ebstein RP, et al: Partial inhibition by lithium of the epinephrine-stimulated rise in plasma cyclic GMP in humans. *Biol Psychiatry* 1980;15:3–8.
221. Berndt S: Lithium as a psychotropic drug. Experimental studies on its mechanism of action. *Fortschr Med* 1982;100:409–413.
222. Meltzer HY, Simonovie M, Sturgeon D, et al: Effect of antidepressants, lithium and electroconvulsive treatment on rat serum prolactin levels. *Acta Psychiat Scand (Suppl)* 1981;290:63,100–121.
223. de la Fuente JR, Rosenbaum AH: Prolactin in psychiatry. *Am J Psychiat* 1981;138:1154–1160.
224. Czernik A, Kleesiek K: Neuroendokrinologische Veranderungen unter Langzeitbehandlung mit lithiumsalzen. *Pharmacopsychiatria Neuropsychopharmakol* 1979;12:305–312.
225. Yamaguchi N, Tarrimoto K, Kuromaru S: Growth hormone (GH) release following tyrotropin-releasing hormone (TRH) injection in manic patients receiving lithium carbonate. *Psychoneuroendocrinology* 1980;5:253–259.
226. Varma SK, Messiha FH, Sharma BB: Neuroendocrine effects of lithium carbonate therapy in Gilles de la Tourette's syndrome. *Res Comm Psychol Psychiat Behav* 1980;5:219–299.
227. Mannisto PT: Endocrine side-effects of lithium, in Johnson FN (ed): *Handbook of Lithium Therapy.* Baltimore, University Press, 1980, pp 310–322.
228. Bagchi N, Brown TR, Mack RE: Effect of chronic lithium treatment on hypothalamic-pituitary regulation of thyroid function. *Horm Metab Res* 1982;14:92–93.
229. Christiansen C, Baastrup PC, Transbol I: Development of "primary" hypoparathyroidism during lithium therapy: Longitudinal study. *Neuropsychobiology* 1980;6:280–283.
230. Davis BM, Pfefferbaum A, Krutzik S, et al: Lithium's effect of parathyroid hormone. *Am J Psychiatry* 1981;138:489–492.
231. Platman SR, Fieve RR: Lithium carbonate and plasma cortisol response in the affective disorders. *Arch Gen Psychiatry* 1968;18:591–594.
232. Devi SP, Hariharasubramanian N, Rao AV: Lithium and the pineal-adrenocorticol axis, in Johnson FN, Johnson S (eds): *Lithium in Medical Practice.* Baltimore, University Park Press, 1978, pp 235–242.
233. Anderson JH, Blackard WG: Effect of lithium on pancreatic islet insulin release. *Endocrinology* 1978;102:291–295.
234. Kajda PK, Birch NJ: Lithium inhibition of phosphofructokinase. *J Inorg Biochem* 1981;14:275–278.
235. Nordenberg J, Kaplansky M, Beery E, et al: Effects of lithium on the activ-

ities of phosphofructokinase and phosphoglucomatase and on glucose-1,6-disphosphate levels in rat muscles, brain and liver. *Biochem Pharmacol* 1982;31:1025–1031.

236. Wehr TA, Goodwin FK: Biological rhythms and psychiatry, in Arieti S, Brodie, HKH, (eds): *American Handbook of Psychiatry*, ed 2. New York, Basic Books, 1981, vol 7, pp 46–74.

237. Kripke DF, Wyborney VG: Lithium slows rat circadian activity rhythms. *Life Sci* 1980;26:1319–1321.

238. McEakron DL, Kripke DF, Wyborney VG: Lithium promotes entrainment of rats to long circadian light-dark cycles. *Psychiatry Res* 1981;5:1–9.

239. Christensen S, Agner T: Effects of lithium on circadian cycles in food and water intake, urinary concentration and body weight in rats. *Physiol Behav* 1982;28:635–640.

240. McEakron OL, Kripke DF, Hawkins R, et al: Lithium delays biochemical circadian rhythms in rats. *Neuropsychobiology* 1982;8:12–29.

241. Kafka MS, Wirz-Justice A, Naber D, et al: Effect of lithium on circadian neurotransmitter receptor rhythms. *Neuropsychobiology* 1982;8:41–50.

242. Friedman E, Yocca FD: The effect of chronic lithium treatment on rat pineal N-acetyltransferase rhythm. *J Pharmacol Exp Ther* 1981;219:121–124.

243. Huey L, Janowsky DS, Bernstein M, et al: Scientific Proceedings of American Psychiatric Association, New Research, 1978, p 31, quoted in Goodnick PJ, Gershon S: Lithium, in Lajtha, A (ed): *Handbook of Biochemistry, Alte, ation of Metabolism in the Nervous System.* New York, Plenum Press, 1983, vol 19 (in press).

244. Johnsson A, Pflug B, Engelman W, et al: Influence of lithium ion on human circadian rhythms. *Pharmakopsychiatrie NeuroPsychopharmakologie* 1979;12:423–425.

245. Kripke DF, Judd LL, Hubbard B, et al: The effect of lithium carbonate on the circadian rhythm of sleep in normal human subjects. *Biol Psychiatry* 1979;14:345–348.

8

Rational Use of Antipsychotic Drugs

Jerrold G. Bernstein

Antipsychotic or neuroleptic drugs are so named because of their ability to alleviate certain symptoms of psychosis and to simultaneously produce extrapyramidal effects. Currently, there are five chemically distinct groups of compounds that exert these actions. The psychotic symptoms most amenable to the beneficial effects of these drugs include disordered thinking, hallucinations, delusions, and agitation, all of which commonly occur during the course of psychotic illness.[1] In terms of numbers of psychotic patients likely to benefit from these drugs, schizophrenia is the most prevalent condition. These drugs are also highly effective in controlling manic psychoses, psychotic symptoms associated with depression, and some of the psychotic manifestations of organic brain dysfunction related to aging or chemical intoxication. Certain atypical psychoses, including decompensation in the borderline patient and the patient with schizoaffective illness, likewise may benefit from antipsychotic drug therapy.

In former times, these compounds were labeled as major tranquilizers. However, this appelation is inaccurate since simple sedation or tranquilization does not account for the beneficial antipsychotic actions seen with the drugs.[2] Indeed, administration of sedatives, whether they be benzodiazepines or barbiturates, may calm an agitated psychotic patient, but they will produce minimal benefit in terms of disordered thinking, hallucinations, or delusions.[1] Unfortunately, unlike the administration of penicillin for the treatment of a susceptible bacterial infection, the antipsychotic drugs are not curative. Although their administration may produce dramatic symptomatic improvement, this beneficial effect eventually terminates following discontinuation of medication and the metabolic disappearance of the administered compound or its active metabolites from the body. Antipsychotic drugs are not always effective in obliterating all manifestations of a psychotic illness, yet their impact on the ability of psychiatrists to manage patients with serious psychotic disturbances has been one of the more dramatic medical advances of the 20th century.

The number of patients requiring custodial care in mental institutions in this country began to drop precipitously with the introduction of the first antipsychotic drug, chlorpromazine, in 1954. Although these drugs were first applied clinically without a clear understanding of their mechanism of action and without much information about the etiology of psychotic disorders, the relationship of their salutory effect and their ability to produce unwanted extrapyramidal movement disorders was recognized very early in the course of clinical experience.[2] This association yielded the two terms, antipsychotic and neuroleptic, which have come to be used synonomously. Unfortunately, all available therapeutic agents of this class do produce some degree of extrapyramidal effects which must be managed when these drugs are administered to patients.[3,4] The connection between these effects has become better understood as dopamine receptor blockade has been recognized as the most likely mechanism of antipsychotic drug action.[1] All currently available, effective antipsychotic drugs appear to act by this mechanism of dopamine blockade, thus suggesting the possibility that in schizophrenia, and perhaps in other psychotic illnesses as well, the underlying disease mechanism may well involve an abnormality of dopamine release or receptor sensitivity. This is discussed in greater detail in Chapter 4 of this volume.

One experimental antipsychotic compound, clozapine, appeared to challenge the necessary connection between antipsychotic efficacy and the production of extrapyramidal effects. Unfortunately, this compound has been largely abandoned because of its ability to produce other more serious and irreversible complications. Clonidine, which acts on noradrenergic receptors rather than dopaminergic sites, has been shown experimentally to have antipsychotic action.[5,6] Perhaps in the future, this compound or others may prove to be therapeutically beneficial in controlling symptoms of psychosis without the production of extrapyramidal effects. At this point in time we do, indeed, have effective therapeutic agents to control psychotic symptoms. A thorough understanding of their pharmacology, and a sophisticated grasp of optimal techniques in their administration, will go a long way to help patients suffering from devastating psychotic illnesses to recover and to return to productive and functional lives. Fears of drug side effects should not prevent physicians and patients from working together toward an appropriate and effective treatment program.

PSYCHOTHERAPY AND PHARMACOTHERAPY IN PSYCHOSIS

In dealing with schizophrenic illness, it is important to recognize that available drugs are far superior to psychotherapeutic treatment. A classic study undertaken a number of years ago divided newly hospitalized schizophrenics into four treatment groups: no therapy, psychoanalytic psychotherapy, phenothiazines alone, and phenothiazines plus psychoanalytic psychotherapy. The group receiving psychotherapy showed no greater improvement than those patients who received no therapy at all. Patients who received antipsychotic medication without psychotherapy showed substantial improvement, with 90% of them being discharged during the study.[7] Those individuals who received combined psychotherapy and pharmacotherapy showed no greater improvement than those who received pharmacotherapy alone.

A subsequent study of schizophrenic patients hospitalized at a major teaching hospital in Boston compared the efficacy of psychoanalytic psychotherapy with and without pharmacotherapy.[8] In that study, no greater improvement was seen in those patients receiving psychotherapy and pharmacotherapy than in patients receiving phenothiazines without psychotherapy. When placebos were substituted for phenothiazine medications in patients who were concurrently receiving psychoanalytic psychotherapy, marked clinical deterioration was noted.[8] Although the antipsychotic efficacy of a variety of medications has been repeatedly demonstrated, such data are lacking with regard to the efficacy of psychotherapy in controlling specific target symptoms of schizophrenia. On the other hand, in patients receiving adequate pharmacotherapy, the coadministration of psychotherapy may help those patients whose hallucinations and delusions are controlled medically to readjust to a more normal pattern of living. Psychotherapy should certainly not be abandoned as a useful technique in helping schizophrenic patients, although the use of this modality in the absence of adequate and appropriate drug therapy is not likely to be beneficial. Likewise, reliance on psychotherapy in the absence of appropriate medication treatment of major affective disorders, including mania and depression, will most often produce a less than optimal therapeutic result.[1]

Patient Evaluation for Pharmacotherapy

Proper use of antipsychotic medication requires a careful evaluation of patients. As much historical data as possible should be obtained prior to instituting treatment. It is important to know whether the patient has had similar episodes in the past. The patient's previous experience with antipsychotic drugs is another useful guideline to planning a strategy of psychopharmacological intervention. Patients who have previously responded well to a given antipsychotic compound are likely to achieve a similar favorable response when the same medication is readministered.[1] Likewise, a history of previous adverse drug effects with specific medication may guide the clinician in choosing that medication most likely to be best tolerated. The presence of coexistant medical conditions, or treatment with medications that may provoke psychotic symptoms, may govern the physician's approach to pharmacotherapy.

Use of alcohol, over-the-counter drugs, or illicit drugs, may precipitate a psychotic episode and may also influence the response to antipsychotic chemotherapy. A patient who develops psychotic symptoms in the course of cocaine or amphetamine abuse will require added caution because low potency phenothiazines, such a chlorpromazine, mesoridazine, or thioridazine, may be particularly likely to provoke a severe hypotensive reaction[1] Proper use of antipsychotic agents demands that physicians know when to avoid their administration, or to be particularly cautious in their use. For example, the patient who develops psychotic symptoms during the course of barbiturate or benzodiazepine withdrawal is more likely to become hypotensive and develop seizures if chlorpromazine is administered.[1] These individuals should generally not receive antipsychotic chemotherapy, but should undergo a pentobarbital tolerance test followed by gradual detoxification using phenobarbital.[1]

When a proper assessment indicates the need for antipsychotic therapy, treatment should be instituted with a single antipsychotic drug. The dose of that medication should be titrated according to the patient's response and the occurrence of side effects. The physician should avoid repeated changes from one neuroleptic to another unless it is absolutely necessary, as in the case of an allergic or other severe adverse reaction to the initial medication. In order to properly administer antipsychotic agents, the physician must become thoroughly familiar with their pharmacology and techniques of clinical application. The clinician must also be familiar with practical approaches that may be helpful in avoiding or managing adverse drug reactions, should they occur.

ANTIPSYCHOTIC DRUGS

Mechanism of Action

There are now on the market almost 20 antipsychotic drugs, divided among five distinct chemical classes. Only eight or nine of these products have widespread clinical use by practitioners. It is certainly unnecessary for any physician to attempt to prescribe all of the marketed antipsychotic drugs in the course of his practice. On the other hand, it is most important that each physician become familiar with the characteristics of each of the five chemical classes of antipsychotic drugs, and learn to recognize the differences among the various antipsychotic drugs in terms of the pattern of side effects likely to be experienced by the patient (see Tables 8-1 and 8-2).

According to current understanding, all chemical compounds with antipsychotic efficacy exert this effect as a result of their ability to block dopamine receptors.[5] The clinical potency of antipsychotic drugs directly parallels in vitro laboratory tests for dopamine receptor binding affinity.[9] Pioneering studies by Snyder's laboratory, utilizing a technique of direct labeling of dopamine receptors, has paved the way, not only for our understanding of some of the underlying biochemical mechanisms of psychosis, but also for concepts regarding the mechanism of action of this important class of therapeutic compounds.[10-12] Indeed, that laboratory has identified two physically distinct dopamine receptors within the brain.[11] The first of these, known as DA-1 is associated with the enzyme adenylate cyclase and is labeled predominantly by the binding of ^{3}H-dopamine and ^{3}H-apomorphine. The DA-1 receptor is blocked by phenothiazine neuroleptics in rough proportion to their clinical potency. However, haloperidol and related nonphenothiazine compounds, which are the most potent antipsychotic agents, act only as weak inhibitors of dopamine cyclase.[11] The other type of dopamine receptor referred to as DA-2 is not linked to adenylate cyclase and is labeled by tritiated butyrophenones such as ^{3}H-spiroperidol and ^{3}H-haloperidol.[11] The clinical potency of all available antipsychotic agents that have been studied thus far correlates well with DA-2 receptor bindings.[9,11] A third receptor, whose function is unclear is known as DA-3. It is relatively insensitive to neuroleptic drugs.

Table 8-1 lists some of the commonly prescribed antipsychotic drugs tabulated in order of their approximate clinical potency. This table also presents data for dopamine receptor binding affinities of these drugs. As can be seen, haloperidol, which is clinically the most potent antipsychotic agent, is also high in dopamine receptor (DA-2) blocking activity, while chlorpromazine and thioridazine are both low potency antipsychotic agents based upon clinical activity and have the lowest affinities as dopamine receptor blocking drugs.

Side Effect Profiles

From this discussion, it can be seen that the available antipsychotic drugs differ in their clinical potency in a way that correlates with their differing dopamine receptor blocking potencies. The other major category of differences between available neuroleptic drugs is in respect to their profile of side effects. As can be seen from Table 8-1, the various

Table 8-1
Characteristics of Commonly Used Antipsychotic Drugs

Clinical Potency of Antipsychotic Action from *Most* to *Least* Potent* [Chemical Class]	Inhibition of (^{3}H) Haloperidol Binding, K_1 (nM)†	Relative Affinity for Muscarinic (Cholinergic) Receptor‡	Anticholinergic Effects Clinically Observed	Parkinsonian Effects Clinically Observed	Sedation Clinically Observed	Hypotension Clinically Observed
haloperidol (Haldol) [butyrophenone]	1.5 ± 0.14	0.21	+	+++++	++	+
fluphenazine (Prolixin) [piperazine–phenothiazine]	1.2 ± 0.12	0.83	++	+++++	++	++
thiothixene (Navane) [piperazine–thioxanthene]	1.4 ± 0.11		++	++++	++	++
trifluoperazine (Stelazine) [piperazine–phenothiazine]	2.1 ± 0.34	0.78	++	++++	+	++
perphenazine (Trilafon) [piperazine–phenothiazine]		0.91	++	++++	+++	+++
molindone (Moban) [dihydroindolone]			+++	+++	+	++

Drug						
loxapine (Loxitane) [dibenzoxazepine]			+++	+++	++	++
chlorpromazine (Thorazine) [aliphatic–phenothiazine]	10.3 ± 0.2	10.0	++++	++	+++++	+++++
thioridazine (Mellaril) [piperidine–phenothiazine]	14.0 ± 0.2	66.7	+++++	+	++++	+++++

*Drugs are listed in order of clinical potency, from most potent to least potent in their action against psychotic symptoms, based upon the author's clinical experience and review of a wide range of published data.

Likelihood of producing various side effects is likewise based upon the author's observations of patients and a review of published information from numerous sources.

†From Creese I, Burt DR, Snyder SH: Dopamine receptor binding predicts clinical and pharmacologic potencies of antischizophrenic drugs. *Science* 1976;192:481–483.

‡From Snyder S, Greenberg D, Yamamura HI: Antischizophrenic drugs and brain cholinergic receptors. *Arch Gen Psychiatry* 1974;31:58–61.

Reprinted with permission from Bernstein JG: *Handbook of Drug Therapy in Psychiatry.* Littleton, MA, John Wright • PSG Inc, 1983.

compounds listed differ considerably in their abilities to produce anticholinergic side effects. The clinical anticholinergic potency of the various antipsychotic drugs closely parallels the laboratory studies measuring the relative affinity of these compounds for muscarinic cholinergic receptors in vitro.[13] Clinically, anticholinergic action is manifested by blurred vision, dry mouth, constipation, urinary retention, increased or decreased sweating, and tachycardia.[1] These peripheral signs of parasympathetic blockade are likely to be uncomfortable for many patients. A severely disturbed schizophrenic patient who becomes constipated and does not receive appropriate treatment, may end up having fecal impaction and perhaps even suffer peritonitis if prompt and effective treatment is not administered. The elderly patient who receives a strongly anticholinergic drug is certainly vulnerable to urinary retention, which may necessitate catheterization and the risk of urinary tract infection.

The central nervous system manifestations of anticholinergic effects may even be more serious than the peripheral manifestations. Blockade of cholinergic sites within the brain is likely to produce a halting or stuttering pattern of speech, memory impairment, confusion, and in some cases a toxic delirium.[1,14,15] Elderly patients are likely to be particularly sensitive to anticholinergic drug effects. They are the ones likely to have the worst complications, not only from peripheral manifestations, but also from central effects of cholinergic blockade. Elderly patients and those with organic brain syndrome are particularly susceptible to the development of increased confusion, hallucinations, paranoia, and agitation in response to excessive anticholinergic drug action.[1] It is for these reasons that the more strongly anticholinergic antipsychotic drugs should be avoided if at all possible in the treatment of elderly individuals, or in those patients suffering from organic brain dysfunction. For the same reason, it is important to try to avoid the administration of antiparkinsonian drugs to elderly patients because of the ability of these compounds to produce anticholinergic toxicity. On the other hand, the positive aspect of the anticholinergic action of antipsychotic drugs is that greater cholinergic blocking potency confers some protection against acute extrapyramidal effects.

Those antipsychotic drugs that are more strongly anticholinergic produce a lower incidence of acute extrapyramidal effects than those compounds possessing lesser anticholinergic action (Table 8-1). The high potency antipsychotic drugs, such as haloperidol, the piperazine phenothiazines, and thiothixene, produce less anticholinergic effect, but more parkinsonian effects than the lower potency antipsychotic agents including chlorpromazine and thioridazine.[1] Available antipsychotic drugs also differ in their sedative action. As was learned many years ago, sedation is not necessary for the control of psychotic symptoms. Sedative drugs lacking dopamine blocking effect have no antipsychotic efficacy, while antipsychotic drugs, even though they may be devoid of sedative effect, may produce profound control of hallucinations, delusions and dis-ordered thinking. Since sedation may interfere with the ability of a pa-tient to participate in varied activities at home, at work, and at school, or even within the therapeutic environment of the hospital, it is most often preferable to prescribe those antipsychotic drugs that possess lower sedative potencies. The patient who is drowsy or readily falls asleep will not participate actively in psychotherapy or in any other aspect of a hospital program. Likewise, that patient will have a difficult time con-vincing his employer that he can function adequately on the job when he demonstrates signs of drowsiness. The patient who falls asleep while sit-ting at home is not likely to be an active participant in family life.

Hypotension is another prevalent antipsychotic drug side effect. This action is the result of alpha-adrenergic receptor blockade in the pe-ripheral vasculature. As a result of this pharmacological effect, there is vasodilation, reduction in peripheral resistance, and a consequent fall in blood pressure.[1] Clinically, drug-related postural hypotension may be manifested by dizziness or fainting. If the patient is elderly or unsteady on his/her feet, the likelihood that postural hypotension may provoke falling and even the occurrence of physical injury must be considered. Among currently available antipsychotic drugs, chlorpromazine, thio-ridazine, and mesoridazine, possess the greatest alpha-adrenergic blocking effect and are the compounds most likely to produce significant hypoten-sive action.[1] The hypotensive effects of these compounds are likely to be worse if they are administered by injection.[16] The piperazine phenothia-zines have much less hypotensive action and haloperidol is least likely to lower blood pressure, among available antipsychotic drugs.[1,16] Certainly in patients with cardiovascular disease, or in those receiving vasodilators or antihypertensive drugs, it is safer to employ antipsychotic medication with low hypotensive activity such as haloperidol.[1,17]

It should also be borne in mind by the clinician that antipsychotic drugs have the ability to lower seizure thresholds, thus increasing the risk of a convulsion occurring in susceptible patients.[18] Chlorpromazine is the compound of greatest concern in this regard and should be avoided in patients who have seizure disorders, particularly if the condition is not well controlled by anticonvulsive medication.[1] Thioridazine and halo-peridol appear to have the least ability to affect seizure threshold, and therefore are safest to use in patients who have convulsive disorders.

The ability of neuroleptic drugs to block dopamine receptor sites ex-plains not only their antipsychotic action and their ability to induce ex-trapyramidal motor effects, but also this mechanism is responsible for the ability of these drugs to elevate plasma prolactin levels.[11] Increased circulating prolactin in response to neuroleptic drugs is a manifestation of the action of these drugs on dopamine receptor sites within the pituitary gland. This prolactin-mediated effect explains the occurrence of amenorrhea and galactorrhea, which are often associated with the

154

Table 8-2
Comparison of Antipsychotic Drugs: Dosage and Special Characteristics

Chemical Class generic name (Trade name)	Daily Dose* Range (mg) (Oral)	Special Characteristics for Clinical Use
PHENOTHIAZINE Aliphatic chlorpromazine† (Thorazine)	100–2000	High sedation and hypotension risk, skin pigmentation, photosensitization. Most likely to lower seizure threshold and produce convulsions, especially at higher dosage.
triflupromazine (Vesprin)	20–150	Similar to chlorpromazine.
Piperidine thioridazine (Mellaril)	100–600	Strongly anticholinergic and hypotensive, prominent EKG changes. Retinal damage and visual loss may occur, especially at high dosage. Minimal effect on seizure threshold.
mesoridazine (Serentil)	100–400	Strongly anticholinergic and hypotensive, avoid IM use because of risk of hypotension.
piperacetazine (Quide)	20–160	Similar to thioridazine.
Piperazine trifluoperazine (Stelazine)	5–60	Low sedation, high potency.
perphenazine (Trilafon)	8–64	Similar to trifluoperazine, somewhat less potent, somewhat more sedating.

Drug	Dose	Comment
fluphenazine (Prolixin)	5–60	Similar to trifluoperazine; may be used orally or IM for rapid neuroleptization. Somewhat more painful at injection site than haloperidol. Enanthate and decanoate are available as long acting IM preparations.
butaperazine (Repoise)	30–100	Similar to trifluoperazine, but lower mg potency.
acetophenazine (Tindal)	20–100	Similar to trifluoperazine, but lower mg potency.
carphenazine (Proketazine)	100–400	Similar to trifluoperazine, but lower mg potency.
prochlorperazine (Compazine)	10–150	Somewhat less potent than trifluoperazine, with greater risk of hypotension and extrapyramidal effects. Primarily used as an antiemetic, although its EPS make this use somewhat problematic.

THIOXANTHENES
Aliphatic

Drug	Dose	Comment
chlorprothixene (Taractan)	100–600	Therapeutic and adverse effects similar to chlorpromazine.
thiothixene (Navane)	5–60	Therapeutic and adverse effects similar to trifluoperazine.

*The dosage ranges presented are intended for medically healthy young or middle-aged adults. In some cases larger doses may be necessary, as in the acutely psychotic, agitated patient who may require larger doses, especially when haloperidol is used in rapid neuroleptization or when doses up to 200 mg/day or more may need to be used. In elderly individuals or those suffering simultaneously from severe medical or metabolic abnormalities, much lower doses should be used. The reader is directed to chapters on children and the elderly elsewhere in this volume for additional dosage guidelines.
†Please refer to the "Selected References" at the end of this chapter. These references provide documentation for the comments made regarding the specific drugs detailed above.

Table 8-2 (continued)

Chemical Class generic name (Trade name)	Daily Dose* Range (mg) (Oral)	Special Characteristics for Clinical Use
BUTYROPHENONE haloperidol (Haldol)	2–100	Somewhat more sedating and more potent than trifluoperazine, least pain when injected IM. Ideally suited to rapid neuroleptization by the oral or IM route. Has been safely used IV in investigational studies. Effective at low doses in maintenance, well tolerated by elderly and patients with cardiovascular disease.
DIBENZOXAZEPINE Loxapine (Loxitane)	30–250	More potent, less sedating and less hypotensive than chlorpromazine. Less potent, produces less EPS than trifluoperazine. May be effective in patients who do not tolerate high potency agents and do not respond to low potency compounds. Low doses may be useful in anxiety and in depression.
DIHYDROINDOLONE molindone (Moban)	10–225	Intermediate potency. Least sedating neuroleptic. Often will decrease appetite and allow weight loss in contradistinction to phenothiazines which promote weight gain. May provoke motor seizures in susceptible patients even at low dosage.

*The dosage ranges presented are intended for medically healthy young or middle-aged adults. In some cases larger doses may be necessary, as in the acutely psychotic, agitated patient who may require larger doses, especially when haloperidol is used in rapid neuroleptization or when doses up to 200 mg/day or more may need to be used. In elderly individuals or those suffering simultaneously from severe medical or metabolic abnormalities, much lower doses should be used. The reader is directed to chapters on children and the elderly elsewhere in this volume for additional dosage guidelines.

†Please refer to the "Selected References" at the end of this chapter. These references provide documentation for the comments made regarding the specific drugs detailed above.

adminitration of these compounds. Although hypersecretion of prolactin appears to parallel dopamine receptor blocking potency of the various neuroleptics, in clinical practice the more potent dopamine blocker, haloperidol, appears to be less often associated with galactorrhea than are some of the weaker dopamine-blocking compounds, such as thioridazine and chlorpromazine.[1]

Having reviewed some of the basic differences among the antipsychotic compounds currently in use, we will now move ahead to consider useful techniques in the administration of these drugs and in their optimal application for the treatment for acute psychosis and the long-term management of persons who suffer from recurrent psychotic conditions.

TECHNIQUES OF ANTIPSYCHOTIC DRUG ADMINISTRATION

Neuroleptics have a therapeutic role in a wide spectrum of psychotic disorders and are useful to control the acute manifestations of psychosis in the schizophrenic, manic, and depressed patient.[1,19] They also have a role in minimizing less overt psychotic symptoms in patients with atypical psychosis, borderline syndrome, and schizoaffective illness.[20,21] Neuroleptics play an important role in the maintenance treatment of schizophrenic patients in which they have considerable ability to reduce the risk of recurrence of acute psychosis.[22,23] Proper selection of medication to be administered is fundamental in achieving the desired result. At the same time, the techniques of administration and dosage titration are critical to achieving an optimal therapeutic response. In the treatment of the acutely ill schizophrenic patient, these drugs should generally be administered in divided doses with the total daily dosage titrated upward in order to achieve optimum control of agitation, paranoia, delusions, and disordered thinking.[1] Although the total resolution of this complex of symptoms may take days, weeks, or months, there is clinical evidence to suggest that dosage titration over the course of the first several days of treatment in the hospitalized acutely ill schizophrenic patient may optimize at least the initial therapeutic response and perhaps allow for a smoother course of recovery.[24,25] A variety of terms has been employed to describe this phase in which antipsychotic medication is instituted. The term I have employed is pharmacolysis of psychosis, wherein the dose of a suitable high-potency dopamine blocking antipsychotic drug is gradually titrated upward so that adequate concentrations of the drug can reach the central nervous system, produce dopamine receptor blockade, and hopefully produce dramatic improvement in the psychotic symptoms.[26]

Pharmacolysis

Two key factors in providing safe and rapidly effective pharmacolysis involve proper evaluation and careful day-to-day monitoring of the patient by the physician and the choice of the most appropriate antipsychotic agent. Low potency neuroleptics are not useful in this technique. The three drugs most extensively studied, using the rapid treatment method, have been haloperidol, thiothixene, and fluphenazine. Some of the clinical studies have employed exceedingly high doses of these drugs.[27] Most of the studies have utilized fairly rigid protocols which at times fall short of meeting the specific clinical needs of each patient. Most of the rapid treatment studies have employed intramuscular medication administration. In reviewing the data from the numerous studies comparing rapid treatment with high dose intramuscular medication to lower dose regimens, in many cases superiority of the former approach could not be proven.[28] On the other hand, those studies employing haloperidol seem to show a more positive therapeutic response to moderate or high dose regimens than to lower dose regimens, suggesting the possible superiority of this agent over either thiothixene or fluphenazine in a rapid treatment model.[25,29]

In my own extensive clinical experience utilizing haloperidol doses which are titrated on a day-to-day basis for each patient, larger doses of antipsychotic medication properly monitored are generally superior to lower dose regimens.[1] In contradistinction to the majority of published studies, I prefer to administer haloperidol by the oral route utilizing a liquid preparation initially and, when clinically appropriate changing to a tablet form of administration. I generally use intramuscular haloperidol for pharmacolysis only in those clinical situations in which the patient is not able to adequately cooperate to take medication orally. Intramuscular administration of haloperidol is most advantageous in those patients who are out of control and require medication for their own safety to help them recover from a devastating psychosis.[1,25]

Although it is true that some time can be saved if antipsychotic drugs are administered intramuscularly,[29] this more invasive approach is usually more upsetting to the patient and may interfere with the physician's attempt to establish an alliance with the patient.[1] In my experience, pharmacolysis utilizing haloperidol can generally be achieved at the daily doses of between 20 and 120 mg of orally administered haloperidol. I infrequently will administer this drug in a higher dosage range, up to 200 mg per day. However, if rapid lysis of the psychosis is going to occur in the course of the first five to ten days of treatment, it generally will occur at doses less than 160 mg per day, so that the much larger doses suggested by some investigators are infrequently necessary.

In treating a typical acutely psychotic young or middle-aged individual, I would generally start with 5 mg of haloperidol administered orally four times daily along with 0.5 to 1 mg of benztropine, also four times daily. Administration of haloperidol in increments of 5 to 10 mg orally is given as frequently as every hour, as necessary, to control agitation, belligerence, and psychotic behavior. Following the first day of this regimen, I would assess the amount of additional haloperidol necessary for that patient and then titrate the dosage upward through the course of the acute phase of psychosis during which time I would observe the patient at least once and preferably several times daily. In general, as the haloperidol dose is increased beyond 60 mg per day, there is less necessity for the coadministration of benztropine or other antiparkinsonian medications, since the increasing anticholinergic effect seen with larger doses of haloperidol will generally antagonize its own acute extrapyramidal reactions.[1]

In the event that acute dystonic reactions occur during the initial phase of dosage titration, diphenhydramine may be administered intravenously, intramuscularly, or orally in a dose of 50 mg. Acute dystonic reactions, should they occur, will, generally, promptly disappear following the intravenous administration of diphenhydramine. Because of the low anticholinergic effect, and minimal hypotensive action of haloperidol, patients receiving moderate to high dosage regimens of this medication during the course of rapid titration are not likely to experience severe adverse cardiovasuclar or anticholinergic complications.[1] The physician should be aware, however, that there is the possibility of anticholinergic complications following the coadministration of benztropine, and may choose to avoid its simultaneous administration, unless acute extrapyramidal reactions do indeed occur. Generally, after a course of two to ten days of treatment, the patient's symptoms will be seen to dramatically diminish and the dosage of antipsychotic medication can then begin to be titrated downward.

This technique of pharmacolysis is equally applicable to the acutely psychotic patient who is suffering from a schizophrenic disorder, as it is to the patient suffering from an acute manic psychosis. In the acutely manic patient, early in the course of antipsychotic chemotherapy the physician should cautiously institute treatment simultaneously with lithium carbonate while carefully monitoring serum lithium concentration. Pharmacolysis is generally not employed in this fashion in patients suffering from psychotic depressive disorders, and in those individuals suffering from drug-induced or other atypical psychoses.

Stabilization

As the acutely psychotic patient begins to improve during the pharmacolysis phase of treatment, the physician should then begin the gradual process of downward dosage titration which I have termed stabilization phase.[26] During this period of treatment, the patient is observed one or more times daily as the dose of antipsychotic medication is gradually diminished. The goal is to allow the patient to be relatively free of symptoms, including hallucinations, delusions, agitation, and disordered thinking. Medication dosage is gradually reduced over a period of one to three weeks during this phase of chemotherapy. In the event that psychotic symptoms re-emerge or worsen, the clinician should temporarily increase the medication dosage and slow the course of downward titration. At the completion of the stabilization phase, even patients who have received 40 to 160 mg of haloperidol per day for pharmacolysis will, in all likelihood, now be receiving a dosage of only 15 to 30 mg per day.

Maintenance

Following stabilization, the patient enters the maintenance phase of antipsychotic chemotherapy, during which time he or she will be receiving the lowest daily dose of an antipsychotic medication capable of controlling the majority of psychotic symptoms. It is not uncommon for patients who have received daily doses of haloperidol in the 40- to 160-mg range to be adequately maintained on a daily dose of only 5 to 15 mg. The frequency of medication administration during the stabilization phase can usually be reduced to a twice-daily regimen. A similar program of twice-daily medication administration may be utilized during the maintenance phase of chemotherapy; however, most patients find it more convenient to take a single dose of antipsychotic medication each evening at bedtime. Most patients will not require long-term administration of antiparkinsonian medication as they recover from their acute psychosis and enter the maintenance phase of chemotherapy.

In manic depressive illness, the maintenance phase of chemotherapy generally entails the administration of lithium carbonate in the absence of antipsychotic medication. Patients with atypical affective disorders and with schizoaffective illness, on the other hand, tend to do best in a maintenance program that includes a relatively low dose of a high potency neuroleptic along with lithium carbonate administered according to standard blood level criteria.[21]

Antiparkinsonian Medications

During the maintenance phase of antipsychotic chemotherapy, a small number of patients will require coadministration of antiparkinsonian medication, particularly because of motor restlessness that is termed akathisia.[30,31,32] Although benztropine is somewhat more effective than trihexyphenidyl in management of muscle stiffness and dystonic reactions, trihexyphenidyl is generally more effective than benztropine in the management of persistent akathisia.[1] In the management of akathisia, even in the presence of a single daily dose regimen of antipsychotic medication, it is preferable to divide antiparkinsonian medication into at least two daily doses, since the half-life of trihexyphenidyl and similar compounds is generally much shorter than that of the various neuroleptic drugs.[33]

It must be borne in mind by the clinician that the occurrence of acute parkinsonian reactions, akathisia, dystonic reactions, and other extrapyramidal manifestations, does not imply that patients so affected are more likely than other patients to develop tardive dyskinesia.[34] The implications of one research study that suggests that thioridazine is safer than haloperidol and other high potency antipsychotic agents, from the standpoint of the risk of tardive dyskinesia, has been discredited. According to that study, it was suggested that thioridazine differed from other antipsychotic agents in producing a site-specific blockade of limbic dopamine receptors, implying that other neuroleptics had a relatively greater effect on striatal dopamine receptors, thereby increasing the risk of developing movement disorders and tardive dyskinesia.[35]

A recent report in the literature found no evidence of site selectivity for the action of thioridazine as compared to the actions of haloperidol and chlorpromazine.[36] It is important for physicians who prescribe antipsychotic medication to be able to recognize, differentiate, and treat the abnormal movement disorders that may occur during the course of antipsychotic therapy.[31,32]

AMBULATORY TREATMENT OF ACUTE PSYCHOSIS

The technique of rapid neuroleptization by the oral or intramuscular route is applicable to the acutely psychotic patient in the inpatient hospital setting. The pharmacological principles that govern this technique are, however, applicable to the treatment of the acutely psychotic patient in the ambulatory nonhospital treatment setting.[1] In the latter situation, the rapidity of dosage titration will be slower in most cases, depending upon the severity of symptoms and the frequency of outpatient visits. Also, in the ambulatory treatment of the acutely psychotic patient, dosage of medication administered will be lower than those employed in the hospital. Nevertheless, high potency piperazine phenothiazines and haloperidol are the antipsychotic agents of choice in the acute treatment and maintenance of ambulatory patients suffering from psychotic illnesses. It is generally good clinical practice to institute antiparkinsonian medication along with neuroleptics and, after the first two or three weeks of treatment, attempt to withdraw the former medication gradually as tolerated by the patient.[1]

Once the acute psychosis has resolved, through either inpatient or ambulatory treatment, it is absolutely critical to maintain the patient on a course of antipsychotic medication in order to avoid relapse in schizophrenic illness.[22,23] Certainly, in affective psychoses lithium is generally the maintenance treatment of choice. In maintenance antipsychotic chemotherapy, use of minimal effective daily doses of a high potency agent is the preferred course, with coadministration of antiparkinsonian medication only if clinically necessary. In some cases, long-acting injectable preparations, such as fluphenazine enanthate or decanoate, are of great value in preventing relapse of psychotic symptoms. These agents are ordinarily administered in a dose of 25 to 50 mg intramuscularly at intervals that may vary from once weekly to once every six weeks, although they are more commonly given at intervals of every two to three weeks.[1]

The frequency and dose of long-acting injectable preparations must be tailored to the needs of each specific patient and will vary from time to time in a given individual. The use of these long-acting drugs should not be instituted until the patient first has been tried on oral medication. In most cases, oral maintenance antipsychotic medication is preferred because it is less invasive and perhaps less threatening to most patients. It is also conceivable that persistent maintenance with injectable medication may in the long range present a greater risk of complications, such as tardive dyskinesia, because the patient is prevented from interrupting his own course of maintenance medication, thus ensuring a fairly constant and high degree of dopamine receptor blockade, and perhaps increasing the likelihood of the development of dopamine receptor supersensitivity, which may well be at the root of the process that causes tardive dyskinesia.[1]

DYSTONIC REACTIONS AND THEIR TREATMENT

Dystonic reactions characterized by acute torsion spasms, primarily affecting the neck muscles, jaw, and tongue, occur fairly commonly when potent neuroleptic drugs are initially administered. They are very rarely associated with dystonic spasms of the larynx and pharynx, and on those occasions acute dystonic reactions may be associated with difficulty in speaking, swallowing, or breathing.[37] The vast majority of acute dystonic reactions are simply manifested by a tightness in the jaw with associated retroflexion and twisting of the neck, but without associated difficulty in breathing and swallowing.[38] Among the potent neuroleptic agents, there is no evidence that any one of them is more or less likely to produce acute dystonic reactions. The most immediate and dramatic treatment for acute dystonic reactions is the intravenous administration of 50 mg of diphenhydramine.[38,39] If the dystonic reaction is severe, the patient is likely to be very frightened; therefore, the most rapid and effective therapeutic response possible utilizing intravenously administered diphenhydramine is to be recommended.

Alternately, benztropine in a dose of 1 to 2 mg intravenously or intramuscularly may also be highly effective, and if an intravenous injection cannot be immediately given, diphenhydramine could alternatively be administered intramuscularly.[38] Patients who have had dystonic reactions during prior courses of antipsychotic chemotherapy are likely to have a recurrence of these reactions during the initial phases of subsequent courses of chemotherapy. Not uncommonly, a patient will have several acute dystonic reactions if an initial reaction has occurred. Therefore, following the initial dystonic reaction, it is preferable to begin the patient on a course of antiparkinsonian medication or to increase the dose of prophylactic antiparkinsonian medication if the patient has been receiving such treatment prior to the acute dystonic reaction.[38] Benztropine, in a dose of 1 to 2 mg orally three to four times daily may provide effective prophylaxis against recurrent dystonic reactions. Trihexyphenidyl appears to be less effective in preventing dystonic reactions than benztropine, although the former drug is more efficacious in the treatment of persistent akathisia. Oculogyric movements occasionally accompany an acute dystonic reaction and respond favorably either to benztropine or diphenhydramine.[39]

Once the patient is established on a regular antipsychotic and antiparkinsonian regimen, in all likelihood there will not be a persistence of recurrent dystonic reactions.[38]

MANAGEMENT OF PARKINSONIAN EFFECTS

Less dramatic than the acutely occurring dystonic reactions or the potentially late occurring dyskinetic reaction to neuroleptic drugs, is the appearance of an extrapyramidal syndrome in the form of parkinsonism, probably the most common neurological sequella of neuroleptic treatment. The patient gradually develops parkinsonian signs marked by a flattening of facial expression, muscular rigidity, and a reduction and slowing of voluntary movement. Patients with parkinsonism often have stuped posture, festinating gait wherein small steps are taken, and there is a reduction in assessory movements of the arms. Patients with this syndrome will often salivate excessively and drool, and will generally show a coarse, "pill-rolling" tremor of the thumbs and fingers at rest.[1] These parkinsonian reactions to neuroleptics are not likely to occur in the first few days of treatment, but occur with increasing frequency as treatment is continued.[40] They are less apt to be severe in patients receiving simultaneously administered antiparkinsonian medication.[30] In association with the parkinsonian manifestations, the patient is likely to experience akathisia or restlessness and, at times, akinesia or a reduction in total movement.[31,32]

The use of the lowest effective dose of neuroleptic medication, once the acute symptoms of psychosis have diminished, is apt to be one of the best approaches to limiting the severity and persistance of acute parkinsonian reactions.[33] In most situations, except in the elderly or in the patient with organic brain dysfunction, the simultaneous administration of benztropine in a dose of 0.5 to 1.0 mg, or trihexyphenidyl in a dose of 2 mg two to four times daily, are likely to produce significant improvement in parkinsonian reactions to antipsychotic chemotherapy.[1] These medications diminish both the muscular rigidity and the tremor of drug-induced parkinsonism. Since their anticholinergic effect may enhance confusion or produce delerium in the elderly, these drugs should generally be avoided in older patients or those with organic brain dysfunction. In such patients, the use of diphenhydramine in a dose of 10 to 25 mg two to four times daily may be useful and produce fewer unwanted effects.[1] Alternately, the use of amantadine in a dose of 50 to 100 mg two to three times daily may be useful in controlling drug-induced extrapyramidal symptoms.[41]

WITHDRAWAL DYSKINESIA: RECOGNITION AND MANAGEMENT

Patients who have been treated with neuroleptic drugs and have the medication abruptly discontinued may experience a variety of withdrawal symptoms including nausea, vomiting, diarrhea, excessive perspiration, restlessness, insomnia, rhinorrhea, headache, increased appetite, and giddiness. Additionally, patients whose neuroleptic treatment is abruptly discontinued may experience a variety of abnormal movements of the extremities, neck, face, and mouth. These abnormal movements associated with neuroleptic withdrawal clinically are indistinguishable from those observed in patients developing tardive dyskinesia during long-term administration of neuroleptic drugs.[42] Dyskinesia associated with withdrawal of these drugs is undoubtedly related to increased cholinergic activity and changes in the dopamine-acetylcholine balance within the basal ganglia.[42] The administration of antiparkinsonian medication is generally of no more value in the treatment of withdrawal dyskinesia than in the treatment of tardive dyskinesia.

The treatment of choice for withdrawal dyskinesia is to reinstitute neuroleptic treatment at a dosage approximating the previously maintained dosage, and then to very gradually reduce the neuroleptic dosage over a period of several weeks while observing the patient for signs of dyskinesia. The neuroleptic tapering procedure may well require one to three months to safely remove the drug without the reappearance of withdrawal symptoms. In those patients with reappearance of dyskinesias even following a very gradual drug withdrawal schedule, it may be necessary to continue observation over a period of months without drug therapy before the dyskinesia symptoms gradually disappear.[42]

TARDIVE DYSKINESIA (TD)

Risk Factors

Tardive dyskinesia is, unfortunately, a potential risk of long-term neuroleptic drug therapy. The complication is related to the ability of neuroleptic drugs to block a variety of receptor sites, including dopamine sites.[43] In view of the link between the therapeutic actions of neuroleptics and the potential development of TD, it must be stated at the outset that there is no evidence that any particular, clinically effective neuroleptic drug is free of the liability of producing TD.[34,44] Research has failed to demonstrate that any particular neuroleptic drug is more apt to produce this complication and has also failed to show that any known neuroleptic is less likely to produce tardive dyskinesia.[34] The unfortunate suggestion in some pharmaceutical advertising that a particular neuroleptic by virtue of its lesser ability to produce acute extrapyramidal effects is more benign from the standpoint of production of TD, is, as far as can be determined from the available information, a distortion of fact.

The prevalence of TD varies considerably and one review of 44 epidemiologic studies has revealed that this syndrome may occur in anywhere from 24% to 56% of chronic neuroleptic users.[44] There appears to be a correlation of the likelihood of TD developing with the total amount of neuroleptic drug that the patient has received over time, thus suggesting, but not proving, that the use of the lowest possible maintenance dosage of neuroleptic drugs would reduce risk of TD and also that minimizing the duration of such treatment would likewise reduce the risk. Since the majority of large studies of TD have involved patients receiving neuroleptic drugs in state mental health programs, it is conceivable that more careful and conservative management of neuroleptic maintenance therapy, as well as more frequent dosage evaluation and dosage reduction, may reduce the overall risk of TD. Studies of the prevalence of tardive dyskinesia have revealed that its likelihood of occurring in neuroleptic-treated patients may vary from zero to 86%.[44] Some investigators have claimed that the use of drug holidays, wherein neuroleptic chemotherapy is interrupted for one to two days each week, may reduce the risk of TD, while others have suggested that drug holidays may actually increase the risk.[34] It has been claimed by some that the continuous administration of antiparkinsonian medication concommitantly with neuroleptics may increase the risk of TD. This finding has been challenged by other investigators, and there is no adequate data to support or deny this contention. Most studies of TD do agree that its incidence is higher in the elderly and in females, although no other predisposing factors for TD have been conclusively demonstrated thus far.[44]

Recognition

The typical clinical appearance of TD involves abnormal movements of the mouth, the presence of persistent chewing motions, peculiar movement of the tongue, often termed "fly-catcher's tongue," as well as sucking, licking, lip pursuing, and blowing movements of the mouth.

The movements of TD are choreiform, coordinated, involuntary, stereotyped, and rhythmic, and continue as long as they are not disturbed by other events.[34,46] Patients with TD may also have choreiform movements and rapid, unpredictable, often dramatic, thrusts of the extremities or neck. Respiratory dyskinesias occur rarely in association with TD and may be manifested by an irregular respiratory rate, shortness of breath, and chest discomfort.[47-49] Patients who have abnormal mouth movements in association with TD most often will salivate and drool excessively. Generally, patients who are in contact with reality are disturbed by the symptoms to TD and family members complain of the unsightliness as well as the abnormal sounds and excessive salivation. Patients with TD may grunt or make strange sounds, thus calling further attention to their unfortunate plight.[34,46]

Management

Several years ago the administration of increased doses of neuroleptic drugs was often recommended as the preferred treatment of TD. The potential that TD would persist or perhaps worsen when the larger doses of neuroleptics were eventually discontinued apparently was not always taken into account. Currently, there is no basis for recommending the administration of large doses of neuroleptics to control TD. Unfortunately, this syndrome has often been considered permanent and untreatable and, therefore, clinicians managing such patients have become alarmed and indeed have not made attempts to treat what was thought to be an irreversible condition. Furthermore, the awareness of the potential for TD to occur has led many clinicians to be frightened of the long-term administration of neuroleptic drugs and has yielded a situation wherein many individuals with treatable psychotic illness failed to receive the necessary course of antipsychotic chemotherapy. Although the risk of TD is very real and it may in some cases be irreversible, this risk must be seen in the context of the risk of serious psychotic illness.[46] In view of the fact that large numbers of individuals suffer from permanent psychotic illnesses that make them dysfunctional or require long-term custodial hospital care, the potential that drugs may alleviate the psychosis and allow the patient to be more functional must be recognized as not infrequently overriding the risk of a possible abnormal movement disorder. The unfortunate and irreversible risk of death by suicide among psychotic patients must be borne in mind by any clinician who is reluctant to prescribe antipsychotic drug maintenance, when clinically indicated, because of concerns about long-term medication complications.

There is certainly no general agreement as to the specific, most effective treatment of TD, nor is its absolute etiologic mechanism fully understood. The mechanism of TD has been suggested to be based upon dopamine receptor supersensitivity following administration of dopamine-blocking agents; another proposed mechanism is that of deficient cholinergic transmission.[43,46] Although both of these explanations may be important, or indeed an interaction between them, it must be borne in mind that a variety of other neurotransmitters may be affected during the course of psychotic illness and its treatment. It is quite possible that some presently unknown neurotransmitter may play a pivotol role in the etiology of late-occurring dyskinetic syndrome associated with neuroleptic treatment. The physician who is willing to embark on a course of treatment for a patient with TD must be flexible, imaginative, and willing to tolerate frustration as well as success. One standard approach to the treatment of TD which was recommended in the past was to discontinue the use of more potent neuroleptics and stabilize the patient on a low potency neuroleptic, since the low potency agents produce less acute extrapyramidal reactions.[50] The thinking was that these agents would be more benign in the presence of TD. There is increasing scientific evidence that this approach is not clinically desirable.[34,43,50] Often, discontinuation of the potent neuroleptic agent in favor of a less potent agent will give rise to the addition of withdrawal dyskinesia on top of an already present TD.[42] Furthermore, the low potency neuroleptics tend to be more strongly anticholinergic, and recent studies suggesting the therapeutic value of cholinergic stimulants or precursors in TD would further favor the potential that the low potency, strongly anticholinergic neuroleptics may actually produce a real or apparent worsening in the symptoms of TD.

When TD develops, the clinician must first decide upon the necessity of continuing neuroleptic therapy. If it is necessary, then therapy should most often continue with the employment of the same neuroleptic agent that the patient has been receiving, preferably in a very gradually diminishing dose rather than an abruptly decreased dose. Amantadine in a dose of 100 mg two to three times daily will, in some patients, produce mild to dramatic improvement in the symptoms of TD. Amantadine is not an anticholinergic, but exerts its beneficial effects on extrapyramidal movement disorders presumably because of its ability to produce a direct stimulation of dopamine receptor sites.[41] Amantadine is available commercially and generally has relatively mild side effects except for the potential that it may exacerbate psychotic symptoms in some patients.

Levodopa, widely used in the treatment of spontaneously occurring parkinsonism, has been reported to improve, worsen, or produce no change in TD.[46] Reports in the literature and my own successful treatment of TD using low dose levodopa suggests its potential value in the treatment of some patients. I would initially start levodopa at 100 mg daily and work up very slowly over a period of several weeks to 2 g daily or more, if clinically necessary. A preliminary report has suggested that clonidine in a dose of 0.3 to 0.7 mg per day may produce marked improvement in TD symptoms and may also exert an antipsychotic effect.[6]

Although more information is necessary to support the value of clonidine, this compound is worthy of consideration in the treatment of TD.

Mechanisms and Therapeutic Advances

The possibility that TD is based upon a deficiency in cholinergic
transmission has been suggested, and this hypothesis has been tested by
the use of experimental techniques that enhance central cholinergic activity. Although physostigmine, a cholinestrase inhibitor, increases central
cholinergic activity, its action is of too short a duration to be practically
employed in the routine management of TD. Experimentally, the intravenous administration of physostigmine has been demonstrated to improve the abnormal movements of TD.[51] Several investigators using
open and double-blind studies have attempted to evaluate the efficacy of
deanol, an orally administered acetylcholine precursor, in patients with
TD. The initial report suggested a favorable effect. However, subsequent
studies have failed to document an improvement in TD symptoms produced by oral deanol therapy which appears to have only limited ability
to increase central nervous system concentration of acetylcholine.[52]

One of the more practical ways of enhancing brain concentration of
acetylcholine is the oral administration of choline or lecithin, which are
precursors that give rise to increased endogenous acetylcholine synthesis.[53,55]
Health food stores sell what is labeled as 100% pure lecithin. Although
this product is pure from the standpoint of its content of phosphatides, in
reality it contains only approximately 20% lecithin and is therefore not
of practical value in the treatment of patients who may require at least 10
to 30 g of pure lecithin per day to achieve a clinically significant increase
in acetylcholine snythesis. Choline in pure form is available as 500 mg
tablets in health food stores; it may be administered in a dose of 2 to 10 g
daily orally, generally without major adverse effects. It will enhance central nervous system synthesis of acetylcholine and may thereby improve
symptoms of TD.[54,55] Choline has a bitter taste and may cause the patient
taking it to emit a rather foul fishy odor. Therefore, it is aesthetically
somewhat less pleasing than the use of lecithin.

It is important to inform the patient that the efficacy and safety of
this treatment is not fully proven. If the patient wishes to receive this
form of treatment, the clinician can supervise the administration of
choline, starting at a dose of 2 g daily and gradually increasing it over a
period of several weeks while the abnormal involuntary movements are
being assessed clinically. Although acetylcholine precursors appear to be
the most promising approach to the treatment of TD, presently the other
previously mentioned treatments may certainly be considered, as well as
a therapeutic trial of lithium carbonate which some investigators have
suggested may diminish signs and symptoms of TD.[1,50]

ELECTROCARDIOGRAPHIC EFFECTS OF NEUROLEPTIC DRUGS

Electrocardiographic abnormalities have long been associated with phenothiazines.[1] The electrocardiographic changes produced by antipsychotic drugs are not necessarily indicative of their ability to produce myocardial disease and tend to be reversible after discontinuation of the offending agent.[1] There is some conflict in the literature as to whether they are dosage-dependent or may occur at any dose of a specific therapeutic agent. There is evidence to support a strong association between the administration of thioridazine and abnormalities of the electrocardiogram, even in patients receiving fairly low doses of this compound. One study reported that 90% of a group of 30 patients receiving less than 300 mg of thioridazine per day had EKG changes.[56] The EKG changes most frequently associated with phenothiazines are repolarization changes resembling those produced by quinidine and by myocardial ischemia. These changes include depression, widening, notching, inversion, and flattening of the T wave, the presence of U waves, and prolongation of QT intervals.

In a study of patients receiving thioridazine in doses of 150 to 400 mg per day, only 32% of the patients had normal electrocardiograms, while 44% had low voltage T waves, and 23% had T wave widening. In patients receiving 150 to 900 mg per day of thioridazine, the incidence of electrocardiographic abnormalities exceeded 70%.[57] Similar electrocardiographic abnormalities have been noted in patients receiving chlorpromazine, trifluoperazine, mesoridazine, and fluphenazine.[58] The presence of first degree atrioventricular block with conduction delay, nonconducted premature atrial beats, and atrial flutter with varying degrees of block have also been reported in patients receiving thioridazine.[58,59] Phenothiazine therapy, particularly thioridazine, is also likely to be associated with ST segment flattening or depression.[56,57] Recurrent unifocal and multifocal ventricular premature beats, ventricular tachycardia, and ventricular fibrillation have also been described in healthy individuals receiving phenothiazines. In one study, patients receiving combined oral and intramuscular fluphenazine had a 91% incidence of abnormal electrocardiograms.[58] In patients with previous histories of cardiovascular disease and in those without evidence of heart disease, haloperidol has repeatedly been demonstrated to be the antipsychotic agent least likely to produce electrocardiographic change or abnormalities in cardiac function.[1]

NEUROLEPTIC MALIGNANT SYNDROME

A rare syndrome described as the neuroleptic malignant syndrome (NMS) characterized by muscular rigidity, hyperthermia, altered consciousness, and autonomic dysfunction, was first recognized in 1960. Initially, this syndrome was described in the French literature. This may be more than coincidence, since French clinicians tend more often than those elsewhere to utilize a combination of multiple neuroleptic drugs simultaneously in the treatment of a given patient. There seems to be some evidence to suggest that the combination of multiple neuroleptics would increase the risk of adverse effects and perhaps the risk of the development of the syndrome.

Since NMS is very serious and potentially fatal, it is of utmost importance to the clinician to recognize the syndrome, diagnose it early, discontinue neuroleptic medication, and institute supportive therapy as quickly as possible. Although some controversy exists as to the likelihood of this syndrome being produced by various neuroleptic drugs, the evidence does not clearly support a statement that the syndrome is any more or less likely to occur with any particular neuroleptic or class of neuroleptic medication.[60,61,62] Reports on NMS in the United States literature have primariy implicated long-acting fluphenazine derivatives as the causative agent, although the world literature fails to support a definitive preeminent position of depot phenothiazines as the causative agent for NMS.[61,63]

Clinical Signs and Symptoms

In NMS there is generalized muscular hypertonicity. Rigidity and akinesia develop simultaneously with or shortly before temperature elevations which may be as high as 41 °C. Consciousness fluctuates from an alert but dazed mutism through stupor and coma. There is excessive salivation, which is most commonly associated with difficulty in swallowing. Patients with NMS have marked tachycardia, labile blood pressure, profuse sweating, dyspnea, and are often incontinent.[61] Patients suffering from this syndrome often will remain in bed for long periods of time with little movement, thus increasing their risk of developing pneumonia and secondary infections as well as pulmonary emboli. Although there is no specific laboratory test that is diagnostic, leukocytosis ranging from 15,000 to 30,000 has been reported, and CPK elevations as high as 15,000 units have been observed. Electroencephalograms may show findings consistent with a diffuse metabolic encephalopathy.

Many patients develop this syndrome over a period of one to three days. Patients who develop NMS may well have had prior courses of antipsychotic medication without developing the syndrome, and once they recover from the syndrome may be treated with the same or different antipsychotic drug without the recurrence of NMS.[61] Although the potent antipsychotic agents have more often been associated with the development of NMS, this syndrome also has occurred in association with thioridazine therapy, and in patients receiving lithium in combination with a variety of neuroleptics.[62] Patients with organic brain dysfunction appear to be more likely to develop NMS when exposed to neuroleptics.[61] There is no particular predilection of any age group or disease category for this syndrome. The symptoms of NMS generally persist for five to ten days after the neuroleptics are discontinued. They are more apt to be even more persistent following long courses of neuroleptic therapy or the use of depot phenothiazines. Fatalities have been reported occurring three to 30 days after the onset of symptoms and generally in association with respiratory or renal failure, or the presence of severe cardiovascular disturbances. A review of 60 cases in the literature revealed 12 deaths, a mortality rate of 20%. Six of the 12 patients that died had been treated with depot fluphenazine preparations.[61,63]

Treatment of NMS

Clearly, the most critical approach to the patient who appears to have NMS is to discontinue all psychotropic medications, most importantly, neuroleptics. A patient's cardiovascular and renal function should be monitored clinically and adequate hydration maintained with the administration of intravenous fluids, if orally administered fluids and nutrients are not tolerated.[61] Although the stiffness and rigidity of the syndrome may respond somewhat to cautious administration of antiparkinsonian medication, these agents are by no means a specific therapy for NMS and may complicate the picture further by adversely affecting autonomic nervous system function. Use of short-acting benzodiazepines, such as oxazepam, may produce some muscle relaxation and allow the patient to be more comfortable, provided that the patient is carefully observed and fluid replacement maintained. Once the patient recovers from NMS, if continued antipsychotic chemotherapy is necessary, it may be reinstituted with the same agent or a different agent generally at a low dose, with cautious monitoring and very slow titration of neuroleptic agent as clinically necessary.[61]

LITHIUM-NEUROLEPTIC INTERACTION

Several years ago, a specific toxic syndrome was attributed to the combined use of haloperidol and lithium carbonate. Patients were described as showing leukocytosis, fever, and neurological symptoms, including lethargy, tremulousness, confusion and extrapyramidal as well as cerebellar dysfunction. There were initially four cases reported, and the authors attributed this to a specific toxic interaction between haloperidol and lithium.[64] Subsequent review of this report and of the rather extensive clinical experience with a combination of lithium carbonate and haloperidol, strongly suggests that this combination of medications is safe and is not the cause of a specific toxic syndrome. One extensive review of a series of 425 patients treated with haloperidol and lithium in combination failed to reveal a single case of the presumed lithium–haloperidol syndrome.[65]

My own extensive use of this combination as the preferred therapeutic approach to the treatment of acutely manic patients has failed to reveal the recurrence of this syndrome as described by Cohen and Cohen.[64] Several investigators reviewing the initial report of four cases suggested the possibility that this cluster of patients within a single institution in a short time span was consistent with a viral encephalomyelitis rather than a specific toxic syndrome. On the other hand, the possible similarlity between this syndrome and the neuroleptic malignant syndrome should be considered, particularly in light of the fact that a similar constellation of signs and symptoms were reported to occur when thioridazine was used in combination with lithium.[66] Of particular note in the patients treated by Cohen and Cohen is the fact that lithium levels reported were above the generally acceptable therapeutic range of 0.6 to 1.2 mEq/L and the contribution of lithium toxicity to the signs and symptoms reported by these authors cannot be denied.

REFERENCES

1. Bernstein JG: *Handbook of Drug Therapy in Psychiatry.* Littleton, MA, John Wright • PSG, 1983.
2. Deniker P: Introduction of neuroleptic chemotherapy into psychiatry, in Ayd RJ, Blackwell B (eds): *Discoveries in Biological Psychiatry.* Philadelphia, J.B. Lipincott, 1970, pp 155–164.
3. Kruse W: Treatment of drug induced extrapyramidal symptoms. *Dis Nerv Sys* 1960;21:79–81.
4. Freyhan FA: Psychomotility and parkinsonism in treatment with neuroleptic drugs. *Arch Neurology* 1957;78:465–472.
5. Freedman R, Bell J, Kirch D: Clonidine therapy for coexisting psychosis and tardive dyskinesia. *Am J Psychiatry* 1980;137:629–630.
6. Freedman R, Kirch D, Bell J, et al: Clonidine treatment of schizophrenia: Double-blind comparison to placebo and neuroleptic drugs. *Acta Psychiatr Scand* 1982;65:35–45.
7. May PRA: *Treatment of Schizophrenia.* New York, Science House, 1968.
8. Grinspoon L, Ewalt JR, Shader RI: Psychotherapy and pharmacotherapy and chronic schizophrenia. *Am J Psychiatry* 1968;124:1645–1652.
9. Creese I, Burt DR, Snyder SH: Dopamine receptor binding predicts clinical and pharmacologic potencies of antischizophrenic drugs. *Science* 1976;192:481–483.
10. Snyder SH: The dopamine hypothesis of schizophrenia: Focus on the dopamine receptor. *Am J Psychiatry* 1976;133:197–202.
11. Snyder SH: Dopamine receptors, neuroleptics and schizophrenia. *Am J Psychiatry* 1981;138:460–464.
12. Snyder SH: Receptors, neurotransmitters, and drug responses. *N Engl J Med* 1979;300:465–472.
13. Snyder S, Greenberg D, Yamamura HI: Antischizophrenic drugs and brain cholinergic receptors. *Arch Gen Psychiatry* 1974;31:58–61.
14. Quader SE: Dysarthria: An unusual side effect of tricyclic antidepressants. *Brit Med J* 1977;2:97.
15. Tune LE, Strauss ME, Lew MF, et al: Serum levels of anticholinergic drugs and impaired recent memory in chronic schizophrenic patients. *Am J Psychiatry* 1982;139:1460–1462.
16. Klein DF, Gittelman R, Quitkin F, et al: *Diagnosis and Drug Treatment of Psychiatric Disorders: Adults and Children,* ed 2. Baltimore, Williams and Wilkins, 1980.
17. Sos J, Cassem NH: Intravenous use of haloperidol for acute delirium in intensive care unit settings, in Speidel H, Rodwald G (eds): *Psychic and Neurological Dysfunctions After Open Heart Surgery.* Stuttgart, Georg Thieme Verlag, 1980, pp 196–199.
18. Borenstein P, Dongier M, Fink M, et al: Clinical and experimental encephalography, in Bobon DP, Janssen PAJ, Bobon J (eds): *Modern Problems in Pharmacopsychiatry: The Neuroleptics.* Basel, S. Karger, 1970, pp 109–125, vol 5.
19. Shopsin B, Gershon S, Thompson H, et al: Psychoactive drugs in mania. *Arch Gen Psychiatry* 1975;32:34–42.
20. Brinkley JR, Beitman BD, Freidel RO: Low dose neuroleptic regimens in the treatment of borderline patients. *Arch Gen Psychiatry* 1979;36: 319–326.
21. Beiderman J, Lerner Y, Belmaker RH: Combination of lithium carbonate and haloperidol in schizo-affective disorder. *Arch Gen Psychiatry* 1979;36: 327–333.
22. Hogarty GE, Goldberg IC: Drugs and social therapy in the aftercare of schizophrenic patients. *Arch Gen Psychiatry* 1973;28:54–64.

23. Davis JM: Overview: Maintenance therapy in psychiatry. I. Schizophrenia. *Am J Psychiatry* 1975;132:1237–1245.
24. Anderson WH, Kuehnle JC: Treatment of psychosis by rapid neuroleptization: Update 1980, in Ayd FJ (ed): *Haloperidol Update: 1958–1980;* Baltimore, Ayd Medical Communication, 1980, pp 31–39.
25. Donlon PT, Hopkin J, Tupin JP: Overview: Efficacy and safety of the rapid neuroleptization method with injectable haloperidol. *Am J Psychiatry* 1979;136:273–278.
26. Bernstein JG: Chemotherapy of psychosis, in Bernstein JG (ed): *Clinical Psychopharmacology*. Littleton, MA, PSG Publishing, 1978, pp 40–51.
27. Rifkin A, Quitkin F, Carrillo C, et al: Very high dosage fluphenazine for non-chronic treatment refractory patients. *Arch Gen Psychiatry* 1971;25:398–403.
28. Cole JO: Psychopharmacology update: Antipsychotic drugs. Is more better? *McLean Hosp J* 1982;7:61–87.
29. Settle EC: Haloperidol regimens in treatment of acute psychosis: How much and how often, in Ayd FJ (ed): *Haloperidol Update: 1958–1980.* Baltimore, Ayd Medical Communications, 1980, pp 40–52.
30. Rifkin A, Quitkin F, Kane J, et al: Are prophylactic antiparkinsonian drugs necessary? *Arch Gen Psychiatry* 1978;35:483–489.
31. Rifkin A, Quitkin F, Klein DF: Akinesia. *Arch Gen Psychiatry* 1975;32:672–674.
32. Maltbie AA, Cavenar JO Jr: Akathisia diagnosis: An objective test. *Psychosomatics* 1977;18:36–39.
33. Tune L, Coyle JT: Acute extrapyramidal side effects: Serum levels of neuroleptics and anticholinergics. *Psychopharmacology* 1981;75:9–15.
34. Anath J: Tardive dyskinesia: Myths and realities. *Psychosomatics* 1980;21:389–396.
35. Borrison RL, Fields JZ, Diamond BI: Site specific blockade of dopamine receptors by neuroleptic agents in human brain. *Neuropharmacology* 1981;28:1321–1322.
36. Reynolds GP, Cowley L, Rossor MN, Iversen LL: Thioridazine is not specific for limbic dopamine receptors. *Lancet* 1982;2:499–500.
37. Flaherty JA, Lahmeyer HW: Laryngeal-pharyngeal dystonia as a possible cause of asphyxia with haloperidol treatment. *Am J Psychiatry* 1978;135:1414–1415.
38. Garver DL, Davis JM, Dekirmenhian H, et al: Dystonic reactions following neuroleptics: Time course and proposed mechanisms. *Psychopharmacology* 1976;47:199–201.
39. McGreer PL, Boulding JE, Gibson WS, et al: Drug-induced extrapyramidal reactions. *JAMA* 1961;1777:665–670.
40. Calne DB: Advances in the neuropharmacology of parkinsonism. *Ann Intern Med* 1979;90:219–229.
41. Fann WE, Lake CI: Amantadine versus trihexyphenidyl in the treatment of neuroleptic-induced parkinsonsim. *Am J Psychiatry* 1976;133:940–943.
42. Gardos G, Cole JO, Tarsy D: Withdrawal syndromes associated with antipsychotic drugs. *Am J Psychiatry* 1978;135:1321–1324.
43. Klawans HL: The pharmacology of tardive dyskinesia. *Am J Psychiatry* 1973;130:82–86.
44. Tepper SJ, Haas JF: Prevalence of tardive dyskinesia. *J Clin Psychiatry* 1979;40:508–516.
45. Cohen S: Tardive dyskinesia. *Drug Abuse and Alcoholism Newsletter* 1975;4(8):1–3.
46. Tarsey D, Baldessarini RJ: The tardive dyskinesia syndrome, in Klawans HL

(ed): *Clinical Neuropharmacology.* New York, Raven Press, 1976, pp 29–61, vol 1.

47. Weiner WJ, Goetz CG, Nausieda PA, et al: Respiratory dyskinesias: Extrapyramidal dysfunction and dyspnea. *Ann Intern Med* 1978;88:327–331.

48. Jackson IV, Volavka J, James B, et al: The respiratory component of tardive dyskinesia. *Biol Psychiatry* 1980;15:485–487.

49. Casey DE, Rabins P: Tardive dyskinesia as a life threatening illness. *Am J Psychiatry* 1978;135:486–488.

50. Kobayashi RM: Drug therapy of tardive dyskinesia. *New Engl J Med* 1977; 296:257–260.

51. Weis KJ, Ciraulo DA, Shader RI: Physostigmine test in the rabbit syndrome and tardive dyskinesia. *Am J Psychiatry* 1980;137:627–628.

52. Penovich P, Morgan JP, Kerzner B, et al: Double-blind evaluation of deanol in tardive dyskinesia. *JAMA* 1978;239:1997–1998.

53. Wurtman RJ: Nutritional and precursor control of brain acetylcholine synthesis. *Psychopharmacol Bull* 1978;14:53–55.

54. Growdon JH: Effects of choline on tardive dyskinesia and other movement disorders. *Psychopharmacol Bull* 1978;14:55–56.

55. Gelenberg AJ, Wojcik JD, Growdon JH, et al: Lecithin for the treatment of tardive dyskinesia: Preliminary results from a double-blind study, in DeVeaugh-Geiss J (ed): *Tardive Dyskinesia and Related Involuntary Movement Disorders.* Littleton, MA, John Wright • PSG, 1982.

56. Branchey MH, Lee JH, Amin R, et al: High and low potency neuroleptics in elderly psychiatric patients. *JAMA* 1978;239:1860–1862.

57. Hutson JR, Bell GE: The effect of thioridazine hydrochloride and chlorpromazine on the electrocardiogram, *JAMA* 1966;198:16–20.

58. Fowler NO, McCall D, Chou T, et al: Electrocardiographic changes and cardiac arrythmias in patients receiving psychotropic drugs. *Am J Cardiol* 1976; 37:223–230.

59. Khan MM, Lopan KL, McComb JM, et al: Management of recurrent ventricular tachyarrhythmias associated with Q-T prolongation. *Am J Cardiol* 1981;47:1301–1308.

60. Morris HH III, McCormick WF, Reinarz JA: Neuroleptic malignant syndrome *Arch Neurol* 1980;37:462–463.

61. Caroff SN: The neuroleptic malignant syndrome. *J Clin Psychiatry* 1980; 41:79–83.

62. Haberman M: Malignant hyperthermia. An allergic reaction to thioridazine. *Arch Intern Med* 1978;138:800–801.

63. Grunhaus L, Sancovici S, Rimon R: Neuroleptic malignant syndrome due to depot fluphenazine. *J Clin Psychiatry* 1979;40:99–100.

64. Cohen WJ, Cohen NH: Lithium carbonate, haloperidol, and irreversible brain damage. *JAMA* 1974;230:1283–1287.

65. Baastrup PC, Hollnagel P, Sorenson R, et al: Adverse reactions in treatment with lithium carbonate and haloperidol. *JAMA* 1976;236:2645–2646.

66. Spring GH: Neurotoxicity with combined use of lithium and thioridazine. *J Clin Psychiatry* 1979;40:135–138.

SELECTED REFERENCES

Chlorpromazine

Rivera-Calimlin L, Nasrallah H, Strauss J, et al: Clinical response and plasma levels: Effects of dose, dosage schedules, and drug interactions on plasma chlorpromazine levels. *Arch Gen Psychiatry* 1976;133:636–642.

176

Thioridazine

Smith GR, Taylor CW, Linkous P: Haloperidol versus thioridazine for the treatment of psychogeriatric patients: A double-blind clinical trial. *Psychosomatics* 1974;15:134–138.

Trifluoperazine

Wijsenbeek H, Steiner M, Goldberg SC: Trifluoperazine, A comparison between regular and high doses. *Psychopharmacologia* 1974;36:147–150.

Perphenazine

Vestre ND, Dehnel LI, Schiele BC: A sequential comparison of amitriptyline, perphenazine, and the amitriptyline-perphenazine combination in recently admitted anergic schizophrenics. *Psychosomatics* 1969;10:269–303.

Fluphenazine

Rifkin A, Quitkin F, Carrillo C, et al: Very high dosage fluphenazine for non-chronic treatment-refractory patients. *Arch Gen Psychiatry* 1971;25:398–403.

Groves JE, Mandel MR: The long-acting phenothiazines. *Arch Gen Psychiatry* 1975;32:893–900.

Butaperazine

Simpson GM, Lament R, Cooper TB, et al: The relationship between blood levels of different forms of butaperazine and clinical response. *J Clin Pharmacol* 1973; 13:288–297.

Thiothixene

Ban TA (ed): *Psychopharmacology of Thiothixene.* New York, Raven Press, 1978.

Haloperidol

Ayd FJ Jr (ed): *Haloperidol Update: 1958–1980.* Baltimore, Ayd Medical Communications, 1980.

Loxapine

Zisook S, Click MA Jr: Evaluations of loxapine succinate in the ambulatory treatment of acute schizophrenic episodes. *Int Pharmacopsychiatry* 1980;15: 365–378.

Molindone

Binder R, Glick I, Rice M: A comparative study of parenteral molindone and haloperidol in the acutely psychotic patient. *J Clin Psychiatry* 1981;42: 203–206.

General

Kurland AA, Hanlon TE, Tatom MH, et al: The comparative effectiveness of six phenothiazine compounds, phenobarbital and inert placebo in the treatment of acutely ill patients: Global measures of severity of illness. *J Nerv Ment Dis* 1965;133:1–18.

Zavodnick S: A pharmacological and theoretical comparison of high and low potency neuroleptics. *J Clin Psychiatry* 1978;38:332–336.

Sriwatanakul K, Weis O: Using antipsychotic drugs during pregnancy. *Drug Therapy* 1982;12:97–100.

9

Insomnia:
Diagnosis and Treatment

Ernest Hartmann

DEFINING INSOMNIA

Insomnia, from the Latin, means "not sleeping" or "no sleep;" however, insomnia is *not* no sleep. Occasionally, one reads in the newspaper about someone in Scandinavia or in Canada who never sleeps. Twenty years of experience in my laboratory and in other sleep laboratories has proven that the condition of not sleeping is nonexistent. No one does not sleep. The closest anyone came is a man in France who slept 15 minutes a night. This was carefully documented. His sleep was cut down from normal nights to one hour, then to 15 minutes; he kept this up for a year or so. He did not seem overly tired, but he had daily hallucinatory periods lasting approximately 15 minutes. No one knew quite what was wrong, but obviously something was wrong; he died after a year. Even at autopsy, there was no clearcut diagnosis, but the staining of his brainstem — the areas that contain serotonin — was unusual.[1] This is the only person who came close to not sleeping in the recorded annals of human sleep.

Insomnia then is not "no sleep." Second, insomnia is not short sleep. It would be convenient if one could say, "Insomnia is sleeping less than six hours." It is not. My laboratory did an extensive study of people who always slept less than six hours and people who always slept more than nine hours. There is quite a variation in normal sleep time. A group of people was found who always slept five or six hours per night, never "caught up," and had no particular complaint; other people who slept between nine and ten hours a night and had no particular complaint.[2] Some physiological differences in sleep were found which are not relevant here, and psychologically, the groups were quite different.

The short sleepers were Napoleon types — they were very active and involved. They seemed somewhat hypomanic, which means happy, keeping busy, sometimes avoiding emotional problems. When they had reasons to be sad and upset, their defense was to push their problems away, to keep busy and not worry about them. These were the short sleepers: they were busy, nonworriers, perhaps hypomanic. The point is that these were not insomniacs; there are many people who sleep less than six hours a night and feel fine. There was some familial tendency in their sleep length patterns; they may be partly genetic. But that is not insomnia. The long sleepers, again, were basically a group of normal people, but they tended to be worriers or reprogrammers. The short sleepers were doing things the way they liked and they kept doing them the same way; the long sleepers gave the impression of worrying, or reprogramming, of changing their lives.[3]

Insomnia is not short sleep. In fact, in a study by Carskadon[4] a large number of people who came to their physicians complaining of insomnia (either a serious problem with falling asleep or with staying asleep) showed that their actual sleep time in the laboratory was on the average considerably longer than they thought. The mean, in fact, was over six hours, but there was a wide distribution. Insomnia, then, is a complaint of sleeping poorly.

Finally, insomnia is *not an illness* for which a sleeping pill is the cure; insomnia is a symptom that can have many causes. This seems fairly obvious, but it is one of those things that is more honored in the breach than in the observance. An insomniac comes to a physician and says, "Can I have a sleeping pill?" Or an insomniac goes to the drugstore and the pharmacist says, "Take a Sominex." Insomnia is treated as though it were an illness for which a sleeping pill is the cure and, of course, it is not. Insomnia is a symptom. It is a symptom produced by a number of underlying causes.

CAUSES OF INSOMNIA

Insomnia is one of four basic symptoms commonly found in sleep disorders medicine. Presently, there are 80 or 90 different sleep disorders classified in many ways, but with few symptoms: 1) *insomnia*, the most common symptom, which will be discussed in further detail; 2) *hypersomnia*; and 3) *excessive daytime sleepiness*, which will not be discussed here. Together, they are sometimes called "hypersomnolence," and occasionally have serious causes such as narcolepsy or sleep apnea. The last group of symptoms is 4) *episodic events*, such as, night terrors, night-mares, enuresis, epilepsy, and painful erections. There are approximately 20 episodic events which are not really part of sleep, but which often occur during sleep and cause problems.[5]

Insomnia is by far the most common symptom. In fact, there are various studies from several countries suggesting that 15% to 30% of the population complain to physicians about insomnia in the course of a year; over 5% to 10% take medication for it. Sleeping pill use increases with age and is higher in women than in men.[6]

How is insomnia approached clinically? Table 9-1 is the Association for Sleep Disorders Centers' classification of insomnia. This is one way of looking at many different causes or conditions associated with insomnia.

Table 9-1
Outline of Diagnostic Classification of Sleep and Arousal Disorders

DIMS: Disorders of Initiating and Maintaining Sleep (Insomnias)
1. Psychophysiological
   a. Transient and Situational
   b. Persistent
2. *associated with* Psychiatric Disorders
   a. Symptom and Personality Disorders
   b. Affective Disorders
   c. Other Functional Psychoses
3. *associated with* Use of Drugs and Alcohol
   a. Tolerance to or Withdrawal from CNS Depressants
   b. Sustained Use of CNS Stimulants
   c. Sustained Use of or Withdrawal from Other Drugs
   d. Chronic Alcoholism
4. *associated with* Sleep-induced Respiratory Impairment
   a. Sleep Apnea DIMS Syndrome
   b. Alveolar Hypoventilation DIMS Syndrome
5. *associated with* Sleep-related (Nocturnal) Myoclonus and "Restless Legs"
   a. Sleep-related (Nocturnal) Myoclonus DIMS Syndrome
   b. "Restless Legs" DIMS Syndrome
6. *associated with* Other Medical, Toxic, and Environmental Conditions
7. Childhood-Onset DIMS
8. *associated with* Other DIMS Conditions
   a. Repeated REM Sleep Interruptions
   b. Atypical Polysomnographic Features
   c. Not Otherwise Specified*
9. No DIMS Abnormality
   a. Short Sleeper
   b. Subjective DIMS Complaint without Objective Findings
   c. Not Otherwise Specified*

*This entry is intended to leave place in the classification for both undiagnosed ("don't know") conditions and additional (as yet undocumented) conditions that may be described in the future.

Reproduced with permission from Association of Sleep Disorders Centers: Diagnostic classification of sleep and arousal disorders. *Sleep* 1979;2:17.

180

Table 9-2 lists the same groups of causes, but they are arranged in a way that seems more useful clinically — when a patient presents with serious insomnia.

First, insomnia is basically one of two major symptoms: people either complain of *difficulty falling asleep* or *difficulty remaining asleep*, occasionally both. Some textbooks speak of a third kind — early morning awakening; but, both clinically and in the laboratory, people with early morning awakening also awaken a great deal during the night and vice

Table 9-2
Causes of Insomnia*

	Insomnias Secondary to Medical Conditions	Insomnias Secondary to Psychiatric or Environmental Conditions
Difficulty in Falling Asleep	Any painful or uncomfortable condition Brain stem lesions Conditions listed below, at times	Anxiety Anxiety, chronic neurotic Anxiety, prepsychotic Tension anxiety, muscular Environmental changes Conditioned (habit) insomnia Phase shift Non-24-hour cycles
Difficulty in Remaining Asleep	Sleep apnea Nocturnal myoclonus and restless legs syndrome Dietary factors Episodic events Direct drug effects (including alcohol) Drug withdrawal effects (including alcohol) Drug interactions Endocrine abnormalities Metabolic abnormalities Brain stem or hypothalamic lesions Aging	Depression, especially primary depression Environmental changes Phase shift Non-24 hour cycles Dream interruption insomnia

*The boundaries between the columns are not entirely distinct. In the column "Insomnia Secondary to Psychiatric and Environmental Conditions" are listed the illnesses and syndromes that are currently classified as psychiatric and that are most frequently seen by psychiatrists and conditions that, in the present state of knowledge, are best conceptualized by using psychiatric terms. However, all or most of those psychiatric illnesses will probably be understood eventually in terms of brain biological mechanisms and interactions with the social and physical environment, so that the distinction between the two columns may no longer be necessary in the future.

Reproduced with permission from Hartmann E: Sleep disorders, in Friedman AM, Kaplan HI, Sadock BJ (eds): *A Comprehensive Textbook of Psychiatry III.* Baltimore, Williams & Wilkins Co, 1980, pp 2014-2029.

versa. It therefore is not really a separate group. People either have difficulty falling asleep or remaining asleep, each for many different reasons. Any *painful or uncomfortable condition* can produce insomnia, usually trouble falling asleep. Some people do not notice the pains and discomforts in the daytime; they notice them at night. Other people do not even notice them at night; they just say, "I can't sleep," and not until one takes a history are they aware of why they are having trouble sleeping.

Sleep apnea can be a cause of insomnia as well as of hypersomnia. In sleep apnea breathing and airflow ceases; with obstructive sleep apnea something is blocking airflow, often but not always at the level of the pharnyx. In obstructive sleep apnea, nasal airflow stops, but thoracic or abdominal respiration keeps up and, in fact, increases as a person tries to force air through the block; oxygen saturation goes down, and usually the sleeper awakes after 20 to 30 seconds, takes a few breaths and goes back to sleep. The process is repeated several hundred times a night in a serious case, and the patient obtains little good sleep. Central sleep apnea means the impulses from the brainstem are not being sent out by nerve impulses so that both nasal airflow and respiratory movements cease. In adults, obstructive sleep apnea is the more common type, and often occurs in an older male whose wife says he snores a lot, gasps, etc. He may or may not actually complain of insomnia, he may just complain of being sleepy all day — hypersomnia.

There are a number of other medical conditions that cause insomnia. *Nocturnal myoclonus* consists of repetitive muscle jerks — usually jerks of the tibial musculature. This is not an uncommon cause of insomnia. Again, the bedpartner will be more aware of this problem than the patient. *Episodic events*, on the other hand, can wake people up.

Drug effects are quite serious causes of insomnia, and there are two types of effects: 1) *direct drug effects*: obviously, stimulants (eg, amphetamines, methylphenidate) can make sleep difficult. Some of the antidepressants, especially the MAO-inhibitors, can act as stimulants producing difficulty in sleeping. 2) *Drug withdrawal* is equally or even more important. Any medication, such as a sleeping pill and most tranquilizers (anything that depresses the central nervous system), will, when it is withdrawn, produce insomnia for a few days and sometimes for a few weeks afterwards. This is hardly surprising, but it is often forgotten. The patient or the physician will stop the medication, and the patient again has trouble sleeping. The danger is that the conclusion is often drawn that this is someone who needs a sleeping pill and cannot get along without it. The person is put back on the sleeping pill and sometimes takes it for the rest of his life. The chances are that if he had been able to wait a few days or a few weeks to get over the withdrawal period, he would not need further medication. This does not mean that it is easy to get along without it or stop when someone has been taking medication for years, but one must at least be aware of insomnia expected during the withdrawal period.

Alcohol as a cause of insomnia is very much worth keeping in mind. Alcohol is magnificently paradoxical: it is, of course, used as a hypnotic medication. Some people have estimated that it is used more than anything else. At the same time, it produces insomnia. Unfortunately, it is quite a serious cause of insomnia, both while one is drinking and after one stops. In talking to any serious drinker, whether the person thinks of himself as an alcoholic or simply as a heavy social drinker, he will tell say, "Yes, it puts me to sleep. Alcohol knocks me out, but I wake up sooner and sooner; I can't stay asleep." Sometimes the awakenings include uncomfortable withdrawing feelings, almost like the beginnings of DTs, and sometimes night terrors. EEG recordings have shown that sleep stages are greatly altered when one has been drinking heavily. So alcohol, even while one is drinking (this may be a matter of rapid withdrawal) produces insomnia. And then, of course, alcohol is a depressant and like any other depressant, after withdrawing alcohol, one can have days or weeks of insomnia as a withdrawal phenomenon.

Aging should not really be listed as a cause of insomnia. Normal aging causes reduced sleep and more waking during the night. This usually is a normal phenomenon, but if an aging person complains a great deal about sleep, one has to think about all of the other causes of insomnia, as well as the possibility of exaggerated or accelerated age changes.

PSYCHIATRIC CAUSES OF INSOMNIA (TABLE 9-2)

Anxiety keeps people from falling asleep, but anxiety is a complex thing. *Simple anxiety*, such as occurs for an important job interview or an exam coming up, will produce trouble falling asleep at night, but there are many other kinds. For example, *prepsychotic anxiety*. Often, when examining a psychotic patient in the emergency room (eg, an acute schizophrenic episode or a suicide attempt) and in obtaining a careful history of the weeks prior to the event, insomnia is often one of the first symptoms of the impending psychosis. Therefore, when someone complains of insomnia, which is not chronic, but has just arisen in the past two weeks and is getting worse, this could be a person who will present with a psychiatric emergency in the hospital two weeks hence.

Chronic muscular anxiety occurs in some people who become more intense and worried about not sleeping: "I've got to sleep, I've got to get up tomorrow." Their muscles become tense, which makes them nervous. This builds up, not just over one night, but sometimes over a long period of time. Chronic muscular anxiety occasionally responds to biofeedback, relaxation techniques, or meditation.

Another cause of insomnia is *chronic neurotic anxiety*. Some psychiatrists think that all insomnia is related to neurotic anxiety; this is not the case. However, there are people who have insomnia on the basis that falling asleep is "letting go." And letting go is not easy for everyone. Letting go represents loosening up the usual ways of dealing with the world — becoming defenseless. For some people, if they do not hold on tight, they are in danger, for example, of either being killed or hurt, or killing or raping someone, or of being raped. In this case, letting go is a danger. Thus, falling asleep becomes a danger and one develops insomnia. This is the type of insomnia that often responds to psychotherapy; most of the others do not.

Depression is quite common as a cause of insomnia. Among middle-aged (40- to 60-year old) persons, especially women, who have difficulty remaining asleep, but often fall asleep all right, depression is worth considering. This difficulty remaining asleep with early morning awakening is one of the major symptoms of depression. In a person with this clinical presentation, if medication is necessary, often an antidepressant will work better than a simple sleeping pill.

There are a series of possible causes of insomnia involving *unusual cycles*. Jet lag is the best known, in which a person's cycle is thrown off balance. He or she trys to get to sleep at a time when the body is not accustomed to sleeping. Some people give themselves jet lag without flying simply by disrupting their normal cycles by going to bed at odd times. Others do indeed have something wrong with their basic, probably hypothalamic, cycling mechanisms. These are all causes of insomnia.

Again, insomnia is a symptom for which there are many causes. The physician must try to determine the cause and treat it. Does this mean that hypnotic medication is never needed and should be banned? There *are* uses for sleeping pills, which may be useful, but they have often been overused, and occasionally used prior to doing a differential diagnosis.

HYPNOTICS

Hypnotic medications can be dangerous drugs for several reasons (see Table 9-3). As the Greeks said, "Sleep is the younger sister of death." If sleep is produced, it is producing a little bit of death in a number of ways. The benzodiazepines are somewhat better in that they do not produce severe respiratory depression in normals. There is evidence, however, that in apneic patients benzodiazepines can produce some respiratory depression when respiration is already compromised. Thus, they are not entirely safe, and they do have other dangers and problems as listed in Table 9-3.

Sleeping Pills and Other Approaches to Inducing Sleep

Sleeping pills are a heterogeneous group of compounds with very different chemical structures that seem to produce sleep. It is not known

Table 9-3
Hypnotic Medication: Major Problems

1. Low therapeutic index (respiratory depression)
2. Dangers in specific illnesses (porphyria, apnea)
3. Abuse
4. Withdrawal reactions
5. After-effects (hangover, performance deficits)
6. Allergy, hypersensitivity
7. Interactions with other depressants (alcohol)
8. Interactions because of enzyme induction
9. Distortion of normal sleep patterns

exactly how they work. A number of compounds could be considered in this category that are not ordinarily called sleeping pills. For example, bromides do produce the same kind of effect; they were used for quite a while as sedatives. Ether and nitrous oxide produce an unconscious state and slow waves on the EEG. Perhaps these examples should be called sleeping pills as well. Pharmaceutical companies and physicians have been mistakenly considering any medication that sedates as a sleeping pill. In fact, the basic test used by pharmaceutical companies for evaluating sleeping medications is the loss of "righting reflex" in the mouse.

Sleeping pills are more accurately called CNS depressants because they bear no known relationship to the biology of sleep. Medications have been developed as though nothing was known about sleep. There are other approaches, perhaps some better sleeping pills, related to our knowledge of the biology of waking and sleeping. A considerable amount is known about the serotonin systems and there is good evidence that the brain serotonin systems are necessary (though not sufficient) for normal sleep. Thus, increasing serotonin levels or activity would be one possible approach. Dopamine activity has a lot to do with wakefulness and alertness; reducing dopamine activity would be expected to promote sleep. And there are some interesting natural peptides about which not very much is known—the nonapeptide, called "delta sleep-inducing peptide," discovered by Monnier's group in Switzerland[7] and the muramyl dipeptides studied by Pappenheimer and Karnovsky in Boston.[8] These naturally occurring peptides produce sleep in minute amounts. The peptides themselves or their analogs might be developed as sleeping medications.

These are all possible approaches to new and more natural, physiological sleeping pills, instead of simply CNS depressants. Our laboratory has done some work on the amino acid, L-tryptophan which of course is a natural food substance. It takes part in protein synthesis within the body and in a number of other pathways. But probably the most important for the purposes of this discussion is that it is a precursor of brain serotonin, 5-hydroxytryptamine. Interestingly enough, brain serotonin can very quickly and actively be influenced by simply feeding tryptophan.[9] Indeed, in a number of our studies on animals and on humans we found that feeding tryptophan produced sleepiness and induced sleep.[6,10] For instance, in investigating the effect of L-tryptophan, using doses of 0.25 g to 15 g, tryptophan did reduce sleep latency (time to sleep). There was a decrease of time to sleep with a 1-g dose and no further change with higher doses. This has been confirmed in a number of other studies, though there are also some contradictory data. It cannot be said at this point that tryptophan is a useful treatment for the world's insomniacs, but it is something to be considered for at least some insomniac patients. In a recently completed summary of 40 different studies of the world literature comparing tryptophan and placebo (author's unpublished data), most, but not all, showed a positive effect. The positive results were found expectedly in normal subjects with long latencies and in mild insomniacs. The results were more mixed in studies of normal subjects (in which there is little room for any improvement) and in serious insomniacs or patients with psychiatric problems. Tryptophan, then, is at least one possibility for a more rational hypnotic.

MEDICATION FOR INSOMNIA

When sleeping pills do need to be used — in other words, when symptomatic treatment is necessary — what current sleeping medication is best? When medication is required for one week or a few weeks for sleep, the most widely used one — flurazepam — is often a reasonable choice. An initial dose of 15 mg is preferred rather than the 30 mg recommended by the manufacturer. This has been found in my laboratory to be adequate in at least one half of the cases and is easier to discontinue.

The most frequent problem is prolonged effects or after-effects the following morning. Perhaps one-quarter of my patients taking flurazepam complain of grogginess the next morning. In those cases, one of the shorter acting benzodiazepines is a more reasonable choice. None of my patients has experienced "rebound insomnia" (increased wakings late during the night with a short-acting benzodiazepine, which suggests a CNS depressant effect followed by a rebound activation).

Several of the benzodiazepines are especially useful in certain situations. For instance, in patients who awaken with severe night terrors, no medication is usually required; but when medication is necessary, diazepam 5 mg at bedtime appears to be most effective. In some patients disturbed by repeated awakenings related to nocturnal myoclonus, clonazepam at bedtime usually is the drug of choice.

Editor's Note: The shorter acting benzodiazepines including alprazolam, lorazepam, oxazepam, and temazepam have elimination half-lives of approximately 12 hours, and thus may produce less daytime grogginess following nighttime administration for insomnia. A more recently marketed benzodiazepine, triazolam, has a rapid onset of action and an elimination half-life of two to three hours, two factors which are likely to enhance its clinical value as a hypnotic agent.[11] Continuing clinical experience with triazolam supports its efficacy as a hypnotic drug with less likelihood of accumulation and daytime sedation following repeated doses.[12] The very short half-life of this drug is an apparent advantage in the older patient who requires pharmacological intervention for insomnia. As with all benzodiazepines, long-term administration and abrupt discontinuation after a prolonged period of use is to be avoided because of the risk of physical dependence and the potential occurrence of withdrawal symptoms.

With the advent of newer drugs, barbiturates have become less important hypnotic medications, although one older drug, chloral hydrate, is still occasionally useful for insomnia. L-tryptophan, discussed above, as well as the antihistamines, should definitely be kept in mind for mild insomnia. I have obtained favorable reports from some physicians using tryptophan in several different situations. For example, in persons with insomnia after withdrawal from alcohol or addicting drugs, the physicians wanted to avoid giving an addict a new drug and were able to use tryptophan since it is a food substance. Many people are using tryptophan in place of over-the-counter medications for occasional difficulty in falling asleep. And, a number of nursing homes are using tryptophan in their elderly patients in preference to stronger medication, finding doses of 2 g to 4 g rather than 1 g to be necessary, but they are reporting positive results at these doses. In older patients, one should also consider the use of an antihistamine, such as diphenhydramine, before turning to long-term use of benzodiazepines, which may produce side effects in older patients, even at low doses.

One final point with regard to treatment: When is it necessary to treat insomnia at all? My detailed discussion of differential diagnoses may have given the impression that insomnia is a horrible problem which requires 10 hours of detailed work by a sleep specialist. Of course, this is not so! Insomnia often can be a very minor symptom of a minor anxiety, psychological disturbance or environmental change, or simply an exaggerated awareness by the patient of a normal aging process. When is insomnia worth taking seriously? One important guide is to pay special attention not to how sleep at night is described, but to how the person functions in the daytime. Someone can say, "I only sleep five hours a night and I wake five times every night." This may or may not be serious. If they also say that everything is going fine in the daytime, there is no need to be concerned. But if someone complains "I'm tired all day. I can't do my work; I'm irritable; I've lost interest in sex," this is something to worry about.

SUMMARY

In summary, the most important point is that insomnia is a symptom which has many causes and treatments. A wide range of treatments — some of them involving psychopharmacological agents — are appropriate in certain cases of insomnia. There are cases of insomnia (obstructive sleep apnea) in which surgery is the proper treatment. Others involve medical treatment for endocrine conditions. In thinking of the list of causes of insomnia, it will also be obvious that antipsychotic medication and antidepressant medication are sometimes the best treatment. Schedule changes, environmental changes, psychotherapy, and providing daytime activity for an elderly person are important as well.

Thus, treatment for insomnia should be treatment aimed at the cause, whenever possible. This can involve a number of treatment modalities, including at times psychopharmacology. When this is not possible — usually in short-term situations and symptomatic treatment — hypnotic medication becomes necessary, and the possibilities have been reviewed.

REFERENCES

1. Fischer-Perroudon C: *Insomnie Totale Pendant Plusieurs Mois et Métabolisme de la Sérotonine.* Lyon, Imprimerie des Beaux-Arts, 1973.
2. Hartmann E, Baekeland F, Zwilling GR: Psychological differences between long and short sleepers. *Arch Gen Psychiatry* 1972;26:463–468.
3. Hartmann E: *The Functions of Sleep.* New Haven, Yale University Press, 1973.
4. Carskadon M, Dement W, Mitler M, et al: Self-report vs. sleep laboratory findings in 122 drug-free subjects with complaints of chronic insomnia. *Am J Psychiatry* 1976;133:1382–1388.
5. Association of Sleep Disorders Centers: Diagnostic classification of sleep and arousal disorders. *Sleep* 1979;2:1–137.
6. Hartmann E: *The Sleeping Pill.* New Haven, Yale University Press, 1978.
7. Monnier M, Schoenberger GA: Characterization, sequence, synthesis and specificity of a delta (EEG) sleep-inducing peptide, in Koella WP, Levin P (eds): *Sleep 1976.* Basel, Karger, 1977, pp 257–263.
8. Pappenheimer JR, Koski G, Fencl V, et al: Extraction of sleep-promoting factor S from cerebrospinal fluid and from brains of sleep-deprived animals. *J Neurophysiol* 1975;38:1299–1311.
9. Fernstrom JD, Wurtman RJ: Brain serotonin content: Physiological dependence on plasma tryptophan levels. *Science* 1971;173:149–152.
10. Hartmann E: L-tryptophan: A rational hypnotic with clinical potential. *Am J Psychiatry* 1977;134:366–370.
11. Eberts FS Jr, Philopoulos Y, Reineke LK, et al: Triazolam disposition. *Clin Pharmacol Ther* 1981;29:81–93.
12. Settle EC Jr: Triazolam: The latest FDA approved hypnotic. *Int Drug Ther Newsletter* 1983;18:1–4.

10

Overview of Clinical Psychopharmacology in Childhood Disorders

Rachel Gittleman
Andres Kanner

In the pharmacologic treatment of childhood behavior disorders, the practitioner is faced with a tactical dilemma: should the treatment be determined by the presence of specific symptoms or behaviors — such as hyperactivity, anxiety, and temper tantrums, to name only a few, or should the therapeutic endeavor be targeted towards the amelioration of a constellation of symptoms which form a syndrome or diagnostic entity — such as hyperkinetic reaction or schizophrenia, childhood type? In other words, do we treat traits or illnesses?

In adult psychiatry, there is growing evidence that predictive validity for drug effects is enhanced by the use of a diagnostic approach. Thus, the treatment of "anxiety" will follow different patterns depending on whether one is dealing with anxious schizophrenic, anxious depressive, or anxious phobic patients. The observed relationship between treatment outcome and diagnosis has given support to the use of diagnostic classification.

The remaining challenge is often to refine criteria to maximize the usefulness of diagnostic entities in the prediction of treatment response. The degree to which we are able to determine therapeutic strategies for a specific diagnosis is a function of our state of knowledge. The fact that much of adult psychopharmacologic therapeutics is still aimed at discrete symptoms reflects a failure to understand fully, so far, the phenomenology and the diagnostic significance of these symptoms.

The above issues are most pertinent in childhood psychiatric disorders and in their psychopharmacologic management. In some cases, chemotherapy is clearly indicated on the basis of the diagnostic group (eg, attention deficit disorder); in others, it is directed at symptoms in a particular diagnostic group (eg, hyperactivity among "psychotic" children); and, in yet other instances, chemotherapy may be attempted for single-symptom removal (eg, temper tantrums). Consequently, the judicious use of medications in children requires consideration of the diagnostic process.

ATTENTION DEFICIT DISORDER WITH HYPERACTIVITY

The new diagnostic term "Attention Deficit Disorder with Hyperactivity" (ADDH) has substituted DSM-II's "Hyperactive reaction of childhood."[1] The redefinition of this disorder has introduced a set of clinical criteria which allows the clinician to discriminate a more homogeneous entity characterized by overactivity, impulsivity and poor attention span from a multiplicity of conduct and learning disorders.

The clinical characteristics of Attention Deficit Disorder with Hyperactivity (ADDH)[2] include:

1. Excessive motor activity: It was previously believed that children diagnosed as hyperactive were not more active, but that their activity was not goal oriented. This behavioral characteristic was believed to give the impression of overactivity. Recently, several investigators have documented that children diagnosed as hyperactive move more than other children. Rapoport[3] even has demonstrated that hyperactive children have increased motor activity during sleep. Excessive motor activity is more apparent at younger ages and, by the time the child reaches 7 or 8 years, it may be expressed in a more subtle form: the child is described as fidgety and restless, and older children can report verbally subjective feelings of restlessness. It is important to stress that this symptom needs to occur in different settings, but not in all, and it may not persist under certain circumstances, (ie, when alone with a parent who sets limits). Furthermore, the presence of this symptom is necessary but not sufficient for the diagnosis.

2. Attentional problems: The main characteristic of this symptom does not lie in the child's capacity to turn his attention to a task but, rather, it consists of the difficulty or incapacity in maintaining his attention once it is engaged. As with the problem of overactivity, poor attention need not be present in all situations.

3. Impulsivity: This term refers to a lack of forethought and planning in the regulation of behavior. We consider this symptom to be of central importance for the diagnosis of ADDH, for it discriminates true hyperactive children from normal children with a variant of motor activity at the high end of the spectrum.

Situational variability in the above mentioned symptoms – hyper-activity, poor attention, impulsivity is the rule. It is felt that children with ADDH are worse in situations that make demands for sustained effort, and that provide little structure.

Aside from these characteristics, children suffering from ADDH often have secondary symptoms such as poor frustration tolerance, poor peer relations, aggressivity, and poor academic performance. Aggression in these children is often different from that seen in children suffering from conduct disorder wherein aggressive, hyperactive children are frequently over-reacting to distressing or frustrating experiences. In conduct disorders, aggressive acts are often initiated by the child. The interaction of the secondary symptoms with the primary symptoms creates a vicious cycle which induces a spiralling effect and thus enhances the severity of the child's problems.

Contrary to prevalent beliefs, abnormal findings in EEG, in neurological examinations, or in psychometric tests are not helpful to the diagnosis of ADDH.

Psychopharmacologic Treatment

The pharmacologic armamentarium available today for the treatment of ADDH includes agents from the families of psychostimulants, neuroleptics, and tricyclic antidepressants.

Stimulants Since Bradley[4] in 1937 described the therapeutic effects of amphetamine in hyperactive children, the psychostimulants have remained, up to the present time, the treatment of choice for this disorder. The clinician can choose among the stimulants methylphenidate (Ritalin), dextroamphetamine (Dexedrine) or magnesium pemoline (Cylert). Their short-term usefulness has been demonstrated in several controlled studies, and a critical perusal of the literature clearly points to the conclusion that the therapeutic value of stimulants has been established for the amelioration of hyperactivity, impulsivity and short attention span. Furthermore, when children selected for treatment are considered hyperactive in several settings, the rate of success with stimulants has been reported to reach up to 90%. When treatment is fully effective, the hyperactive child becomes undistinguishable from normal children; not only does his behavior improve, but the teacher–child and parent–child interactions "normalize."

A note of caution is in order: Until 1978, it was believed that a positive response to a stimulant drug confirmed a diagnosis of ADDH. This was challenged by the demonstration that, following a single oral dose of dextroamphetamine, a group of normal boys showed decreased motor activity, increased vigilance, and improvement on a learning task.[5] Therefore, the nature of the drug effect cannot be construed as a diagnostic test.

Although the effectiveness of stimulant drugs in improving the child's hyperactivity and short attention span cannot be doubted, much debate exists regarding the effect of these drugs in improving cognitive functions and academic performance. In 1976, Gittelman et al[6] found that methylphenidate improved performance on psychometric tests in children with pure learning disorders. Nevertheless, such improvements were not reflected in the teachers' ratings of academic achievement, or in objective measures of achievement. It was concluded that the observed improvement in attention following stimulant treatment does not automatically ameliorate the acquisition of specific skills, such as reading, arithmetic, or memory.

Barkley and Cunningham[7] believed that the major effects of stimulants consist of an improvement in classroom manageability, not in the enhanced development of academic skills.

In a comprehensive review, Gadow[8] came to similar conclusions. In some hyperactive learning-disabled children, stimulants can enhance academic performance by increasing on task behavior, accuracy, and productivity. On the other hand, psychostimulants should not be used in nonhyperactive learning-disabled children.

Since the introduction of methylphenidate in the early 1960s, no clinical differences have been reported between this drug and dextroamphetamine. Both dextroamphetamine and methylphenidate are now available in two presentations: as a short-acting agent and in a sustained-release formulation. The sustained-release preparations do not always provide an even clinical effect throughout the day. However, the use of a single administration may be a real advantage in cases in which daytime dosage is problematic. Moreover, the simpler the regimen, the better the compliance. Dextroamphetamine is given at doses ranging from 5 to 40 mg/day and methylphenidate at doses ranging from 10 to 80 mg/day. Both drugs show immediate clinical effect, when given in appropriate doses.

Magnesium pemoline (Cylert) begins showing an effect two weeks after its initiation and induces maximal effect as late as the fifth or sixth week of treatment. Effective dosage ranges from 37.5 to 112.5 mg/day. It has a half-life of 12 hours, which should make it possible to be given in one single dose daily. However, multiple dosages may be necessary in some cases.

Unfortunately, magnesium pemoline has not been shown to be as consistently effective as the other two stimulants.

Pharmacokinetics The last four to five years have witnessed a great interest in the pharmacokinetics and clinical relevance of plasma levels of methylphenidate and dextroamphetamine. Recent studies have addressed one of the shortcomings of methylphenidate — its very short half-life. Hungund and Perel[9] explained that the short half-life of the drug (one- to three-hours) was related to its low protein binding, which resulted in rapid access to the CNS and a high percentage of its being available for metabolism into inactive compounds.

In looking at the clinical relevance of blood levels of these drugs, Brown et al[10] in 1979 reported that clinical response to dextro-amphetamine was not related to plasma levels. Winsberg et al[11] found a linear relationship between plasma levels, oral dose, and behavioral improvement in 14 hyperactive children.

On the other hand, Gualtieri,[12] in a study with 28 hyperactive children, did not find any relationship between plasma level and clinical response. Furthermore, he found marked inter- and intra-individual variability in plasma levels, the significance of which, at this point, is unclear.

In summary, at this time the plasma levels of psychostimulants are of no relevance to clinical practice.

Side effects In choosing a stimulant drug, the clinician takes into consideration clinical effectiveness and side effects. Loss or reduction of appetite and delay in onset of sleep occurs in 30% of children treated with moderately high doses of stimulants. More rarely, mood changes, consisting of interpersonal sensitivity, touchiness, and a sad demeanor, may occur. These side effects are present mostly in the beginning of treatment and often diminish over time. In a child who responds well, the untoward effect should not lead to a premature termination of treatment. At these times, the dosage should be lowered and subsequently increased very gradually.

The three stimulants differ in their degree of inhibiting growth in height and weight. Since Safer et al[13] identified this problem in 1972, much research has been underway to elucidate the drug's underlying mechanisms causing such effect.[14-18] Unfortunately, the literature on this issue is difficult to interpret because of the lack of uniform methodology in the different studies. Nevertheless, the following tentative conclusions can be suggested:

1. Dextroamphetamine and methylphenidate can decrease weight gain and it may also depress height velocity.

2. Dextroamphetamine seems to have more growth inhibiting effect than other psychostimulants.[18]

3. The growth-inhibiting effect seems related to total cumulative dose.[18]

4. Rebound growth acceleration for height and weight occurs following the discontinuation of the drugs. Thus, drug holidays during weekends and summer vacations are advisable when clinically feasible.[20]

5. The mechanisms by which psychostimulants affect growth are not yet known. Human growth hormone secretion does not seem to be affected. On the basis of in vitro studies, Kilgore[21] has suggested that psychostimulants may affect growth through the inhibition of somato-

medins. In vivo investigations of this issue have not been carried out as yet.

6. The final height of children treated with methylphenidate does not appear compromised.

Length of therapy Although the short-term effectiveness of the stimulants has been widely accepted, the ultimate benefits of treatment are debated. Several studies have looked at the relationship between the length of time on stimulants and the outcome of behavioral and social problems, as well as of academic achievement. In general, their observations suggest that treatment does not appear to modify the long-term outcome of hyperactive children. One has to consider with caution such conclusions, since many of these studies suffer from serious methodological flaws.

It is our recommendation that children should be maintained on their medication for as long as they need it. Following the discontinuation of the stimulant during a summer vacation, the clinician can assess the adjustment of the child upon return to school after the first month. The recurrence of symptoms will indicate the need to continue treatment.

The old theory which postulated that ADDH constituted a maturational lag that did not linger beyond puberty has been shown to have been overoptimistic. Recent studies in adolescents and adults who had a history of ADDH in childhood suggest that: 1) the symptoms may diminish over time, but they often persist into adulthood.[22] Thus, the pharmacologic treatment of this disorder should not be considered only for prepubertal children; 2) the use of psychostimulants may be effective in adolescents with ADDH. Unfortunately, there are no controlled trials to confirm this clinical observation; and 3) the use of psychostimulants during childhood has not been associated with increased drug abuse during adolescence. In cases in which the clinician is concerned about such potential, magnesium pemoline may be tried since it is devoid of the euphoric effect that the other two stimulants may have.

Neuroleptic drugs Total refractoriness to the treatment with psychostimulants is rare — about 10% to 20%. In these instances, the clinician will have to choose among the drugs belonging to the families of neuroleptics or tricyclic antidepressants.

In general, the experience with neuroleptics in the treatment of ADDH has shown that these drugs are effective in improving the child's behavior, but their overall effect is much less broad than that of the stimulants. Chlorpromazine and thioridazine have been the drugs most widely used in clinical trials. In separate studies, Rapoport et al[23] and Werry et al[24] found chlorpromazine to decrease overactivity but not to improve distractibility. On the other hand, Gittelman-Klein et al[25] found that thioridazine was effective in improving hyperactivity and short attention, but this effect was mostly apparent during the first four weeks of treatment and it decreased thereafter.

Werry and Aman[26] used haloperidol in a group of hyperactive children and, although the response to the drug was favorable, it was not impressive.

The dosage of chlorpromazine and thioridazine often needs to be increased up to 200 mg/day. Usually, no clinical advantage is accrued beyond this level and side effects increase considerably. Drowsiness is the most common side effect. A change in schedule of drug administration may reduce this problem, but it is often difficult to eliminate it.

The concern that neuroleptics impair cognitive function in hyperactive children is not based on objective data.

Finally, in using neuroleptic drugs, the clinician must be aware of the potential long-term side effects such as tardive dyskinesia. Although tardive dyskinesia has not been identified yet in nonretarded children, withdrawal dyskinesias have been described. This problem is addressed in the discussion on conduct disorders.

Tricyclic antidepressants Tricyclic antidepressants have been found to be superior to placebo in different studies of hyperactive children. Nevertheless, in a review of the literature, Gittelman[2] suggests that, as with the neuroleptic drugs, their effectiveness is not very consistent. Furthermore, studies by Gittelman,[27] and Quinn and Rapoport[28,29] noted that, even when children treated with imipramine showed as good an initial response as with methylphenidate, such effects often disappeared or decreased after a short time (about six weeks or so).

In treating hyperactive children with tricyclics, the clinician must consider the cardiotoxic effects of the medication. A series of precautions, which are described in the section on depression, must be followed.

Finally, the determination of the dose to be used should follow the same principles as outlined for the treatment of depression.

Nontreatment factors influencing drug response Empirical findings in regard to the contention that medications have a selective effect on brain-damaged hyperactive children are ambiguous. Satterfield et al[30] have reported greater improvement with drug treatment in those children with minimal brain dysfunction who show both electroencephalographic and neurologic abnormalities than in those children with minimal brain dysfunction who show neither of these abnormalities. However, the proportions of children who improved in each group did not differ statistically. It is conceivable that children with both electroencephalographic and neurologic abnormalities were more behaviorally disturbed, so that the difference in degree of improvement might reflect differences in symptomatology

A similar problem exists in a study on dextroamphetamine which reports a relationship between clinical neurologic signs and treatment response.[31] The actual contribution of organicity to outcome remains unclear since there was a positive relationship between organicity and the initial level of hyperkinesis.

There is some, but not conclusive, evidence that neurologic dysfunction plays a role in mediating the response of hyperkinetic children to stimulants. The clinical lesson to be derived from the studies seems to be that neurologically impaired children with a less than clear-cut pattern of hyperkinesis should be given a trial of stimulant administration. On the other hand, no child who displays the symptoms of a hyperkinetic reaction, without neurologic signs, should be deprived on that basis of the opportunity to receive a trial of stimulant treatment.

In addition to the role of brain dysfunction in mediating drug response, the relationship of clinical improvement to other physiologic characteristics, such as skin resistance and central nervous system evoked potentials, has been examined. The work has considerable theoretical importance but little clinical significance, and there is no reason to recommend that physicians obtain these technologically difficult measures.

Aspects of psychopathology not related to diagnosis, such as severity or stability of symptoms, do not discriminate between responders and nonresponders. Environmental factors, such as quality of home and mother–child relationship, have also failed to relate to drug therapy outcome.

There is a disproportionate number of boys among hyperkinetic youngsters, but sex has not been found to be associated with improvement. On the other hand, young, preschool hyperactive children show a more variable response to the stimulants. The lack of drug effect in a large proportion of very young children as compared to older ones may reflect greater diagnostic ambiguity, and therefore diagnostic inaccuracy, among the younger group. At the same time, it is conceivable that there is an age-related physiologic variability that affects drug response.

In summary, it appears that brain dysfunction and the level of physiologic reactivity may be relevant dimensions in the prediction of drug effects among hyperactive children, but these factors are of no practical value for clinical management. Much controversy surrounds the use of medications for the management of behavior disorders in children. Behavior therapy has been suggested as an effective alternative to drugs. Indeed, some investigators have demonstrated the clinical efficacy of behavioral techniques in hyperactive children. The therapeutic impact of methylphenidate is much superior to that of behavior therapy. Therefore, though the behavioral techniques may be useful, they are not the most effective interventions in hyperkinetic children.[32]

AFFECTIVE DISORDERS OF CHILDHOOD AND ADOLESCENCE
Depressive Disorder

Over the past four years, researchers have been attempting to answer one of the most controversial questions in child psychiatry: Do prepubertal children suffer from major depressive disorders? In 1978, Puig-Antich et al[33] published a pilot study which suggested that children displayed a disorder similar to the major depressive disorders of adulthood. Using the Research Diagnostic Criteria (RDC) as a screening instrument, the authors identified 13 prepubertal children as depressed. All suffered as well from separation anxiety disorder and five of them also had conduct disorder.

Carlson and Cantwell,[34] using the same approach, identified 28 children and adolescents (7 to 17 years) with major depressive disorders among a population of 102 consecutive admissions to a child psychiatric service. Eight of these depressed children presented a concomitant conduct disorder. Kupferman and Stewart[35] found that among 175 consecutive admissions, 13% of the girls and 5% of the boys met adult criteria for major depressive disorder.

The acceptance of major depressive disorder of childhood and adolescence as a diagnostic entity is reflected by its definition in the DSM-III as similar to the disorder in adults. The incidence of depressive disorder in prepubertal children is less than that in adolecents. In an epidemiological survey in the Isle of Wight, Rutter[36] identified three depressed children among 2193 prepubertal subjects and 35 depressed adolescents among 2303 14-year-olds.

In the last three years, Puig-Antich et al[37,38] have tried to establish the validity of the diagnosis by attempting to replicate neuroendocrine and polysomnographic findings reported in adults suffering from major depressive disorders. Among the neuroendocrine tests shown to be associated with major depressive disorder of adults are the following: 1) circadian rhythms of plasma cortisol and, 2) growth hormone response to insulin-induced hypoglycemia. Puig-Antich et al[38] have reported that two of four depressed prepubertal children showed hypersecretion of cortisol when measured during a 24-hour period. Poznansky[39] reported the same phenomenon in five of nine children with major depressive disorder, as reflected by a nonsuppressive response of the dexamethasone suppression test. This test was abnormal in 50% of her sample, a frequency similar to that described for adolescents[40,41] and adults.[42] Others have published similar data. The levels of growth hormones in response to insulin-induced hypoglycemia were found to be decreased (below 4 ng/mL) in nine of 10 endogenous depressed, four of 10 nonendogenous depressed children and in none of seven nondepressed emotionally ill children.[37] These results are still preliminary. If sustained, they will provide evidence supporting the existence of major depressive disorder in childhood.

Pharmacologic Treatment

The pharmacologic literature of the depressive disorder of childhood up to 1977 is difficult to interpret because the reported studies lack consistent standards for diagnosis and used vastly different treatment procedures. Recent studies have been more satisfactory. In 1978, Puig-Antich[33] reported an open trial with imipramine in eight children with an average age of 9.6 years (range 6 to 12). The children received an average dose of 4 mg/kg/day. Seven of the eight patients responded over six to eight weeks. Following this open trial, Puig-Antich[43] and his group undertook a five-week, double-blind placebo-controlled study. He reported an overall drug response rate of 60%, equal to the placebo response. Children with total plasma levels (imipramine and desipramine) above 142 ng/mL had a 100% response rate to the drug versus 33% for those children who had lower levels. This clinical finding, if replicated, will support the usefulness of imipramine at certain plasma concentrations, in prepubertal depression.

On the other hand, Puig-Antich failed to replicate this finding in a study of 33 depressed adolescents. (Personal communication.)

Petti et al[44] conducted a six-week placebo controlled trial with imipramine among six prepubertal children who met diagnostic criteria for major depressive disorder. On a dose equivalent to 5 mg/kg/day, two of the three children on the active medication responded favorably versus one of three on the placebo. Unfortunately, the sample is too small to permit even tentative conclusions.

The paucity of good psychopharmacologic studies does not allow yet for definite claims that tricyclic medication is clinically effective. The clinician may start with a dose of 25 mg/day and increase it by 50 mg every fourth day until an adequate clinical response is obtained, significant side effects occur, or a maximum dose equivalent to 5 mg/kg/day (or a total maximum dose of 300 mg/day) is reached.

In administering imipramine, the clinician must be aware of the following potential EKG changes which have been reported to occur with this drug and which could elicit arrhythmias if not monitored appropriately: increase in the PR interval and widening of the QRS complex. It is helpful to obtain an EKG before treatment and again at the time the dose is increased beyond the equivalent dose of 3.5 mg/kg/day (Saraf et al[45]). Dosage should be lowered in the presence of a PR interval >0.21 sec, or QRS widening exceeding 30% of pretreatment duration. Increased heart rate often occurs, but is not a source of concern unless tachycardia is observed. This is a rare phenomenon. Imipramine may also cause postural hypotension. If mild orthostatic hypotension occurs, it can be avoided by instructing the patient not to stand up abruptly. Other side effects to keep in mind include dry mouth, drowsiness, constipation, and, more rarely, changes in appetite. In most cases, the drug trial should be continued for three months, after which the dose should be tapered off slowly over a two- to three-week period.

Manic Disorders

It has been a general consensus that manic disorders are extremely rare in prepubertal children and only occasional single case reports have been published. On the other hand, mania has been described more frequently during adolescence, but not as frequently as during adult life. Recent studies suggest that the frequency of mania in adolescence has been underestimated. This has been manifested by the overdiagnosis of psychotic episodes as schizophrenia, that, when reviewed retrospectively, consisted of mania.[46,47] The differentiation of the two conditions may at times be very difficult and the correct diagnosis may have to await a subsequent psychotic break. Nevertheless, the presence of periodicity in the manifestation of the symptoms and a marked affective component in the clinical picture should alert the clinician to the possibility of mania during adolescence.[48] The pharmacologic treatment of a manic episode is aimed at inducing its remission and providing prophylaxis to avoid further psychotic breaks.

From a review of the literature, Puig-Antich[48] suggested "that youngsters with bipolar illness may be as responsive to lithium as adults with the same diagnosis." After reviewing 46 records of children and adolescents treated with lithium, Youngerman and Canino[49] concluded that the presence of affective illness in the child's family predicted a good response to lithium. Furthermore, when parents and their offspring suffer from bipolar illness, a favorable response to lithium in one may predict effectiveness of lithium in the other.[50]

For prescribing lithium, the clinician should titrate the dose to blood levels between 0.6 and 1.2 mEq/L. Since children have higher lithium renal clearance than adults, they need to be given larger oral doses to reach the same serum level. When using lithium, the clinician should be aware that our experience with this drug is limited in children and some questions remain unanswered. For instance, we know that lithium accumulates in bone tissue, and it has been reported to have an inhibitory effect on the bone size of growing rats.[51] The issue of growth in lithium-treated children is still unresolved. In all other respects, the monitoring of lithium-treated adolescents should follow the procedures applied to adults.

ANXIETY DISORDERS OF CHILDHOOD AND ADOLESCENCE

Severely disturbed, psychotic children who often display anxious mood and behavior are excluded from consideration here. There are four basic types of anxiety that may occur singly or in combination in children and adolescents.

The first, social anxiety, is related to a sense of embarrassment and fear of humiliation and ridicule, and is described in DSM-III under the diagnostic term of "Avoidant Disorder of Childhood and Adolescence."

A second pattern of anxiety in children, labeled "Overanxious Disorder" in DSM-III, relates to a performance anxiety, which stems from a fear of failure and incompetence.

The third form of anxiety disorder includes the different phobias (animals, insects, etc), which when transitory and occurring around the age of four may not be of pathologic significance.

Separation anxiety is the fourth type of anxiety and consists of the fear of losing a beloved one or a close attachment. This is the only childhood anxiety disorder whose psychopharmacologic treatment has been studied in a controlled manner and, therefore, will be considered here in more detail. In moderation, this anxiety is not pathologic, but it may become so severe that the child experiences marked difficulties separating from the parents or home. Such children may become dysfunctional. In the extreme, they cannot attend school or participate in many activities, such as visiting friends, going shopping, or going to camp, which calls for separation.

The genesis of pathologic separation anxiety is very different from that of most of the other childhood disorders that tend to be chronic. In contrast, separation anxiety may come on quite suddenly, in a matter of a few weeks, in children whose adjustment was previously unremarkable. In about 80% of the cases, it follows a change in the child's environment, such as a move, school change, illness, or loss of a relative. The disorder tends to be self-limiting and spontaneous remissions occur regularly. Nevertheless, in some instances the affected period may be extended and last for years. The disorder occurs equally often in boys and girls. The clinical syndrome has been described widely; children with the disorder experience anxiety to the point of panic when separation is attempted. They are plagued with morbid fears and worries concerning their parents' welfare, or sometimes their own. They tend to be clinging, demanding children. During the acute phase of the illness, they are extremely manipulative and may become incensed, even aggressive, if they are forced into situations that make them anxious. The anxiety often has marked diurnal fluctuations, worsening in the morning and evening. Psychophysiologic symptoms are common and usually consist of stomachaches, nausea, or vague aches and pains.

Children with severe separation anxiety are often described as depressed. They do not, however, exhibit the anhedonia or the pessimism typical of adult depressives. The sad look they regularly present when seen professionally can be viewed as being a reaction to being confronted with their difficulties. When no demands or threats of separation are made, the children can enjoy themselves easily. Therefore, it is felt that it is diagnostically erroneous to consider pathologic separation anxiety the equivalent of adult depressive disorder. Some argue that the onset of this disorder in adolescence is a harbinger of severe pathology such as schizophrenia. We have found no evidence for this clinical claim. Age is not associated with a differential drug response.

School phobia is the expression of the most severe form of separation anxiety. A clinical study with 28 school phobic children reported good effects with imipramine.[52] In a subsequent double-blind, placebo-controlled six-week study, among 45 children who refused to go to school, imipramine was clearly superior to placebo.[53]

The effects of imipramine can be very marked among children and adolescents with severe separation anxiety. In some cases the effect is noticeable within as little as a week, but most children required three to four weeks of treatment before symptom amelioration clearly occurred. Good clinical results may be very dramatic; the child becomes totally free of morbid preoccupations. However, the child still retains the conviction that the previous worries will return to plague him, and he will continue to resist separation. Therefore, the pharmacologic treatment of this childhood disorder regularly needs to be combined with a vigorous therapeutic effort aimed at reducing anticipatory anxiety.

Dosages up to 5 mg/kg per day of imipramine are typically necessary with treatment of the severe forms of separation anxiety. The clinician may use up to the equivalent dose of 5 mg/kg/day, and should follow the same guidelines and precautionary steps described in the section on depressive disorders. Many patients treated with imipramine require six to eight weeks of treatment to attain clinical amelioration. Following this period, imipramine dosage usually can be lowered to a maintenance level approximately one-half that of the maximum therapeutic dose. Further, if a patient has not responded to imipramine at higher doses within six to eight weeks, it is quite unlikely that there will be response to continued imipramine treatment.

The use of imipramine in children with severe separation anxiety can be of relatively short duration. In most cases administration of imipramine need not be long term, and frequently children remain symptom-free after a three- or four-month treatment period. Since children are susceptible to withdrawal symptoms from imipramine (nausea, stomachache), the dosage should be reduced gradually over a two-week period.

OBSESSIVE COMPULSIVE DISORDER

Obsessive compulsive disorder is a rare illness which occurs in about 1% of child psychiatric populations. In the last decade, pharmacologic treatment in adult patients suffering from this condition has gained increasing interest. The use of chlorimipramine has yielded positive results in decreasing the severity of obsessive and compulsive symptoms, allowing patients to function in spite of them. Tricyclic antidepressants such as imipramine, doxepin, amitriptyline,[54,55] as well as MAO inhibitors have also have been reported to be successful in isolated cases. On the other hand, in the only controlled study done with adolescents, Rapoport[56] did not find chlorimipramine or desipramine to be superior to placebo among a sample of nine adolescents. Each drug was given for three to five weeks and at a maximum dose of 150 mg/day. The short treatment period and relatively low doses may have been limiting factors, as suggested by Insel and Murphy,[57] who, in reviewing all the pharmacologic studies available up until 1981, concluded that "these patients need to be treated longer and with larger dosages than depressed patients, there being few responders in the early weeks of treatment."

We treated a 14-year-old adolescent with amitriptyline at a dose of 300 mg/day (equivalent to 5 mg/kg/day) for eight months and observed a disappearance of his compulsions and a partial decrease in his obsessions after six to eight weeks of treatment at this dose.

The pharmacologic treatment in obsessive-compulsive disorder of childhood and adolescence needs to be studied further. Meanwhile, the clinician should be aware of the potential benefit of pharmacologic agents in the treatment of this condition. Since chlorimipramine is not yet available in the United States, amitriptyline may be used in doses up to 5 mg/kg/day. The same precautions outlined for imipramine in the section on depressive disorders should be followed when using amitriptyline.

PERVASIVE DEVELOPMENTAL DISORDERS

The disorders grouped in this class include those reflecting difficulties in several developmental functions such as communicative language, social skills, intellectual functions and emotional development.

They replace the DSM-II classifications of schizophrenia, childhood type. The entities comprising the pervasive development disorders include infantile autism and pervasive developmental disorder of childhood onset. Schizophrenia is a very rare condition in children and usually is not manifest before the age of 8. The diagnostic evaluation and treatment of such children should follow the same principles as those of adult schizophrenia.

Infantile autism begins very early in life; usually well before the age of 30 months, and is characterized by lack of response to other people (autism) and gross deficit in language development. If present, speech is abnormal, consisting of patterns such as immediate and delayed echolalia, metaphorical language and pronominal reversals. Finally, the child may show an interest in or fascination with unusual objects and refuses to allow any changes or disruptions from his/her attachment to them.

The clinical characteristics of childhood onset pervasive developmental disorders include impaired social and emotional functioning as well as the presence of bizarre behaviors, including illogical anxiety, unexplained fears and panics, lack of appreciation of realistic dangers, lack of appropriate fears, extreme sudden rage reactions, extreme mood changes, self-mutilations, peculiar mannerisms, hyperactivity, and lethargy. It differs from infantile autism in that its onset occurs after 30 months of age, and from childhood schizophrenia by the absence of delusions, hallucinations, and of formal thought disorders.

The pharmacologic treatment for these conditions consists of the use of neuroleptics aimed at controlling the marked agitation, hyperactivity, and destructive behavior of the child. Successful pharmacotherapy can prevent institutionalization by making the child more manageable so he/she can remain at home. The doses of neuroleptics used in these conditions may be higher than those given to children suffering from attention deficit disorder with hyperactivity or conduct disorders; these high doses are often well tolerated. Thus, chlorpromazine and thioridazine have been given in doses of up to 400 mg/day, haloperidol and fluphenazine up to 20 mg/day.

Campbell et al[58,59] reported that haloperidol combined with behavioral therapy was more effective than placebo in decreasing stereotypy and withdrawal in autistic children aged 4 years or older. Haloperidol did not affect other behaviors (activity level, angry affect, abnormal object relations). Dosages were low (the average dose was below 2 mg/day); higher doses might result in better effects.

The clinician should remember that children with pervasive developmental disorders present sterotypies, mannerisms, or tics which may disappear when neuroleptics are started. Upon withdrawal of the drug, the same movements may reappear. Thus, the clinician should not confuse them with withdrawal emergent symptoms or tardive dyskinesias.

CONDUCT DISORDERS

The literature on the pharmacotherapy of conduct disorders should be considered with caution since aggressive and nonaggressive conduct disorders appear in children and adolescents who suffer from different psychiatric and/or neurological disorders. Aggressive behavior can be associated with depressive disorders, attention deficit with hyperactivity, mental retardation, or with nonspecific organic brain dysfunction. In a recent report, Puig-Antich et al[60] described 16 children diagnosed as having both a major depressive disorder and conduct disorder. In the 13 cases who had a full response to imipramine, the conduct disorder disappeared in 11 cases following the antidepressant response. Therefore, in trying to determine the appropriate treatment, a comprehensive psychiatric evaluation is essential.

The drugs used in the treatment of aggressive disorders include lithium, neuroleptics, and psychostimulants. In the last two years, propranolol, given in high doses, has been reported effective in rage attacks.

To summarize the evidence:

1. Psychostimulants are indicated in children with conduct disorders if an attention disorder with hyperactivity is also present.[2]

2. Lithium has been reported to decrease aggressiveness in autistic and mentally retarded children[61] as well as in nonpsychotic children of normal intelligence.[62,63] In a recent study, Campbell et al[64] found lithium to be as effective as haloperidol in decreasing aggressive behaviors in children with undersocialized aggressive conduct disorder. Furthermore, lithium was found to have less disturbing side effects than haloperidol. Lithium may be considered as a potential drug in treating aggressive children since, when administered at appropriate doses and monitored carefully, it is devoid of the long-term side effects of neuroleptic drugs.[65-68] The dosages and precautions to be followed when using this drug are described in the section on manic disorder.

3. The neuroleptics are the drugs more commonly used today for the treatment of aggressive children and adolescents in psychiatric hospitals and outpatient clinics. An adequate response may be obtained with doses equivalent to 200 to 300 mg/day of chlorpromazine, although higher doses may be necessary. Despite the effectiveness of neuroleptics, the presence of drowsiness, weight gain, dermatosis, and acute, as well as potential long-term extrapyramidal side effects, should alert the clinician to using these drugs for extended periods only when other approaches have failed.

Gualtieri et al,[69] in a review of the literature, suggested that

> Tardive dyskinesia may occur in children and adolescents of all age groups and it can be seen with low doses and short term treatment; it is not always reversible and its manifestations are more varied than in adult groups — ie, facial tics and grimaces, choreoathetoid, ballistic and myoclonic movements of the extremities and trunk, ataxia; the involuntary movements usually do not involve the buccolingual area, in contrast to what occurs in adults. . . .

Withdrawal symptoms with or without dyskinetic movements seem to occur more frequently in children and adolescents than in adults.

The dyskinetic movements appear within one to 15

days after withdrawal of the drug. In 50% of the cases, the symptoms remit spontaneously within one to two weeks, and they are regularly reversible with reinstitution of treatment. It is very difficult to differentiate them from tardive dyskinesia, except for the concomitant presence of other symptoms of withdrawal, such as nausea and vomiting,[70] and the fact that they disappear within six months after cessation of the drug. Their incidence is related to total dose exposure and length of treatment. Drugs seem to vary in their contributions to neurologic withdrawal symptoms. These symptoms seem more likely to occur with the use of high-potency neuroleptics such as fluphenazine or thiothixene (50% to 80% of cases) than with the low-potency ones such as chlorprothixene or thioridazine (10% to 30%).

4. In a clinical study, Williams et al[71] reported improvement in more than 75% of 30 patients — of which 11 were children and 15 adolescents — who were treated with high doses of propranolol (range 50 to 960 mg/day). All had uncontrolled rage outbursts over a period of at least six months. All of these patients had concomitant organic brain dysfunction ranging from minimal brain dysfunction (MBD) to severe uncontrolled seizures, and all of them had been refractory to different pharmacologic trials, including neuroleptics, psychostimulants, anticonvulsants, or a combination of these. Despite the relative high doses of propranolol used, the side effects observed were transitory and reversible and mainly included drowsiness and hypotension.

GENERAL CLINICAL CONSIDERATIONS

Certain practices that are extremely helpful yet often neglected in the pharmacologic treatment of childhood disorders deserve mention. For example, sources of information regarding a child's response to treatment should not be limited to the parents. Schools should always be consulted if the child's symptoms are manifest in the classroom setting, as well as at home. In some cases, even if there are no complaints from school, teachers should be queried to ascertain that side effects such as drowsiness are not interfering with the child's academic performance. Input from the school also is often helpful in formulating a diagnosis.

Dosage levels are variable and there are no guidelines (such as age, weight, or body surface) to indicate a specific dosage range. Therefore, a flexible approach is necessary. If a child who has obtained good results with a drug deteriorates, it should not be asumed that the medication is no longer effective. Often, increments in dosage will reestablish a positive response. Children on medication should be followed on a regular basis to evaluate their status as regards side effects and continued need for drug treatment. (Many children who have been prescribed low dosages of medication are kept on these for extended periods of time and are never examined again.) Also, children should be given "off-drug" periods, or "drug holidays," to determine the ongoing clinical usefulness of the drug and to minimize whatever deleterious effects might potentially be associated with the medication.

Parents should never be left to regulate dosage or to make decisions to terminate or continue treatment. They may overreact to minor or temporary changes in behavior; they may underestimate the degree of the child's difficulty, or they may use the medication in a punitive fashion. Therefore, medication adjustments should reflect a consensus between the family and the physician.

Finally, it is unusual for medication to be the sole intervention necessary (except in some cases of hyperkinesis in which stimulants completely eliminate symptoms and the parent–child relationships are good). Medication can rarely be viewed as a total treatment in children with behavior disorders.

This summary of childhood psychopharmacology is not exhaustive. Consultation of a fuller review is recommended for further information.

REFERENCES

1. *Diagnostic and Statistical Manual of Mental Disorders*, ed 3. Washington DC, American Psychiatric Association, 1980.
2. Klein DF, Gittelman R, Quitkin F, et al (eds): Diagnosis and drug treatment of childhood disorders, in: *Diagnosis and Drug Treatment of Psychiatric Disorders: Adults and Children*. Baltimore, Williams & Wilkins, 1980, pp 590–775.
3. Rapoport J, Porrino L, Behar D, et al: *Twenty-four Hour Activity in Hyperactive and Control Boys. A Naturalistic Study*. Presented at the annual meeting of the American Academy of Child Psychiatry, Dallas, Texas, October 17, 1981.
4. Bradley C: The behavior of children receiving benzedrine. *Amer J Child Psychiatry* 1937;94:577–585.
5. Rapoport JL, Buchsbaum MS, Weingartner H, et al: Dextroamphetamine: Its cognitive and behavioral effects in normal and hyperactive boys and normal men. *Arch Gen Psychiatry* 1980;37:933–943.
6. Gittelman-Klein R, Klein DF: Methylphenidate in learning disabilities. *Arch Gen Psychiatry* 1976;33:655–664.
7. Barkley RA, Cunningham CE: Do stimulant drugs improve the academic performance of hyperkinetic children? *Clin Pediatr* 1978;17:85–92.
8. Gadow KD: Effects of stimulant drugs on academic achievement in hyperactive and learning disabled children. (Submitted for publication.)
9. Hungund BL, Perel JM, Hurwic MC, et al: Pharmacokinetics of methylphenidate in hyperkinetic children. *Br J Clin Pharmacol* 1979;8: 571–576.
10. Brown GL, Ebert MH, Mikkelsen EJ, et al: Behavior and motor activity response in hyperactive children and plasma amphetamine levels following a sustained release preparation. *J Am Acad Child Psychiatry* 1980;19:225–239.
11. Winsberg BG, Kupietz SS, Sverd J, et al: Methylphenidate oral dose plasma concentrations and behavioral responses in children. *Psychopharmacology* Berlin, 1982;76:329–332.
12. Gualtieri T, Wargin W, Kanoy R, et al: Clinical studies of methylphenidate serum levels in children and adults. *J Am Acad Child Psychiatry* 1982;21: 19–26.
13. Safer D, Allen R, Barr E: Depression of growth in hyperactive children on stimulant drugs. *N Engl J Med* 1972;287:217.
14. Puig-Antich J, Greenhill LL, Sassin J, et al: Growth hormone, prolactin and cortisol responses and growth patterns in hyperkinetic children treated with dextroamphetamine. *J Am Acad Child Psychiatry* 1978;17:457–475.
15. Greenhill LL, Puig-Antich J, Chambers W, et al: Growth hormone, prolactin and growth responses in hyperkinetic males treated with d-amphetamine. *J Am Acad Child Psychiatry* 1981;20:84–103.
16. Greenhill LL, Puig-Antich J, Sachar E: Hormone and growth responses in hyperkinetic children on stimulant medication. *Psychopharm Bull* 1977;13: 33–35.
17. Schultz FR, Hayford JT, Wolraich ML, et al: Methylphenidate treatment of hyperactive children: effects on the hypothalamic-pituitary-somatomedin axis. *Pediatrics* 1982;70(6):987–992.
18. Greenhill LL: Stimulant-related growth inhibition in children: A review. In Gittelman R (ed): *Strategic Interventions for Hyperactive Children*. Armonk NY, ME Sharpe, 1981, pp 39–63.
19. Mattes JA, Gittelman R: Growth of hyperactive children on maintenance regimen of methylphenidate. Arch Gen Psychiatry 1983;40:317–321.

20. Safer DJ, Allen RP, Barr E: Growth rebound after termination of stimulant drugs. *J Pediatr* 1975;86(1):113–116.

21. Kilgore B, Dickinson L, Burnett CR, et al: Alterations in cartilage metabolism by neurostimulant drugs. *J Pediatr* 1979;94:542.

22. Weiss G, Hechtman L, Perlman T, et al: Hyperactives as young adults. *Arch Gen Psychiatry* 1979;36:675–681.

23. Rapoport JL, Abramson A, Alexander D: Playroom observations of hyperactive children on medication. *J Am Acad Child Psychiatry* 1971;10:524–534.

24. Werry JS, Weiss G; Studies on the hyperactive child III. The effect of chlorpromazine upon behavior and learning ability. *J Am Acad Child Psychiatry* 1966;5:292–312.

25. Gittelman-Klein R, Klein DF, Katz S, et al: Comparative effects of methylphenidate and thyroidazine in hyperkinetic children. *Arch Gen Psychiatry* 1976;33:1217–1231.

26. Werry J, Aman MG: Haloperidol and methylphenidate in hyperactive children. *Acta Paedopsychiatr (Basel)* 1976;42:26–40.

27. Gittelman-Klein R: Pilot clinical trial of imipramine on hyperkinetic children, in Conners CK (ed): *Clinical Use of Stimulant Drugs on Children*. The Hague, Excerpta Medica, 1974, pp 192–201.

28. Quinn PO, Rapoport JL: One year follow-up of hyperactive boys treated with imipramine or methylphenidate. *Am J Psychiatry* 1975;132:241–245.

29. Rapoport JL, Quinn PO, Bradbard G, et al: Imipramine and methylphenidate treatments of hyperactive boys: A double-blind comparison. *Arch Gen Psychiatry* 1974;30:789–793.

30. Satterfield JH, Cantwell DP, Lesser LJ, et al: Physiological studies of the hyperkinetic child. *Am J Psychiatry* 1972;128:102–108.

31. Steinberg GS, Troshinsky C, Steinberg HC: Dextroamphetamine-responsive behavior in school children. *Am J Psychiatry* 1971;128:174–179.

32. Gittelman-Klein R, Klein DF, Abikoff H, et al: Relative efficacy of behavior modification and methylphenidate in hyperkinetic children: An interim report. *J Abnorm Child Psychol* 1976;4:361–379.

33. Puig-Antich J, Blau S, Marx N, et al: Prepubertal major depressive disorder. Pilot study. *J Am Acad Child Psychiatry* 1978;17:695–707.

34. Carlsson G, Cantwell D: Unmasking masked depression in children and adolescents. *Am J Psychiatry* 1980;137:445–449.

35. Kupferman S, Stewart MA: The diagnosis of depression in children. *J Affective Disord* 1979;1:213–217.

36. Rutter M, Tizard J, Whitmore K: *Education, Health and Behavior*. London, Longman, 1970.

37. Puig-Antich J, Gittelman R: Depression in childhood and adolescence. in Paykel ES (ed): *Handbook of Affective Disorders*. New York, Guilford Press, 1981.

38. Puig-Antich J, Chambers W, Halpern F, et al: Cortisol hypersecretion in prepubertal depressive illness. *Psychoneuroendocrinology* 1979;4:191–197.

39. Poznanski E, Carrol B, Benegas M, et al: The dexamethasone suppression test in prepubertal depressed children. *Am J Psychiatry* 1982;139:321–324.

40. Crumley FE, Clevenger J, Steinfink D, et al: Preliminary report on the dexamethasone suppression test for psychiatrically disturbed adolescents. *Am J Psychiatry* 1982;139:1062–1064.

41. Robbins DR, Alessi NE, Yanchyssyn GW, et al: Preliminary report on the dexamethasone suppression test in adolescents. *Am J Psychiatry* 1982;139: 942–943.

42. Carrol BJ: The dexamethasone suppression test for melancholia. *Br J*

Psychiatry 1982;140:292–304.

43. Puig-Antich J, Perel JM, Lupatkin W, et al: Plasma levels of imipramine and desmethylimipramine and clinical response to prepubertal major depression. *J Am Acad Chil Psychiatry* 1979;18:616–627.

44. Petti TA, Law W: Imipramine treatment in depressed children. *J Clin Psychopharmacol* 1982;2:107–109.

45. Saraf KR, Klein DF, Gittelman-Klein R, et al: EKG effects of imipramine treatment in children. *J Am Acad Child Psychiatry* 1978;17:60–69.

46. Bellanger JC, Reur VL, Post RM: The atypical presentation of adolescent mania. *Am J Psychiatry* 1983 (in press).

47. Cast CD: The under and over diagnosis of mania in children and adolescents. *Comprehensive Psychiatry* 1982;23:552–559.

48. Puig-Antich J: Affective disorders in childhood: A review and perspective. *Psychiatr Clin North Am* 1980;3:403–424.

49. Youngerman J, Canino IA: Lithium carbonate use in children and adolescents. *Arch Gen Psychiatry* 1978;35:216–224.

50. McKnew DH, Cytrin L: Lithium in children of lithium responding parents. *Psychiatry Res* 1981;4:171–180.

51. Birch NJ: Bone side effects of lithium, in Johnson FN (ed): *Handbook of Lithium Therapy*. Lancaster, England, MTP Press, 1980, pp 310–322.

52. Gittelman-Klein R, Klein DF: Controlled imipramine treatment of school phobia. *Arch Gen Psychiatry* 1981;25:204–207.

53. Gittelman-Klein R: Pharmacotherapy and management of pathological separation anxiety. *Int J Mental Health* 1975;4:225–271.

54. Snyder S: Amitriptyline treatment of obsessive-compulsive neurosis. *J Clin Psychiatry* 1980;41:8.

55. Freed A, Kerr TA, Ruth M: The treatment of obsessional neurosis. *Br J Psychiatry* 1972;120:590–591.

56. Rapoport JL, Elkins R, Mikkelsen E: Clinical controlled trial of chlorimipramine in adolescents with obsessive-compulsive disorder. *Psychopharm Bull* 1980;16:61–63.

57. Insel TR, Murphy D: The psychopharmacologic treatment of obsessive compulsive disorder: A review. *J Clin Psychopharmacol* 1981;1:304–311.

58. Campbell M, Anderson LT, Meier M, et al: A comparison of haloperidol and behavior therapy and their interaction in autistic children. *J Am Acad Child Psychiatry* 1978;17:640–655.

59. Cohen IL, Campbell M, Posner D, et al: Behavioral effects in young autistic children. *J Am Acad Child Psychiatry* 1980;19:665–677.

60. Puig-Antich J: Major depression and conduct disorders in prepuberty. *J Am Acad Child Psychiatry* 1982;21:118–128.

61. Dostal T, Zvolsky P: Antiaggressive effect of lithium salts in severely mentally retarded adolescents. *Int Pharmacopsychiatry* 1970;5:203–207.

62. Lena B: Lithium therapy in hyperaggressive behavior in adolescence, in Sandler M (ed): *Psychopharmacology of Aggression*. New York, Raven Press, 1979, pp 98–103.

63. Lena B, Surters SJ, Maggs R: The efficacy of lithium in the treatment of emotional disturbances in children and adolescents, in Johnson FN, Johnson S (eds): *Lithium in Medical Practice*. Baltimore, University Park Press, 1978, pp 79–83.

64. Campbell M, Cohen IL, Small AM: Drugs in aggressive behavior. *J Am Acad Child Psychiatry* 1982;4:107–117.

65. Steinberg D: The use of lithium carbonate in adolescence. *J Child Psychol Psychiatry* 1980;21:263–271.

210

66. Sheard MH: The effect of lithium and other ions on aggressive behavior. *Neurol Probl Pharmacopsychology* 1978;13:53–58.
67. Worral EP: The antiaggressive effects of lithium, in Johnson FN, Johnson S (eds): *Lithium in Medical Practice.* Baltimore, University Park Press, 1978, pp 84–90.
68. Jefferson JW: The use of lithium in childhood and adolescence: An overview. *J Clin Psychiatry* 1982;43:174–177.
69. Gualtieri CT, Bainhill J, McGimsey J, et al: Tardive dyskinesia and other movement disorders in children treated with psychotropic drugs. *J Am Acad Child Psychiatry* 1980;19:491–510.
70. Polizos P, Engelhardt DM: Dyskinesia phenomena in children treated with psychotropic medication. *Psychopharmacol Bull* 1978;14:65–68.
71. Williams DT, Mehl R, Yudofsky S, et al: The effects of propranolol on uncontrolled rage outbursts in children and adolescents with organic brain dysfunction. *J Am Acad Child Psychiatry* 1982;21:129–135.

11

Psychotropic Medications and Mentally Retarded Patients

Mai-Lan Rogoff

SCOPE OF THE PROBLEM

Mentally retarded people are as likely as their nonretarded peers to experience emotional distress. They are environmentally more likely to experience stresses and constitutionally less able to cope adaptively with these experiences. The problem of optimal use of drug therapy with mentally retarded people is exacerbated by communication difficulties, a higher incidence of associated neurological abnormalities, and constraints imposed on the prescribing physician by other agencies (such as the prohibition of prn medication schedules or of certain medications). Many of the specific problems in prescribing medication for retarded people are the result of difficulties in making appropriate diagnoses and evaluating side effects. It is common to find response to minimal doses of medication or lack of response to seemingly very high doses of medications, calling for flexibility on the part of the prescribing physician. Flexibility and creativity seem to be generally necessary for diagnosis and prescribing for this group.

The Diagnostic and Statistical Manual (DSM-III) defines the essential features of mental retardation as: 1) significantly subaverage intellectual functioning; 2) resulting in, or associated with, deficits or impairments in adaptive behavior; and 3) with onset before the age of 18. This definition contains the elements contributing to the vulnerability of mentally retarded children and adults to emotional and behavioral disturbance. Subaverage intellectual function compromises the individual's ability to comprehend events and their consequences. Judgment, insight, the ability to learn from mistakes, and flexibility may be compromised in the retarded person because of the deficit in adaptive ability. Mental retardation is a disorder of the developmental stages of life. The other conditions of the disorder, subaverage intellectual functioning and deficits in adaptive behavior, thus affect the child as he or she grows up, forms a sense of self, and develops ways of coping and interacting with the world.

Mentally retarded people are often at greater risk for disorders associated with loss of self esteem, as they may be subject to repeated experiences of failure at school, difficulty competing successfully with age peers, ridicule, and sometimes rejection by parents or other members of their social milieu. The mentally retarded person must cope with these stresses despite difficulties in verbalizing feelings and a relatively limited and inflexible repertoire of coping behaviors.

Unknown prenatal influences that are often associated with mental retardation may contribute to increased central nervous system vulnerability, and thus to major psychiatric syndromes or side effects of medications that are suspected to be associated with organic brain damage. If the mentally retarded person has been placed in an institution, additional behavioral complications of "institutionalization" may be present. Institutionalized mentally retarded patients are also more likely to be severely or profoundly retarded, or to have other handicaps that further compromise their ability to react to situations, and which limit the observers' ability to interpret their reactions.

The incidence of mental illness in mentally retarded children and adults is difficult to determine. Previous studies are beset with methodological flaws such as use of clinic rather than randomly selected populations, lack of agreement on definitions of essential terms (such as the criteria for diagnosis of mental illnesses or even of mental retardation), and the problems associated with retrospective and chart studies. Studies of institutionalized retarded people give a falsely elevated incidence of mental illness because of the lower level of functioning associated with placement in an institution, and because behavioral disturbance is, in itself, a common reason for institutionalization. Most studies agree, however, that there is an increased incidence of emotional disturbance in mentally retarded people, with reported incidence varying from 30% to 60%.[1-3] The type of reported disturbance varies.

Frequently seen reasons for consultation in the nonmentally retarded population, such as depression, are also seen in the retarded population. Other problems also may be presented, depending on the situation in which the retarded individual finds him or herself. In the case of institutionalized mentally retarded residents, problems such as oppositional behavior, refusal to cooperate in activities of daily living (eg, feeding and dressing), socially inappropriate behaviors (eg, undressing or masturbating in public), rumination, or fecal smearing, may be the reason for consultation. Approximately 90% of mentally retarded people, however, function in the mild to moderate range, and present with symptoms and syndromes similar to those seen in nonretarded populations.

Perhaps the most significant problem in prescribing medications for mentally retarded people is the temptation to see drug intervention as the only treatment alternative, ignoring the possibilities of individual and group psychotherapy, behavior therapy, and manipulation of the environment. Therapy needs to be directed generally to issues appropriate to the mentally retarded person's chronological age, as emotional issues in mildy and moderately retarded persons tend to go more with chronological than with mental age. Thus, a retarded adolescent will probably be coping with issues of identity formation, acceptance by a peer group, and sexuality, regardless of mental age. Many behavioral disturbances in institutionalized people respond well to increased stimulation and attention, and both "talking" psychotherapy and play therapy are extremely useful modes of treatment, especially in mild-to-moderately retarded people.

EFFICACY OF MEDICATION IN MENTALLY RETARDED PATIENTS

Despite the fact that the majority of mentally retarded patients do not live in institutions, most studies of drug efficacy have been done on institutionalized people. Other methodological problems, such as lack of placebo control or lack of random assignment, also make the assessment of studies complex. Several excellent reviews of the literature, however, do exist. Freeman[4] reviewed available studies in 1970, and this was followed in 1971 by Sprague and Werry[5] who reviewed 180 drug studies, classifying them with regard to the methodology employed. Lipman et al[6] reviewed 147 studies, focusing on major tranquilizers and stimulants and eliminating from their review studies of primarily schizophrenic or autistic children who were functioning in the retarded range. These reviews were reexamined and updated by Rivinus,[7] who reviewed 166 studies. The present chapter will examine these and other reviews, major papers contained in these reviews, and current literature in psychopharmacology with mentally retarded patients.

Two major conclusions emerge from the studies reviewed. First, no drug has been shown to cause a specific increase in intellectual functioning of mentally retarded persons. There is, in fact, some evidence that neuroleptics may decrease learning and response to behavioral programming, especially if injudiciously used.[4-7] The effect of antipsychotics on learning and on speed of information processing is not clear, however. In schizophrenic subjects, chlorpromazine actually aided certain types of information processing.[8] It may be that use of neuroleptics for nonspecific behavior control in mentally retarded patients has "required" doses associated with oversedation and decreased attention due to this side effect. Second, several drugs, including neuroleptics, lithium, antidepressants, minor tranquilizers, stimulants, and propranolol, have been shown to be quite effective when used to treat specific psychiatric syndromes. These drugs continue to be effective over the long term, frequently with recurrence of symptoms if discontinued.[9] Medications indirectly benefit learning in those instances wherein learning was interfered with by incompatible states such as depression, withdrawal, short attention span, and competing thoughts.

The implication of these studies is that psychotropic drugs must be prescribed with a psychiatric syndrome in mind and not prescribed to treat specific symptoms, although "target" symptoms may be very useful in monitoring progress. Psychotropic drugs are also misused if they are used in lieu of adequate staffing, to induce a state of "pseudo-appropriate" social behavior by creating a quieted but nonfunctional state, for staff convenience, or for punishment. Hopefully, these practices, as well as the widespread use of polypharmacy, may be decreasing with the increased availability of psychiatric consultation and increased awareness of social and psychological needs of retarded persons.[7] Unfortunately, patterns and effectiveness of psychotropic drug use have not been as well studied in noninstitutionalized as they have in institutionalized mentally retarded persons.

DIAGNOSIS AND MENTALLY RETARDED PATIENTS

Differential diagnosis of emotional and behavioral disturbance is not especially problematic in verbal mild to moderately retarded people, in whom DSM-III criteria may be used. There are some general strategies for interviewing retarded people, however, that have been described in depth by Szymanski.[3] Retarded people are perhaps more likely to view the psychiatric examination as an anxiety-provoking "test" that they may fail. It is also important not to confuse a patient's misunderstanding of the situation, due to diminished intellectual functioning, with psychotic delusional misunderstandings. Careful, simple explanations of the purpose and nature of the examination, including reassurances that there are no right and wrong answers, or that this doctor does not give "shots," are helpful. It may be necessary and is often helpful to see the retarded person with his or her major caretaker as well as individually. The examiner may also need to be more directive and to provide more structure, encouragement and limits than usual in order to compensate for the retarded person's expectation of criticism and failure, the passive-dependent presentation often seen, and the tendency for the retarded person to withdraw into silence and anxiety.

Some estimate must be made during the early part of the interview regarding the retarded person's use and comprehension of language, to allow the examiner to address the mentally retarded person on his or her communicative and emotional level. Interpretations of observations made during the interview must also be modified, depending on the mentally retarded person's level. Some verbal productions, such as mild echolalia and inability to interpret proverbs, may be a result of intellectual compromise rather than psychosis. Severely and profoundly retarded people may show self-stimulatory behaviors, such as rocking, in the absence of psychosis.

The problems of diagnosis become more formidable when the individual is nonverbal or has severely compromised communicative function. Techniques borrowed from child psychiatry such as play interviews or drawing may be helpful, especially in younger retarded persons. Care must be taken, however, to make the retarded adult feel that he or she is being treated respectfully, and that he or she is not being infantilized. With severely and profoundly retarded people, the history obtained from the caretakers (preferably from different caretakers who see the individual in several settings such as residence, workshop, and day program) becomes of paramount importance. The interview is more limited and the value of a "team" approach more evident. Some thought processes may need to be inferred rather than obtained from verbal exchange, such as the possible existence of delusions or hallucinations on the basis of sudden unexplained changes in affect or periods of apparent attention to nonexistent stimuli. Standard or modified assessment scales are helpful in interpreting the initial information provided by caretakers and may be repeated to assist in determining response to medications.

SPECIFIC SYNDROMES

Psychoses

Diagnosis As with nonretarded persons, several psychiatric and medical syndromes are capable of producing psychotic symptoms. Correct differential diagnosis is essential to treatment. Differentiation of psychosis due to schizophrenia from that due to affective disorder or atypical psychosis is complicated in the absence of verbal production; consideration of whether or not delusions are mood congruent then becomes quite difficult. Other clues to the presence of affective disorder may be helpful. The presence of hyperactivity, elated mood, and cyclicity of symptoms are valuable in differentiating manic psychosis from other psychoses. Marked social withdrawal and biological signs of depression are useful in differentiating depressive psychosis. Newer laboratory tests, such as the dexamethasone suppression test and the thyrotropin stimulation test, offer some promise in the problem of differential diagnosis, although there have not been reports of their use in mental retardation. The "periodic" psychoses associated with abnormalities of electrolytes should also be considered.[10]

The differential diagnosis of organic brain syndrome such as dementia or delerium is especially difficult in the mentally retarded person. Dementia must be increasingly considered, as mentally retarded people are living longer[11,12] and increased incidence of Alzheimer's disease in people with Down's syndrome has been reported.[13] Behavioral rather than verbal cues to disorientation, such as the patient's inability to find his or her own room, are suggestive of organic brain syndrome. Neurological examination, including EEG and CT scan may also be helpful in making the diagnosis of dementia. Reliable behavioral observations serially over time remain essential for obtaining a reasonable understanding of causes for disturbed behavior.

Pharmacologic Treatment   Treatment of primary psychotic syndromes in mentally retarded people requires a combination of pharmacologic and environmental management. The most commonly studied neuroleptics have been thioridazine (Mellaril), chlorpromazine (Thorazine), and haloperidol (Haldol). There are no good data showing one to be more effective in treatment of psychosis in mentally retarded patients than another. Several studies have demonstrated improvement in behaviors such as hyperkinesis, attention and concentration, aggressiveness, assaultiveness, appetite, and sleep disturbances after treatment with neuroleptics,[6] although some individuals have actually been shown to improve when neuroleptics were discontinued.[14,15] As with nonmentally retarded patients, concerns such as amount of sedation desired, presence or absence of movement disorders prior to administration of medications, and occurrence of other desirable or undesirable side effects will be major influences in drug choice. In the case of preexisting movement disorders, aliphatic and piperidine phenothiazines probably are indicated as they seem to have less tendency to exacerbate these symptoms.[7] Although the evidence for increased incidence of tardive dyskinesia in organic brain damage is controversial, patients should be carefully watched for the development of early symptoms because there is some possibility that brain damage associated with mental retardation may predispose to tardive dyskinesia.[16,17] Youth is not protection against this symptom; tardive dyskinesia has been described in mentally retarded children taking long-term neuroleptics.[18,19] Management of this troublesome side effect, if it occurs, is similar to that in nonretarded persons and has been well reviewed elsewhere.[20-21]

More common side effects may present in uncommon ways. The discomfort of akathisia may, for example, result in aggression[22] or agitation with mood lability and crying. Other concerns about side effects that have been raised especially in mentally retarded people are reports in the British literature of cases of fatal hyperthermia in patients receiving depot preparations of phenothiazines.[23] In these cases of hyperthermia, patients were also taking other anticholinergic drugs, such as antiparkinsonian medications, which contributed to decreased sweating. Another reported side effect appears in a recent report of a high incidence of corneal and lenticular opacities in patients receiving long-term high doses of thioridazine.[24] Yearly slit lamp examinations are recommended to follow possible development of ocular complications. The precaution of being vigilant in watching for side effects and possible drug–drug interactions again becomes apparent when working with mentally retarded persons who may not be able to complain of the early onset of side effects.

Affective Illness

Diagnosis Unipolar and bipolar affective illnesses occur at least as frequently in the mentally retarded as in the general population.[25] The manic phase of bipolar illness has been well described in mentally retarded people.[26-28] Characteristic symptoms of manic hyperactivity and irritability are likely to be more apparent than grandiosity or flight of ideas, especially in less verbal people. Mentally retarded patients not infrequently have rapid cycling variants of bipolar illness, which may be more difficult to diagnose as well as to treat. One problem in making the diagnosis of bipolar illness, manic state in the retarded is that many of the behaviors that characterize the bipolar syndrome may be part of the retarded person's general repertoire of behaviors. Such factors as decreased judgment, hyperactivity, and short attention span may be present before the onset of mania. Increase in intensity rather than appearance of these symptoms may therefore be the most significant clue. Since manic irritability may lead to aggressiveness, it is important to consider mania in differential diagnosis. Aggressiveness is one of the more troublesome symptoms in mental retardation, and manic aggressiveness will often respond well to therapy. Differential diagnosis of mania and depression from other psychoses and from dementia may present problems, as previously discussed.

Factors predisposing mentally retarded people to unipolar affective illness are: 1) interpersonal, eg, difficulty maintaining self-esteem because of repeated experiences of failure and rejection; 2) intrapersonal, including rigid defensive systems often with a passive-aggressive defensive style and view of the self as incapable of causing change; and 3) societal, as a result of environmental deprivation and reinforcement of these views of self. Mentally retarded people often have great difficulty coping with changes in their environment and with the loss of significant caretakers. They are subject to multiple changes of residence and companions at the will of administrators of community and institutional placements, and to multiple changes of caretakers as staff leave for new positions, seek career advancement, or "burn out" and leave the field of mental retardation work altogether. All of these factors may cause adjustment reaction with disturbance of mood, or facilitate the development and expression of major affective illness.

Change in behavior should always raise the possibility of affective disorder in the examiner's mind, and inquiry should be made as to changes in staff, clients, or programs at the various settings in which the mentally retarded person spends his or her day. Criteria that are commonly used for the diagnosis of depression may be used with the retarded, although some may have to be modified for use with nonverbal retarded patients. For example, difficulty concentrating may manifest itself in diminished performance in a program or workshop setting, loss of appetite may become evident in refusal to eat or weight loss, and decreased energy may present as lethargy and fatigue. There may be increased evidence of nonspecific distress and loss of interest in activities usually seen as pleasurable. Suicidal ideation and suicide attempts may be seen more frequently in mildly retarded patients. Even profoundly retarded persons express feelings, often in easily understood ways such as laughing or crying, and almost always in ways that can be understood by regular caretakers. Misery seems to be a potentially universal experience.

Pharmacologic treatment Affective disorders in mentally retarded people respond well to psychotherapy in combination with traditionally used drugs such as antidepressants and lithium.[25] In studies reviewed by Freeman,[4] Sprague and Werry,[5] and Lipman et al,[6] tricyclic antidepressants were not found to have beneficial effects unless prescribed for depressive illness, suggesting that the tricyclics do not have nonspecific beneficial effects. Rivinus[7] has questioned this finding because of recent work in adults with attention deficit disorders who have been shown in some studies to respond to imipramine,[29] and on the work of Rybak[30] in this area. The benefits of the use of antidepressants must be weighed against the risk of side effects, as with all medications, and against the risk of exacerbation of psychotic symptoms, especially in this group of patients in whom differential diagnosis is difficult. The frequency of depressive illness in the mentally retarded population and the clinical finding of improvement with antidepressants in mentally retarded people (Rosefsky and Eissner, personal communication 1983),[25] warrants consideration of pharmacologic as well as psychotherapeutic treatment.

Lithium has been shown to be useful in the treatment and prophylaxis of manic episodes in mentally retarded patients.[28,31] Baldessarini[32] has also suggested the use of lithium in prophylaxis for depressive illness. Lithium must be used with caution in mentally retarded patients who may not be able accurately to describe or complain of side effects, and who may react to discomfort such as gastrointestinal distress by increasing hyperactivity, assaultiveness, self-injurious behavior or other symptoms that led to the original diagnosis of manic depressive illness. The usual problems of therapeutic versus toxic range, possible alterations in renal or thyroid function, and lithium/neuroleptic drug interactions apply also in mental retardation. In additon, mentally retarded patients may have more than the usual problems of maintaining adequate fluid and electrolyte balance while on lithium therapy, especially if the common side effect of pseudodiabetes insipidis develops. The uncommon complication of reversible organic brain syndrome while taking lithium salts in the therapeutic dose range may be more common in patients already suffering from cerebral dysfunction.[33] This suggests that the mentally retarded may be a group more susceptible to this complication. Lithium should therefore be used with caution, adequate monitoring and follow-up. When used with discretion and as indicated, lithium is an extremely useful adjunct to environmental, behavioral and psychotherapeutic maneuvers.

Anxiety Disorders

Diagnosis One of the more frequent presenting complaints in psychiatric patients, mentally retarded or not, is anxiety or agitation. Any of the intrapsychic, intra- and interpersonal or societal factors discussed under "Depression" may also lead to anxiety. The DSM-III lists five general types of adult anxiety disorders: anticipatory, generalized, panic, phobic and obsessive-compulsive disorder, and anxiety disorders of childhood including overanxious and avoidant disorders. Disorders requiring sophisticated defensive systems such as phobias and obsessive-compulsive disorder are more common in mild to moderately retarded people. Generalized anxiety disorder and the anxiety disorders of childhood are frequently seen in more retarded individuals. As in the normal population, differential diagnosis must include organic causes of symptoms of anxiety, rational fears, avoidant behavior caused by a response to delusions, and agitation resulting from affective disorder, either manic or depressed.

Pharmacologic treatment The traditional drugs of choice for simple anxiety disorders have been the benzodiazepines and related compounds. Older studies have referred to the use of barbiturates and meprobamate for control of anxiety.[4,34,35] Generally, the barbiturates are indicated only for seizure control, because of rapid habituation to their calming effect and their potential for eliciting a paradoxial rage reaction. Meprobamate has not been shown to be useful in management of anxiety in mentally retarded patients.

The benzodiazepines have at least short-term effects in relief of anxiety and associated symptoms.[36,37] Use of the benzodiazepines in mentally retarded patients does raise some concerns, however. This group of patients is less likely to be allowed to regulate their own medication schedules and more likely to have deficiencies in judgment, both conditions that increase the potential for abuse, either by staff or by the clients themselves. In an attempt to reduce abuse, use of prescriptions for prn medication is often prohibited in institutions or community residences for mentally retarded people. One unfortunate side effect of such policies is the prescription of regular doses of the benzodiazepines, a practice rarely followed with nonretarded patients, or of avoiding the use of benzodiazepines altogether by using low doses of neuroleptics, exposing these patients to the side effects and decreased anxiolytic effectiveness of neuroleptics used as antianxiety agents. Data on the frequency of development of addiction to "minor" tranquilizers in the general population is unclear and are based on people who tend to self-regulate their dosage, even if it was not originally prescribed on an "as needed" basis.[38,39] On the other hand, the benzodiazepines are very effective medications for the management of anxiety and have the luxury of having few side effects. They remain the preferred group of medications for short-term management of anxiety. Use over a longer term requires frequent review, with attention to the potential for development of tolerance and addiction.

Another group of drugs receiving attention in the management of anxiety are the beta blocking agents such as propranolol.[40] These agents seem to exert their antianxiety effect by blocking the peripheral manifestations of anxiety. It is possible that part of the effect of the beta blockers may be cognitively mediated by decreasing anticipatory anxiety. This raises a question as to how effective these agents might be in reducing anxiety in more retarded individuals.

Small doses of neuroleptics are frequently used for the management of anxiety and agitation in the mentally retarded. These drugs have the advantage of being nonaddicting, nonhabituating, and less likely to produce pradoxical effects than the benzodiazepines. They have the disadvantage of producing potentially more side effects.

The MAO inhibitors have been suggested for the treatment of anxiety manifesting as panic attacks rather than as generalized or anticipatory anxiety.[41,42] Tricyclic antidepressants also have been used with some success. Panic attacks are an uncommon complaint in mentally retarded patients. Tricyclic antidepressants may be of help in the treatment of this syndrome when it does occur. The limited ability of mentally retarded patients to follow a strict diet in either a group care situation or under unsupervised conditions, in which poor understanding of the diet and of the reasons for maintenance of the diet may compromise compliance, and make consideration of use of MAO inhibitors unlikely by the prescribing physician.

Aggressive and Assaultive Behavior

Diagnosis Aggressive and violent behavior in mentally retarded patients is difficult to manage, makes community placement harder to sustain, and is a major cause for seeking psychiatric consultation. Chronic or repeated episodic aggressive behavior is a more common problem than acute violence. The approach to differential diagnosis requires a developmental as well as a psychopathological view. What may be seen as relatively innocuous oppositional behavior in a 2-year-old may become significant potentially dangerous aggressive behavior in a retarded adolescent, although the dynamics of separating and establishing independence in the face of inadequately developed judgment are the same. Similarly, temper tantrums in an adult are more difficult to tolerate than they are in a toddler, and may be frightening or even dangerous to the staff and other clients.

Mentally retarded persons are more likely to resort to defensive maneuvers in the face of perceived inability to cope, because more adaptive ways of responding to stresses are limited. It is unclear, however, whether they are any more prone to resort to violence than to another defense. A comparative study of violent and nonviolent delinquent boys found that while the violent delinquents functioned on a slightly lower level on the WISC, the differences were not significant. The most significant predictors of violent behavior were a combination of familial vulnerability, compromised central nervous system function, physical and psychological abuse from a parent or significant others in the environment, and social deprivation.[43,44] Nonlocalizing neurological signs suggestive of some compromise or immaturity in the central nervous system of violence-prone individuals have been described by other authors.[45] An association between low 5-hydroxyindole levels and a syndrome of increased activity and aggression has also been described.[46] Unfortunately, an adverse combination of constitutional and environmental factors is not that uncommon among mentally retarded individuals, who often have sustained central nervous system insult, may have been difficult infants or children with increased risk of being abused by parents, or have been placed in understaffed institutions with poor supervision of older aggressive clients. Mentally retarded children often have language, communication and sensory difficulties, predisposing them to misunderstandings and difficulties in successfully using words to get their wants or needs met. This may predispose them to act out their conflicts. Aggressive intrusiveness in an attempt to reach out and interact with others may also be an early response to social awareness in a more retarded individual. Aggressive behavior may thus be seen as adaptive as well as maladaptive. It may be more than a little difficult, however, to ask the staff to view a client's increasingly effective aggression as a positive step in socialization while they are busy trying to protect themselves and other clients.

The DSM-III lists at least 20 diagnoses known to be associated with violent behavior. Among the ones ordinarily seen in mentally retarded individuals are manic episodes, adjustment disorder with disturbance of conduct, attention deficit disorder with hyperactivity, oppositional and overanxious disorders, organic personality syndrome, and the psychotic disorders. In addition to these, aggression representing adaptive or previously adaptive behavior (as, for example, in people who have previously lived in dangerous environments), and medical problems causing pain, discomfort or decreased sensory input must be considered. Even an apparently simple matter of decreased hearing due to excess cerumen in ears, or the pain of otitis media may result in a paranoid presentation with aggression. Although the association of violence with temporal lobe seizures as an ictal phenomenon is not generally well supported,[47] some cases have been described.[48] A syndrome of increased interictal tendency to violence and other symptoms of affective lability, possibly on the basis of disconnection of sensory inputs and limbic integrative pathways, has been well described.[44,49]

Psychopharmacologic treatment As in other psychiatric syndromes, an attempt at differential diagnosis and understanding of some of the causes of this multiply determined behavior must be made. Treatment should involve consideration of the client's current environment, possible losses, other clients and staff, consistency of response, amount and quality of stimulation, more appropriate outlets, reward and reinforcement systems, and the client's own understanding of the behavior. Medication will play only a part in treatment.

The oldest medications used in response to aggressive and assaultive behavior in institutions are the barbiturates, used as a "chemical straightjacket." Unfortunately, these medications may themselves produce a behavioral syndrome which includes irritability, mood lability and assaultiveness.[34,50] Barbiturates are therefore not recommended, although on rare occasion their use may be warranted for rapid sedation of a dangerous patient. Specialized training of staff in physical restraint of violent patients followed by tranquilization with other agents is preferable. Benzodiazepines have also been described as causing a reaction of irritability and aggressiveness,[51] although beneficial effects have been described with their use.[52]

There have been several reports of pathologically aggressive behavior as a response to phenothiazines and butyrophenones.[4,53-59] In many of these studies, attempts to differentiate syndromes were not made. It is unclear therefore whether neuroleptics have a primary antiaggressive effect beyond their sedative side effects, or whether they are effective because of their effect on a primary psychotic process that had been causing distortions of perception. Lithium also has been used successfully in treatment of aggressive states.[60] Lithium is described as being of more use in impulsive, explosive, retarded patients than in those determined to do violence, delusionally or otherwise. The mechanism of action is again unclear, especially as lithium tends to be used in hyperactive aggressive clients who may well be manifesting manic symptoms.

One of the more interesting drugs that has been tried in aggressive behavior is propranolol.[61-65] In these reports, propranolol was described as effective in treatment of explosive rage and belligerence in acute and chronic brain syndromes, including in those patients who had been unresponsive to neuroleptics and anticonvulsants. Potential side effects of bradycardia and hypotension were well tolerated. The mechanism of action is unclear. Yudofski[63] speculates that the medication may act centrally by blocking disinhibition of the rage response, or peripherally by blocking somatic responses to stress, anxiety and fear, much as the drug is hypothesized to work in anxiety and panic states. Propranolol is not without its problems, however. There are potential medical complications and medical contraindications to its use in congestive heart failure, bronchospasm, sinus bradycardia and other cardiac abnormalities, and in diabetics taking insulin who are prone to bouts of hypoglycemia. Toxic psychosis recently has been reported with low-dose propranolol therapy[66] and other toxic effects have been reported when propranolol was used in combination with a neuroleptic.[67]

Other medications have been used in treatment of violent discontrol. Amphetamines were reported to be effective in patients with attention deficit disorder with hyperactivity and impulsive violence as part of the syndrome.[68] Anticonvulsants have been used successfully in patients with episodic epileptiform discontrol.[69,70] The syndrome of epileptiform episodic discontrol appears to be rare in mentally retarded people, but anticonvulsants might be considered in selected patients.[7] Therapeutic trials of amphetamines and anticonvulsants in treatment of aggressive behavior in mentally retarded individuals have not yet been reported.

Attention Deficit Disorder

Diagnosis   The syndrome of attention deficit disorder is characterized by a triad of short attention span, impulsivity and distractibility/lack of goal directedness. Attention deficit disorder may be present with or without hyperactivity. Associated features include stubbornness, negativism, low frustration tolerance, temper outbursts, and low self-esteem. Because so many of these characteristics are commonly found in severely and profoundly retarded individuals, the DSM-III recommends that the diagnosis in mentally retarded people only be made in the presence of mild or moderate retardation. Differential diagnosis includes activity appropriate to developmental stage, reaction to inappropriate amounts of stimulation (too much or too little), and hyperactivity as a part of an agitated state in manic or other psychosis, depression, anxiety, or as a paradoxical effect of medication such as phenobarbital.

Pharmacologic treatment   The medication probably most frequently used to treat attention deficit disorder with or without hyperactivity is methylphenidate. Methylphenidate in mentally retarded patients has been shown to increase alertness, attention, and concentration, with associated improvements in tests of memory and cognition as a result.[71,72] No improvement has been found in aggressiveness, noisiness or manageability.[73] Sprague, as cited in Rivinus,[7] found that with high doses of stimulant, learning decreased in the face of decreased activity and suggested that an optimum dosage curve may exist for each patient. The possibility of decreased rather than increased learning response must therefore also be considered if stimulants are prescribed. In addition, stimulant medication may precipitate manic or other psychosis and may increase anorexia or insomnia, both of which are commonly problems for mentally retarded patients. Similar benefits and cautions have been shown for dextroamphetamine.[74,75] Stimulants may be very useful in treatment of attention deficit disorder, especially in children, and should neither be denied nor be indiscriminately prescribed in the presence of mental retardation. Imipramine has also been suggested for use in attention deficit disorder and may be useful, especially in older children and adults.[29] Other modalities for improved attention and learning must also be explored.

Self-Stimulatory and Self-Injurious Behaviors

Diagnosis Self-stimulatory behaviors are commonly seen in retarded individuals, especially those on the lower end of the spectrum of function. These behaviors include finger waving, flapping, rocking, rubbing face or other parts of body, or more socially inappropriate behaviors such as rumination or forced vomiting, and smearing saliva or feces. Stereotypic movements may be self-stimulatory or may be involuntary. Self-stimulatory behaviors may increase in intensity and become self-injurious when, for example, facial or other rubbing is done to the point of producing sores, sucking on fingers macerates hands, or headbanging intensifies to the extent of producing injury. Occasionally, this injury may be quite severe; patients have been known to detach retinas by severe headbanging.

Severe self-injurious behaviors are more often seen in severely and profoundly mentally retarded individuals than in the mild to moderately retarded population.[76,77] Exceptions are found in patients with psychosis, pervasive developmental disorder, and certain types of brain damage such as Lesch-Nyhan syndrome. In severely and profoundly retarded persons, however, this behavior may be seen in patients who do not differ from other severely and profoundly retarded patients in the same setting with regard to their relationship abilities, attention to surroundings, affect, or response to programming. Thus, it appears that self-injurious behavior may be seen in severely and profoundly retarded persons independent of the presence of psychosis.

The origin of self-stimulatory and self-injurious behaviors is unclear.

While self-stimulatory behavior is common in normal 6- to 18-month-old infants, such infants rarely injure themselves. Singh[78] has raised the developmental hypothesis that the prolonged time required to negotiate this developmental stage in severe and profound retardation leads to self-injurious rather than self-stimulatory behavior. Cataldo and Harris[79] reviewed the biological hypotheses and have proposed that stereotypic and other self-stimulatory movements serve to decrease sympathetic arousal following stimulation of the hypothalamic-pituitary-adrenal axis by anxiety or other affective stimuli. L.S. Szymanski (personal communication 1983) has suggested a related hypothesis, currently being studied, that initiation and continuation of self-injurious behavior is related to liberation of endogenous endorphins. Psychological hypotheses include the psychodynamic theory of guilt reduction, which seems more plausible in psychosis than in this developmentally more immature group, and theories based on learning and reinforcement.[80] Self-stimulatory behaviors and, to a lesser extent, self-injurious behaviors tend to increase in the presence of heightened emotion or inadequate external stimulation and to decrease if more appropriate stimulation and interpersonal attention is provided. They also may be used as a means of communicating discomfort from physical illness or emotional pain. Behavioral and environmental interventions are therefore essential.

Pharmacologic treatment   When self-stimulatory behavior is seen in anxious states as a means of self-calming, use of a neuroleptic or minor tranquilizer may help. Self-injurious behavior may be a response to overwhelming anxiety, depression, psychosis, or physical discomfort from, for example, constipation or otitis media. When there are other corroborating symptoms or signs, appropriate treatment of the accompanying condition will often help to relieve self-injurious behavior. Neuroleptics have also been reported to be effective in management of these atypical stereotypic behaviors, although environmental stimulation and manipulation are more effective in the long run.[7] In the case of self-stimulation consisting of rumination and forced vomiting severe enough to cause dehydration, neuroleptics and/or lithium may be of some help.[26] It is important to remember that many behaviors become part of the common struggles over control, diet, and relationships with caretakers that occur in treatment of mentally retarded persons. Careful attention to these and other environmental factors may be more useful than medications in producing remission of undesirable symptoms over the long run. Pharmacologic management is of help in temporary amelioration of symptoms, especially in those cases in which the behavior is part of a larger syndrome.

Behavioral Syndromes Associated with Seizure Disorder

The organic brain dysfunction most commonly associated with mental retardation is seizure disorder. Other central nervous system abnormalities may be present, such as tuberous sclerosis, which may also affect behavior. Several studies have shown some correlation between seizure disorder and behavioral disorders.[81,82] Much attention has been paid to interictal behavior rather than to behavior during the seizures themselves, although the automatisms of complex partial seizures may be mistaken for stereotypic movements, self-stimulatory behavior, oppositional and stubborn behavior, or inappropriate attention-getting maneuvers. Organic personality disorders and dementia may be associated with other central nervous system abnormalities. Anticonvulsants are psychoactive drugs and may themselves produce undesirable symptoms. There is, for example, some possibility that the psychosis associated with epilepsy may be caused by long-term treatment with anticonvulsants.[7,34] Phenobarbital may produce paradoxical excitement and confusion; phenytoin may be associated with organic brain syndrome and dementia.

Disturbances of behavior in the epileptic may be indicative of poor seizure control. The behavioral symptoms may be the result of attention deficits, deteriorated intellectual and social functioning, psychomotor automatisms or the interictal psychotic-like behavior which has been described in psychomotor epilepsy.[83] Bringing the seizure disorder under better control may ameliorate the symptoms. In the case of psychosis as a consequence of a particular anticonvulsant drug regimen, changing the anticonvulsant regimen may help. Flor-Henry[84] has described a syndrome of "alternating psychosis" in which behavior temporarily improves following each seizure and deteriorates as seizure control improves, although evidence for this condition has been contradictory. In general, worsening of behavior in the epileptic patient calls for review of the neurological status and the current medication regime before other medications are considered. If a neuroleptic is added to the treatment plan of a patient with seizure disorder, the tendency for change in dosage (increase or decrease) to lower seizure threshold should be kept in mind and dosage adjustments should be made gradually.

Gilles de la Tourette Syndrome

Clinical characteristics of this interesting and relatively uncommon syndrome have been well reviewed elsewhere.[85] Many of the sufferers from this syndrome have been described as mildly mentally retarded, although a normal IQ distribution has also been described in this disorder.[86] Differential diagnosis may be problematic in mentally retarded people, in whom tics, swearing and grunting vocalizations characteristic of the disorder may be present on a behavioral basis, as primary behaviors or in imitation of the behavior of other institutionalized residents. Not every mentally retarded person who swears has Tourette's syndrome. Some clues to the diagnosis are the patient's behavior prior to the onset of the disorder and physical location of the tics. As the disease progresses in a cephalocaudad direction, the most commonly seen tics are those of the face, head and shoulders. The etiology of the syndrome is unclear, but is thought to be related to catecholaminergic hyperactivity.[87] The classic drug of choice for treatment of the disorder has been haloperidol (Haldol), although recently there have been some reports of the successful use of clonidine to induce remission of symptoms.[88,89]

SUMMARY AND CONCLUSIONS

Mentally retarded people are more susceptible than nonretarded people to emotional and behavioral disturbance because of inter- and intrapersonal issues, societal factors, and biological vulnerability. Communication is frequently impaired, coping mechanisms may be rigid and limited, and environment may contribute to, rather than ameliorate stress. Prescribing medication for mentally retarded people is complicated by difficulties in diagnosis, and in evaluation of effects and side effects.

Previous reviews of psychotropic drug use in the mentally retarded have indicated that drugs may be abused through misuse and polypharmacy and that no drug has been found to improve intellectual functioning per se, but that psychotropic medications can be quite helpful and effective when prescribed for indicated syndromes rather than for specific symptoms. Once medications are prescribed, they must be carefully evaluated for efficacy and side effects, preferably by several observers. Mentally retarded people respond to the same medications prescribed in the nonretarded population, although they may respond to minimal doses or require unusually large doses. The old axiom of "start low, go slow" applies in this population at least as much as in any other.

Finally, medications are not a substitute for evaluation and management of environment, for consideration of intrapsychic processes, or for the need of mentally handicapped people to receive services and to feel accepted as useful members of society.

228

REFERENCES

1. Menaloscino FJ: Emotional disturbance and mental retardation. *Am Mental Defic* 1965;70:248–256.
2. Menaloscino FJ: The facade of mental retardation. *Am J Psychiatry* 1966;122: 1227–1235.
3. Szymanski LS: Psychiatric diagnostic evaluation of mentally retarded individuals. *J Am Acad Child Psychiatry* 1977;16:67–87.
4. Freeman RD: Psychopharmacology and the retarded child, in Menaloscino J (ed): *Psychiatric Approaches to Mental Retardation.* New York, Basic Books, 1970, pp 294–368.
5. Sprague RL, Werry JS: Methodology of psychopharmacological studies with the retarded, in Ellis NR (ed): *International Review of Research in Mental Retardation.* New York, Academic Press, 1971, pp 147–219, vol. 5.
6. Lipman RS, DiMascio A, Reatig T: Psychotropic drugs and mentally retarded children, in Lipman RS, DiMascio A, Killam KF (eds): *Psychopharmacology, A Generation of Progress.* New York, Raven Press, 1978, pp 1437–1449.
7. Rivinus TM: Psychopharmacology and the mentally retarded patient, in Szymanski LS, Tanguay P (eds): *Emotional Disorders of Mentally Retarded Persons.* Baltimore, University Park Press, 1980, pp 195–221.
8. Braff DL, Saccuzzo DP: Effect of antipsychotic medication on speed of information processing in schizophrenic patients. *Am J Psychiatry* 1982;139(9): 1127–1130.
9. Zimmerman RL, Heistad GT: Studies of the long term efficacy of antipsychotic drugs in controlling the behavior of institutionalized retardates. *J Am Acad Child Psychiatry* 1982;21(2):136–143.
10. Carman JS, Wyatt RJ: Calcium: Pacesetting the periodic psychoses. *Am J Psychiatry* 1979;136(8):1035–1039.
11. Reid AH, Aungle PG: Dementia in aging mental defectives: A clinical psychiatric study. *J Ment Defic Res* 1974;18:15–23.
12. Reid AH: Psychiatric disturbances in the mentally handicapped. *Proc Royal Soc Med* 1976;69:509–512.
13. Burger PC, Vogel FS: The development of the pathologic changes of Alzheimer's disease and senile dementia in patients with Down's syndrome. *Am J Pathol* 1973;73:457–468.
14. Marholin D, Touchette PE, Stewart RM: Withdrawal of chronic chlorpromazine medication: An experimental analysis. *J Appl Behav Anal* 1979;12(2): 159–171.
15. Paul GL, Tobias LI, Holly BL: Maintenance psychotropic drugs in the presence of active treatment programs: "Triple blind" withdrawal study with long term mental patients. *Arch Gen Psychiatry* 1972;27:106–115.
16. Jeste DP, Wyatt RJ: Tardive dyskinesia: The syndrome. *Psychiatr Ann* 1980; 10:6–13.
17. Ananth J: Tardive dyskinesia: Myth and realities. *Psychosomatics* 1980;21: 389–396.
18. Gualtieri CT, Breuning SE, Schroeder SR, et al: Tardive dyskinesia in mentally retarded children, adolescents, and young adults: North Carolina and Michigan studies. *Psychopharmacol Bull* 1982;18(1):62–65.
19. Gualtieri TC, Barnhill J, McGinsey J, et al: Tardive dyskinesia and other movement disorders in children treated with psychotropic drugs. *J Am Acad Child Psychiatry* 1980;19(3):491–510.
20. Ananth J: Drug induced dyskinesia: A critical review. *Int Pharmacopsychiat* 1979;14:21–33.

21. Klawans HL, Goetz CG, Perlik S: Tardive dyskinesia: Review and update. *Am J Psychiatry* 1980;137(8):900–908.
22. Kumar BB: An unusual case of akasthisia. *Am J Psychiatry* 1979;136(8):1088.
23. Craft MJ: Toxic effects of depot tranquilizers in mental handicap (letter). *Br Med J* 1977;1(6064):218–227.
24. Gualtieri CT, Lefler WH, Guimond M, et al: Corneal and lenticular opacities in mentally retarded young adults treated with thioridazine and chlorpromazine. *Am J Psychiatry* 1982;139:1178–1180.
25. Reid AH: Psychosis in adult mental defectives: I. Manic-depressive psychosis. *Br J Psychiatry* 1972;120:205–212.
26. Reid AH, Leonard A: Lithium treatment of cyclical commiting in a mentally defective patient. *Br J Psychiatry* 1977;130:316.
27. Hasan M, Mooney RP: Three cases of manic-depressive illness in mentally retarded adults. *Am J Psychiatry* 1979;136:1069–1071.
28. Rivinus TM, Harmatz JS: Diagnosis and lithium treatment of affective disorder in the retarded: Five case studies. *Am J Psychiatry* 1979;136:551–554.
29. Linnoila M, Gualtieri CT, Jobson K, et al: Characteristics of the therapeutic response to imipramine in hyperactive children. *Am J Psychiatry* 1979;136(9):1201–1203.
30. Rybak WS: More adult brain dysfunction. *Am J Psychiatry* 1977;134:96–97.
31. Naylor GJ, Donald JM, LePoidevin D: A double-blind trial of lithium therapy in mental defectives. *Br J Psychiatry* 1974;124:52–57.
32. Baldessarini RJ: Antipsychotic agents, in Baldessarini RJ (ed): *Chemotherapy in Psychiatry*. Cambridge, MA, Harvard University Press, 1977, pp 12–56.
33. Rifkin A, Quitkin F, Klein DF: Organic brain syndrome during lithium carbonate treatment. *Comp Psychiatry* 1973;14:251–254.
34. Reynolds E: Antiepileptic toxicity: A review. *Epilepsia* 1975;16:319–352.
35. Craft M: Tranquilizers in mental deficiency: Meprobamate. *Am J Ment Defic* 1958;2:17.
36. La Veck GD, Buckley P: The use of psychopharmacological agents in retarded children with behavior disorders. *J Chron Dis* 1961;13:174–183.
37. Galambos M: Long-term clinical trial with diazepam on adult mentally retarded persons. *Dis Nerv Syst* 1965;26:305–309.
38. Greenblatt DJ, Shader RI: Dependence, tolerance and addiction to benzodiazepines. *Drug Metab Rev* 1978;8:13.
39. Winokur A, Rickels K: Withdrawal from long-term, low-dosage administration of diazepam. *Arch Gen Psychiatry* 1980;37:101.
40. Cole JO, Altesman RI, Weingarten CH: Beta blocking drugs in psychiatry. *McLean Hosp J* 1979;4:40–68.
41. Sheehan DV: Current concepts in psychiatry: Panic attacks and phobias. *N Engl J Med* 1982;307(3):156–158.
42. Sheehan DV, Claycomb JB, Kouretas N: Monoamine oxidase inhibitors: Prescription and patient management. *Int J Psychiatry Med* 1980–1981;10(2):99–121.
43. Lewis DO, Shanok S, Balla D: Perinatal difficulties, head and face trauma, and child abuse in the medical histories of seriously delinquent children. *Am J Psychiatry* 1979(April);130:419–423.
44. Lewis DO, Shanok S, Pincus J, et al: Violent juvenile delinquents: Psychiatric, neurological, psychological and abuse factors. *J Am Acad Child Psychiatry* 1979;18:307–319.
45. Pincus JH, Tucker GJ: Violence in children and adults. *J Am Acad Child Psychiatry* 1978;17:277–288.
46. Greenberg AS, Coleman M: Depressed 5-hydroxyindole levels associated

with hyperactive and aggressive behavior. *Arch Gen Psychiatry* 1976;33: 331–336.

47. Rodin EA: Psychomotor epilepsy and aggressive behavior. *Arch Gen Psychiatry* 1973;28(2):210–213.

48. Ashford JW, Schulz C, Walsh GO: Violent automatism in a partial complex seizure: Report of a case. *Arch Neurol* 1980:37(2):120–122.

49. Pinel JP, Treit D, Rovner LI: Temporal lobe aggression in rats. *Science* 1977; 197(4308):1088–1089.

50. Kirman B: Drug therapy in the mentally handicapped. *Br J Psychiatry* 1975; 127:545–549.

51. Greenblatt DJ, Shader RI: Psychotropic drugs in the general hospital, in Shader RI (ed): *Manual of Psychiatric Therapeutics*. Boston, Little, Brown & Co, 1975, pp 1–26.

52. Itil TM, Wadud A: Human aggression with major tranquilizers, antidepressants and newer psychotropic drugs. *J Nerv Ment Dis* 1975;160:83–99.

53. Le Vann LJ: Haloperidol in the treatment of behavioral disorders in children and adolescents. *Can Psychiatry Assoc J* 1969;14:217–220.

54. Le Vann LJ: Clinical experience with Tarasan and thioridazine in mentally retarded children. *Appl Ther* 1970;12:30–33.

55. Le Vann LJ: Clinical comparison of haloperidol with chlorpromazine in mentally retarded children. *Am J Ment Defic* 1971;75:719–723.

56. Kaplan S: Double blind study at state institution using thiorizadine in program simulating outpatient clinic practice. *Penn Psychiatry Q* 1969;9:24–34.

57. Tischler B, Patriasz K, Beresford J, Bunting R: Experience with pericyazine in profoundly and severely retarded children. *Can Med Assoc J* 1972;106:136–141.

58. Grabowski SW: Safety and effectiveness of haloperidol for mentally retarded behaviorally disordered and hyperkinetic patients. *Curr Ther Res* 1973;15: 856–861.

58. Grabowski SW: Safety and effectiveness of haloperidol for mentally retarded behaviorally disordered and hyperkinetic patients. *Curr Ther Res* 1973;15: 856–861.

59. Lacny J: Mesoridazine in the care of disturbed mentally retarded patients. *Can Psychiatry Assoc J* 1973;18:389–391.

60. Dale PG: Lithium therapy in aggressive mentally subnormal patients. *Br J Psychiatry* 1980;137:469–474.

61. Elliott FA: Propranolol for the control of belligerent behavior following acute brain damage. *Ann Neurol* 1977;1:489–491.

62. Yorkstone NJ, Zaki SA, Pitcher DR, et al: Propranolol as an adjunct to the treatment of schizophrenia. *Lancet* 1977;2:575–578.

63. Yudofsky S, Williams D, Gorman J: Propranolol in the treatment of rage and violent behavior in patients with chronic brain syndromes. *Am J Psychiatry* 1981;138:218–220.

64. Sheppard GP: High dose propranolol in schizophrenia. *Br J Psychiatry* 1979; 134:470–476.

65. Schreier HA: Use of propranolol in the treatment of post-encephalitic psychosis. *Am J Psychiatry* 1979;136:840–841.

66. Remick RA, O'Kane J, Sparling TG: A case report of toxic psychosis with low-dose propranolol therapy. *Am J Psychiatry* 1981;138:297–309.

67. Miller FA, Rampling D: Adverse effects of combined propranolol and chlorpromazine therapy. *Am J Psychiatry* 1982;139(9):1198–1199.

68. Richmond JS, Young JR, Groves JE: Violent discontrol responsive to d-amphetamine. *Am J Psychiatry* 1978;135:365–366.

69. Maletsky BM, Klotter J: Episodic control: A controlled replication. *Dis Nerv Syst* 1974;35:175–179.

70. Monroe R: Anticonvulsants in the treatment of aggression. *J Nerv Dis* 1975; 160:119–126.
71. Blackridge VY, Ekblad RL: The effectiveness of methylphenidate hydrochloride (Ritalin) on learning and behavior in public school educable mentally retarded children. *Pediatrics* 1971;47:923–926.
72. Blue AW, Lytton GJ, Miller OW: The effect of methylphenidate on intellectually handicapped children. *Am Psychol* 1960;15:393.
73. Levy JM, Jones BE, Croley HT: Effects of methylphenidate (Ritalin) on drug-induced drowsiness in mentally retarded patients. *Am J Ment Defic* 1957;62: 284–287.
74. Anton AH, Greer M: Dextroamphetamine, chatecholamines, and behavior: The effect of dextroamphetamine in retarded children. *Arch Neurol* 1969;21: 248–252.
75. Alexandris A, Lundell F: Effect of thioridazine, amphetamine, and placebo on hyperkinetic syndrome and cognitive area in mentally deficient children. *Can Med Assoc J* 1968;98:92–96.
76. Bartak L, Rutter M: Differences between mentally retarded and normally intelligent autistic children. *J Autism Child Schizophr* 1976;6(2):109–120.
77. Ando H, Yoshimura I: Prevalence of maladaptive behavior in retarded children as a function of IQ and age. *J Abnorm Child Psychology* 1978;6(3): 345–349.
78. Singh NN: Prevalence of self-injury in institutionalized retarded children. *N Z Med J* 1977;86(597):325–327.
79. Cataldo MS, Harris J: The biological basis for self-injury in the mentally retarded, in *Analysis and Intervention in Developmental Disabilities*, Vol 2. Elmsford, NY Pergammon Press, 1982.
80. Carr EG: The motivation of SIB: A review of some hypotheses. *Psychol Bull* 1977;84(4):800–816.
81. Pincus JH, Tucker GJ: Seizure disorders, in *Behavioral Neurology*. New York, Oxford University Press, 1974, pp 25–39.
82. Waxman SG, Geschwind N: The interictal behavior syndrome of temporal lobe epilepsy. *Arch Gen Psychiatry* 1975;32:1580–1586.
83. Glaser GH, Newman RJ, Schafer R: Interictal psychosis in psychomotor temporal lobe epilepsy: An EEG-psychological study, in Glaser GH (ed): *EEG and Behavior*. New York, Basic Books, 1963, p 345.
84. Flor-Henry P: Psychosis and temporal lobe epilepsy. *Epilepsia* 1969;10: 363–395.
85. Woodrow KM: Gilles de la Tourettes's disease – A review. *Am J Psychiatry* 1974;131(9):1000–1003.
86. Lukas AR, Kauffman PE, Morris EM: Gilles de la Tourettes disease: A clinical study of 15 cases. *J Am Acad Child Psychiatry* 1967;6:700–722.
87. Moskowitz MA, Wurtman RJ: Catecholamines and neurologic diseases. *N Engl J Med* 1975;293(7):332–338.
88. Cohen DJ, Detlor J, Young JG: Shaywitz BA: Clonidine ameliorates Gilles de la Tourette Syndrome. *Arch Gen Psychiatry* 1980;37(12):1350–1357.
89. Ferre RC: Tourette's disorder and the use of clonidine. *J Am Acad Child Psychiatry* 1982;21(3):294–297.

12

Pharmacologic Management of the Elderly Patient

Jerrold G. Bernstein

PSYCHOTROPIC DRUGS IN ELDERLY PATIENTS

Aging is synonymous with change and, unfortunately, not always for the better. The aging person encounters many changes: familial, socioeconomic, emotional, and physiologic. Each of these factors influences drug therapy in the elderly patient. Since physiological aging occurs at different rates among people, chronological age cannot be used to define the elderly. As people age, thay are more likely to encounter a variety of medical and emotional problems, and to be exposed to more medications.[1] Surveys have found that 65% to 90% of elderly patients being treated for psychiatric conditions also have at least one physical disorder.[2] Since it has been estimated that four of five elderly persons have at least one chronic illness, it is not suprising that many of them are taking multiple prescribed medications on a regular basis.[3] As a new condition arises, the patient may be given an additional prescription that will interact with an underlying medical problem or with previously prescribed medications. The elderly may also be consuming over-the-counter remedies, alcohol, tobacco, or caffeine which may interact with prescribed medications. Although no age group is immune to adverse drug reactions, studies have found that patients over age 70 have approximately twice as many adverse drug reactions as do people under age 50.[4]

Compliance Problems

Although failure to comply with prescribed therapeutic regimens occurs in all age groups, the problem of noncompliance is likely to be greater in the elderly. Motivation to recover from an illness is a factor governing a patient's willingness to follow a prescribed regime, but the limitations of aging can impair compliance even in a well-motivated individual. Decreased visual acuity in the elderly patient may interfere with the ability to read prescription labels, or recognize and differentiate the various medications that have been prescribed.[2] Impaired hearing, memory, and cognition may decrease the ability to understand spoken instructions, the proper sequence of taking medication,[2] and whether or not a specific dose of medication has been taken. Impairment in manual dexterity and in fine motor coordination may make it difficult for that person to open prescription bottles, particularly those with safety caps, and to handle tablets or capsules or to pour and properly measure doses of liquid medications.

The potential mechanical difficulties of medicating the elderly patient should call the physician's attention to the necessity of prescribing the simplest therapeutic regimen possible with the smallest number of medications,[12] and with clear and understandable instructions. Medication costs may become a clinically important factor in determining compliance in the elderly person with limited financial means. Although people over age 65 comprise about one-tenth of our population, they consume approximately one-fourth of prescribed medications.[2] Clinical investigations of new therapeutic agents primarily are done using young people. Thus, when a new drug is employed in the treatment of geriatric patients it may have unanticipated adverse effects.[5]

Medical Considerations

Although the occurrence of multiple medical illnesses and the likelihood of prescribing multiple medications in the elderly are important factors that may lead to therapeutic misadventures in this population, it must be kept in mind that even in a healthy aging person, numerous metabolic and physiologic changes occur which may have an important impact on the response (both favorable and unfavorable) to psychotropic medications.[1,5] The signs and symptoms of various psychiatric conditions in the elderly may differ somewhat from those seen in young healthy patients.[1] Attitudes held by psychiatrists toward performing physical examinations on their patients and the competence of psychiatrists in conducting these examinations must be kept in mind. For optimal safety in prescribing psychotropic medications for an elderly person, the physician should be willing and able to make appropriate observations. It is often necessary to determine blood pressure and pulse rate, auscultate the heart and lungs, palpate the liver, and observe the patient for evidence of increased cervical venous pressure and pedal edema. These observations and techniques of physical examination should be supplemented when appropriate, with x-ray studies, electrocardiograms, blood counts, blood chemistry determinations, and urinalysis. In situations when the psychiatrist does not feel comfortable using these techniques of general medicine, his management of the elderly patient should include a close working relationship with the patient's internist.

Physiology of Aging

In considering the physiological changes of aging that affect the response to drug therapy, the physician must be aware of changes that occur in drug metabolism as people age.[6] With aging there generally is a decrease in renal blood flow, glomerular filtration rate, and renal tubular secretion of drugs, thus reducing the rate of excretion of medications and their metabolites.[3] Aging may be associated with reduced metabolic enzyme activity in the liver, thus slowing the rate of drug degradation.[3] There may be a decrease in protein synthesis in the aging liver, thus decreasing plasma protein binding of drugs and an increased concentration of pharmacologically active unbound drug.[3] Diminished cardiac output associated with aging increases circulation time and may modify tissue distribution of drugs.[1] As a person ages, there is an increased ratio of fat to lean body mass. Because most psychotropic drugs are lipid soluble, this factor may also contribute to increased plasma and tissue concentration of therapeutic agents.[7] Each of these physiologic changes favors increased serum drug concentration in the elderly, as well as an increased duration of action of any administered medication.[3]

In the aging brain, neurons may be replaced by glial cells which can contribute to increased sensitivity of the brain to any administered medication that crosses the blood-brain barrier.[7] This change, in conjunction with metabolic changes, suggests that elderly patients are likely to require lower doses of any medicine than may be required for the proper treatment of a young individual. The necessity to titrate medication dosage in the elderly patient is an important cornerstone of proper pharmacotherapy, and the proper dosage titration of a medication is better therapeutic technique than adherence to any published dosage recommendation.

Many medications produce minor adverse effects that are insignificant in a young healthy individual, but that are likely to have more serious consequences in an elderly person with or without concurrent medical illnesses. For example, the arrhythmogenic potential of an antidepressant is likely to present a greater risk in a 75-year-old patient with coronary artery disease than in a healthy 30-year-old individual.[1] A young person may briefly feel uncomfortable as a result of postural hypotension produced by an antipsychotic drug, while the same medication in a frail 80-year-old person may cause that individual to faint, fall, and sustain a hip fracture.[1] The possibility that an elderly person with multiple diseases is receiving multiple medications calls attention to the greater risk of drug interaction between psychotropic and nonpsychotropic medications.[3] Some of the important drug interactions likely to be seen in the geriatric patient are illustrated in Table 12-1.

As the psychiatrist evaluates the elderly patient who is suffering from a disorder of cognition, mood, or mentation, the physician must recognize that the symptoms of psychiatric illness in the elderly patient may differ from those observed in younger individuals.

The clinician must not hastily attribute changes in mental function to senility just because the patient is 80 years of age.[1,8] Patience and effort are required of the physician as he evaluates the elderly person. Even though drug therapy in the elderly may be complicated and subject to adverse reactions, the failure to prescribe appropriate medication may be damaging to the patient not only in terms of the lack of recovery, but to an even greater extent if that person is improperly labeled as having senile organic brain disease.[1]

Adverse Drug Reactions

Before adding a new medication in treating the elderly patient, the physician should consider the possibility that some of the patient's symptoms are related to medication that he or she is already taking. Discontinuing a medication may need to be considered before prescribing an additional medication. In the course of pharmacological treatment of the geriatric patient, unexpected behavioral or physiological changes should lead the clinician to assess the possibility that these changes may be drug related and consider temporary discontinuation of the previously prescribed medication.[11] Before prescribing for the elderly patient, a careful drug history must be taken and the physician must evaluate the possibility of the new medication interacting with existing medical conditions or therapeutic agents. Only one medication should be started at a time; if two or more medications are started simultaneously, it will be difficult to ascertain which agent is producing specific beneficial or unwanted effects.[1] When medication is prescribed for the geriatric patient, the initial dose should be smaller than that for a younger individual, and should be below the anticipated therapeutic range so that the physician can carefully and gradually titrate the dosage upward to achieve the desired effect, rather than having to titrate the dosage downward once an unwanted response has occurred.[1]

Table 12-1
Psychotropic Drug Interactions*

	Interacts With	Effect	Mechanism
SEDATIVES			
Ethanol	CNS depressants	CNS depression	Synergistic effect
Barbiturates	Phenytoin	Decreased phenytoin effect	Enzyme induction
		Enhanced phenytoin toxicity upon discontinuing barbiturate	Return of enzyme activity to normal without reducing dose of phenytoin
		Enhanced phenytoin effect ?	Competition for metabolizing enzymes ?
	Anticoagulants (warfarin dicumarol)	Decreased anticoagulant effect	Barbiturates induce liver enzymes
Chloral hydrate	Anticoagulants (warfarin dicumarol)	Enhanced effect of warfarin	Trichloroacetic acid, a metabolite, displaces warfarin from plasma proteins
Phenytoin	Anticoagulants (warfarin dicumarol)	Enhanced phenytoin toxicity	Dicumarol inhibits phenytoin metabolism
		Decreased anticoagulant effect	Phenytoin stimulates dicumarol metabolism
Benzodiazepines (All except: oxazepam, lorazepam, ?alprazolam)	Cimetidine	Increased prolonged benzodiazepine effect	Inhibits benzodiazepine metabolism
Chlorazepate and prazepam	Antacids	Decreased benzodiazepine effect	Impaired gastrointestinal absorption

Table 12-1
Psychotropic Drug Interactions*

	Interacts With	Effect	Mechanism
ANTIPSYCHOTICS			
Antipsychotic drugs (all)	Levodopa	Decreased levodopa effect	Dopamine blockade
Phenothiazines	Antacids	Decreased therapeutic effect of phenothiazines	Antacids decrease absorption
Phenothiazines (especially chlorpromazine, thioridazine, mesoridazine)	Vasodilators: coronary, cerebral, peripheral	Hypotension	Peripheral vasodilation
	Antihypertensive drugs	Hypotension	Peripheral vasodilation
Chlorpromazine	Guanethidine, clonidine	Decreased antihypertensive effect	CPZ inhibits uptake mechanism necessary for drug action
Haloperidol	Methyldopa	Dementia	Dopamine blockade decreased catecholamine synthesis
ANTIDEPRESSANTS			
Tricyclic antidepressants	Direct-acting sympathomimetics (epinephrine, norepinephrine)	Hypertensive effect, arrhythmias	Inhibition of neuronal uptake
	Guanethidine, clonidine	Decreased antihypertensive effect	Inhibition of neuronal uptake
Monoamine oxidase inhibitors	Wine, cheese, other tyramine-containing foods	Hypertensive crisis	Tyramine effects enhanced due to inhibited metabolism; catecholamine release
	Sympathomimetics	Hypertensive crisis	Increased norepinephrine stores, decreased metabolism

MOOD STABILIZER
Lithium carbonate

Meperidine	Severe excitation, hypertension, hypotension, coma, death	Unknown; inhibited metabolism
Tetracyclines	Lithium intoxication	Enhanced lithium absorption ? Impaired lithium excretion ?
Succinylcholine	Prolonged muscle paralysis	Synergism at neuromuscular junction
Carbamazepine	Enhanced lithium effect Possible lithium toxicity	Synergistic effect ? Uncertain
Methyldopa	Lithium toxicity	Uncertain
Phenylbutazone, indomethacin	Lithium toxicity	Increased tubular reabsorption of lithium

*Data for this table were compiled from the following references:
Ayd FJ (ed): Adverse interactions with lithium. *Int Drug Ther Newsletter* 1978;13:31–32.
Desmond PV, Patwardhan RV, Schenker S: Cimetidine impairs elimination of chlordiazepoxide in man. *Ann Intern Med* 1980;93:266–268.
Hansen PD *Drug Interactions.* Philadelphia, Lea & Febiger, ed 4, 1979.
Kenny AD: Designing drug therapy for the elderly. *Drug Therapy* 1979;9:49–64.
McGennis AJ: Lithium-tetracycline: Toxic interaction. *Br Med J* 1978;1:1183.
O'Regan JB: Adverse interaction of lithium carbonate and methyldopa. *Can Med Assoc J* 1976;115:385.
Shader RI, Georgotas A, Greenblatt DJ et al: Impaired absorption of desmethyldiazepam from chlorszepate by magnesium aluminum hydroxide. *Clin Pharmacol Ther* 1978;24: 308–315.
Thornton WE: Dementia induced by methyldopa with haloperidol. *N Engl J Med* 1976;294:1222–1223.

Recommended dosage guidelines for psychotropic agents in the elderly are to be seen in relative rather than absolute terms, and if a clinician errs in selecting an initial dosage, it is better to err by administering too low a dose. As will be discussed later in this chapter, there may be diminished cholinergic activity in the aging brain and since elderly people tend to be excessively sensitive to anticholinergic effects of drugs, it is preferable to choose an agent within a given therapeutic group that has the least possible anticholinergic action.[1,9]

Because many elderly patients have coronary heart disease, the choice of psychotropic drugs with less cardiovascular effect is generally preferable.[1] As previously pointed out, hypotension may produce serious consequences in the elderly patient, thus those psychotropic agents with greater ability to lower blood pressure should generally be avoided.[1] Within some therapeutic groups, such as the benzodiazepines, there are a variety of compounds that differ from each other in their duration of action or plasma half-life. Because of the tendency of drugs to have more persistent effects in elderly patients, it is strongly recommended that drugs with longer half-lives be avoided.[1,3]

Having reviewed some of the general principles of pharmacotherapy in the elderly patient, the remainder of the chapter will focus on some specific psychiatric problems encountered in the geriatric population, and on suggestions for optimal employment of medication in the management of these problems in this ever-increasing segment of our population.

DEMENTIA

A normal concomitant of aging is the development of some slowing of intellectual processes and mild forgetfulness. In the elderly, speed of learning and performance of complex tasks are also reduced. These phenomena of aging may be termed "benign senescent forgetfulness" and do not necessarily herald the development of progressive mental deterioration referred to as "dementia." In dementia the degree of deterioration of intellectual function is likely to interfere with occupational and social performance.[8] Memory function, learning, abstract thinking, and problem solving ability are significantly disturbed in the demented patient. It is estimated that about 10% of people over age 65 suffer from mild dementia while an additional 5% are afflicted with dementia severe enough to make the individual unable to care for himself.[8]

A variety of conditions that occur in the elderly must be differentiated from dementia. Delirium is generally a temporary condition in which there is alteration in the level of consciousness, disorganization of thinking, and fluctuating cognitive impairment.[8] Delirium may occur as a result of metabolic abnormalities secondary to medical conditions such as diabetes, hyperparathyroidism, hepatic encephalopathy, and other organic conditions.

Dementia must also be differentiated from psychosis wherein there may be disordered thinking in the absence of impaired memory. Acute manic psychoses may occur for the first time in persons as late as the eighth decade of life. Toxic psychoses produced by drugs may occur in the elderly.[1]

Elderly persons may suffer from receptive aphasia without derangement of other higher cortical functions. These patients may suffer from an isolated inability to comprehend language and there may be an associated mild hemiparesis.[8]

Depression is one of the most common psychiatric conditions occurring in the elderly and it may readily mimic dementia. Many elderly people who become depressed, and who have a prior history of depressive illness, will also present with abnormalities of mood, sleep disturbance, and loss of appetite and/or weight, which can be clues to differentiating depression from true dementia.[8] The depressed patient will generally remain well oriented. However, the elderly individual who is likely to have some degree of "benign senescent forgetfulness" may appear to be demented when he or she becomes depressed. Since depression, even in the elderly, is a readily treatable condition, it is critical to make a proper diagnosis so that appropriate treatment can be instituted. The term "pseudodementia" has been employed to describe depression in the elderly wherein the clinical presentation strongly resembles a demented state.[10]

Dementia in the elderly may be associated with episodic worsening of memory, followed by partial improvement which may suggest cerebral vascular disease or carotid occlusion as the mechanism of the dementing process.[8] On the other hand, a gradual but steady decline in cognitive function over a period of years is more characteristic of Alzheimer's disease.[8] In evaluating the demented patient, it is important to obtain a careful history and clarify the source of the dementia, and to assess recent drug therapy as a possible clue to the origin of the mental status changes. Laboratory studies will be helpful in pointing out possible metabolic factors such as hyperglycemia, hypercalcemia, pernicious anemia, hypothyroidism, and syphilis.[8] The presence of an irregular cardiac rhythm may point to cardiac factors with decreased cerebral perfusion, which may be responsible for impaired mental function. Auscultation of the carotid arteries may demonstrate a bruit, and suggest further diagnostic studies which may reveal the presence of partial carotid occlusion as a contributor to decreased cerebral perfusion and function.[8] Computerized tomographic scanning may reveal a subdural hematoma or evidence of cortical atrophy. The presence or absence of cortical atrophy on CT scan does not, however, correlate quantitatively in all cases with the clinical symptomatology. Normal pressure hydrocephalus and brain tumors may be other potentially treatable organic causes of dementia.

Unfortunately, perhaps the most common and least treatable form of dementia is Alzheimer's disease, a primary degenerative process of unknown etiology. There is some evidence to suggest that a deficit in cholinergic activity within the brain may partially account for the mechanism of cerebral dysfunction seen in patients with Alzheimer's disease.[9] A reduction in choline acetyltransferase, the synthetic enzyme for acetylcholine, has been found in the cortex of patients with Alzheimer's disease.[7] Anticholinergic drugs, such as scopolamine and atropine, are known to impair learning ability.[11] Administration of physostigmine, an inhibitor of acetylcholinesterase, is capable of reversing anticholinergic drug-induced memory and learning impairment.[11-13]

Oral administration of choline or purified lecithin, both of which act as acetylcholine precursors, are capable of increasing central nervous system synthesis of this neurotransmitter.[14,15] Research endeavors to employ these compounds in the treatment of Alzheimer's disease have yielded inconsistent results; some patients show transitory improvement in mental function while others experience no benefit.[15] Commercially available lecithin, even though it may be labeled "100% pure," is in fact a mixture of a variety of phosphatides and is of no practical value in enhancing acetylcholine synthesis. On the other hand, commercially available choline tablets containing either the chloride or bitartrate salt of choline, when administered in doses of 4 to 15 g per day may provide benefit for some patients and may be worthy of at least limited clinical trials. This compound may be associated with nausea, diarrhea, and the presence of a body odor resembling spoiled fish. Recent clinical studies using choline precursors administered with oral doses of physostigmine have produced some memory improvement generally superior to that observed with administration of precursors alone.[16] One of the more important aspects of the studies of cholinergic function in dementia is that the findings strongly suggest that drugs with potent anticholinergic effect should be avoided wherever possible in the Alzheimer patient whose symptoms are likely to worsen when such compounds are administered.

Ergoloid (Hydergine), which is a combination of hydrogenated ergot alkaloids, may diminish some symptoms of mental dysfunction in demented patients. However, significant improvement in memory associated with this drug is generally not observed.[8] This compound may be more likely to be beneficial in patients with cerebral arteriosclerosis than in those with true Alzheimer's disease. Improvement in sociability, mood and confusion, may be observed in some patients treated with ergoloid.[1] This compound is somewhat more likely to be effective than a variety of other marketed cerebral vasodilators, although it may produce unwanted side effects including postural hypertension, dizziness, and faintness. If the clinician does not present an overoptimistic evaluation of the remedy, a therapeutic trial of 0.5 to 1 mg of ergoloid (Hydergine) three times daily may be useful to consider.

In an Alzheimer patient with agitation, small doses of potent antipsychotic compounds should be considered as the best pharmacologic approach to managing agitation. The preferable antipsychotic agent is haloperidol, starting at a dose of 0.25 or 0.5 mg and gradually titrating the dosage upward as tolerated and needed to control symptoms of agitation or psychosis. Haloperidol doses in excess of 10 mg per day generally are not necessary in patients with dementia. Because of this compound's limited anticholinergic and hypotensive activity, it is likely to be safer than low potency neuroleptic drugs such as chlorpromazine and thioridazine which are more likely to lower blood pressure and to produce complications associated with their potent anticholinergic effects.[1] Patients suffering from Alzheimer's disease may be depressed to the extent that antidepressant drug therapy needs to be considered. Although a more detailed discussion of antipsychotic and antidepressant drug therapy in the elderly will be presented subsequently, clinicians should bear in mind the necessity to avoid strongly anticholinergic antidepressants in the demented patient whose confusional symptoms may worsen before there is an improvement in mood.[1] For this reason, desipramine, amoxapine, doxepin, maprotiline, and trazodone should be considered as the preferred antidepressants in a demented patient.[1]

DEPRESSION

Elderly persons, whether they are demented or not, are likely to suffer from depression. The variety of social, economic, and physiological changes that impinge on the aging individual may contribute to the development of depression. On the other hand, depressive illness as it is currently understood is based upon changes in brain neurotransmission.[17] Patients who retain their mental faculties may be reduced to a severely dysfunctional status by the occurrence of depressive illness. Those persons who become demented may have their capabilities further compromised by the coexistence of a depressive illness. Satisfactory treatment of depression in this latter group of patients can allow for a more tolerable life, even in the absence of their former level of mental acuity. In an elderly person who is both depressed and demented, proper treatment may spell the difference between that individual remaining within a family structure as opposed to being ejected into a custodial environment.

The ability to fall asleep or remain asleep is a common symptom of depression. The occurrence of changes in sleep pattern as a result of depression must be differentiated from those changes that occur normally in the course of aging.[1] The use of more sedating antidepressants given at bedtime may improve the sleep pattern and avoid the coadministration of other sedatives. Among the more sedating antidepressant drugs useful in treating the elderly patient are doxepin, maprotiline, and trazodone.[1] Some patients develop excessive daytime drowsiness when these more sedating antidepressants are employed, thus antidepressant compounds with lower sedative potential may be better tolerated. Desipramine and amoxapine have minimal sedative effects and are very useful in elderly depressed patients.[1] Additionally, amoxapine has the advantage of a rapid onset of action, often producing an initial mood improvement within the first three to five days of treatment.[1] Since elderly patients may also be receiving other nonpsychotropic medications with sedative action, the physician treating the elderly depressed patient must remain vigilant for the development of excessive drug-induced drowsiness which may impair the patient's ability to go about his or her daily routine.

The ability of antidepressant drugs to produce cholinergic blockade may be associated with a variety of peripheral manifestations including blurred vision, dry mouth, urinary retention, constipation, and tachycardia.[1] The likelihood of prostatic hypertrophy occurring in an elderly male must be kept in mind before prescribing a strongly anticholinergic drug. Of even greater consequence in the elderly patient is the central manifestation of anticholinergic action that may appear as reduced ability to concentrate and remember, as well as the appearance of stuttering speech and acute confusion, or the development of a toxic delirium.[1,18,19] The latter is well known to physicians in the form of an atropine-induced toxic brain syndrome. In the elderly patient it is preferable to avoid the more strongly anticholinergic antidepressants such as amitriptyline and imipramine.[20] Desipramine, doxepin, amoxapine, maprotiline, and trazodone have much less anticholinergic activity and are therefore more likely to be better tolerated by the elderly patient.[1]

Because of the ability of antidepressant drugs to precipitate or worsen cardiac arrhythmias and to produce postural hypotension, it is generally preferable to administer these drugs in small divided doses two to three times daily as opposed to the administration of a single larger dose at bedtime.[1,21] Therefore, the combined presence of relatively low sedative effect as well as limited anticholinergic action would be desirable attributes in choosing the ideal antidepressant in an elderly person. For this reason, desipramine and amoxapine are good therapeutic choices in depressed geriatric patients. The possibility of additive interactions with other therapeutic agents must be considered whenever medication is prescribed for an elderly patient. Tricyclic antidepressants may produce a depression of myocardial contractility and may precipitate or worsen congestive heart failure.[21] They may also be associated with the appearance of atrial or ventricular premature beats and may produce abnormalities of cardiac impulse conduction.[21] Electrophysiologic effects of these drugs may be additive to the action of any coadministered antiarrhythmic drug, such as quinidine or procainamide.[22] In contradistinction to the concerns that most experienced clinicians have regarding the safety of tricyclic antidepressants in patients with heart disease, a recent report suggests that these drugs may be safer than previous studies have indicated.[23] With proper caution and drug selection, they have a place in depressed cardiac patients.

Tricyclic and tetracyclic antidepressants inhibit nerve reuptake of norepinephrine and serotonin to a variable degree.[24,25] Inhibition of this reuptake mechanism also inhibits uptake of two commonly used antihypertensive drugs, guanethidine and clonidine.[26] Neither of these compounds should be used concurrently with antidepressant drug therapy since the latter prevents therapeutic action of the former. Furthermore, an attempt to titrate the dose of one of these antihypertensive agents to produce an adequate therapeutic effect in the presence of tricyclic antidepressant drug therapy may eventually lead to a severe hypotensive reaction once the antidepressant is discontinued. In prescribing antidepressants for elderly patients, the dosages employed are generally one-half of the conventional adult dose. Several well-controlled clinical studies have documented plasma concentrations of antidepressant drugs in the elderly at levels approximately twice those seen with comparable dosage in young people.[27] On the other hand, when any medication is prescribed, the dosage must be individualized for that specific patient. Some elderly patients will require doses comparable to the ordinary therapeutic dose employed in younger individuals. Table 12-2 presents suggested dosages of commonly employed antidepressants for elderly patients.

Just as some younger individuals do not respond to tricyclic or tetracyclic antidepressant compounds, a similar finding occurs in some elderly people. In spite of the concern of greater risks of prescribing monoamine oxidase inhibitor-type antidepressants, these compounds are safe and effective therapeutic agents even in elderly individuals.[28] Since MAOI-type antidepressants are free of anticholinergic action, they have an added advantage of not producing the central or peripheral manifestations of cholinergic blockade commonly associated with other antidepressant drugs.[1] As with younger patients, the elderly must be warned to avoid tyramine-rich foods such as fermented cheeses, red wine and beer. Likewise, the coadministration of nasal decongestants, stimulants, and vasconstrictor compounds are to be avoided in the patient being treated with a monoamine oxidase inhibitor. Elderly patients on monoamine oxidase inhibitors should have blood pressure and pulse rate determined at regular intervals. They should be evaluated for the presence of postural hypotension which is a common side effect of these drugs, particularly phenelzine.[1] The occurrence of postural hypotension may be a more serious problem in the elderly since, in these individuals, circulatory homeostasis is more fragile than in younger patients. Likewise, if an elderly patient develops postural hypotension, he or she may be more apt to faint or fall and sustain physical injury.

The combination of MAO inhibitors with tricyclic antidepressants has recently been investigated extensively in younger patients. Limited studies have been done in older people using this drug combination.[29]

Table 12-2
Dosage Guidelines for Psychotropic Drugs in Elderly Patients

THERAPEUTIC CLASSIFICATION Chemical Group Generic Name (Trade Name)	Daily Dosage (mg)	THERAPEUTIC CLASSIFICATION Chemical Group Generic Name (Trade Name)	Daily Dosage (mg)
ANTIANXIETY/SEDATIVE		Dibenzoxazepine	
Benzodiazepine		Loxapine (Loxitane)	10–60
Alprazolam (Xanax)	0.125–0.5	Dihydroindolone	
Lorazepam (Ativan)	0.5–1.5	Molindone (Moban)	10–60
Oxazepam (Serax)	10–30	ANTIDEPRESSANT	
Propanediol Carbamate		Tricyclic/Tertiary Amine	
Meprobamate (Equanil)	200–600	Amitriptyline (Elavil)	30–150
Antihistamine		Imipramine (Tofranil)	30–150
Diphenhydramine (Benadryl)	10–75	Doxepin (Sinequan)	30–150
Hydroxyzine (Atarax)	10–75	Tricyclic/Secondary Amine	
		Desipramine (Norpramin)	50–150

ANTIPSYCHOTIC/NEUROLEPTIC

Aliphatic Phenothiazine	
Chlorpromazine (Thorazine)	25–200
Piperidine Phenothiazine	
Thioridazine (Mellaril)	25–200
Piperazine Phenothiazine	
Trifluoperazine (Stelazine)	2–15
Piperazine Thioxanthene	
Thiothixene (Navane)	2–15
Butyrophenone	
Haloperidol (Haldol)	0.25–15

Tricyclic/Dibenzoxazepine	
Amoxapine (Asendin)	25–150
Tetracyclic	
Maprotiline (Ludiomil)	50–150
Triazolopyridine	
Trazodone (Desyrel)	50–150
Monoamine Oxidase Inhibitor	
Phenelzine (Nardil)	15–45
Pargyline (Eutonyl)	10–30
Tranylcypromine (Parnate)	10–20

Although these studies suggest that the combination may be safe, it is not to be recommended as a routine clinical practice and its application should be reserved for well-selected patients wherein the combination may be employed by physicians who are experienced with its use in younger individuals.[29]

In treating elderly depressed patients, particularly those in whom drug side effects have been problematic or in whom acute suicidal potential has been observed, a consideration of electroconvulsive therapy is appropriate. Electroconvulsive therapy has been documented as being both safe and effective even in individuals who are well into their 80s.[1]

Some depressed individuals who do not tolerate either tricyclic antidepressants or MAOI-type antidepressants may have a temporary mood improvement when treated with methylphenidate (Ritalin) in doses of 5 mg two to three times daily.[30] One of the newer benzodiazepines, alprazolam, has been reported to produce some mood improvement in patients with mild depression.[1] This compound does not produce significant anticholinergic effect or postural hypotension. It may be beneficial in doses of 0.125 to 0.25 mg two to three times daily in elderly individuals with mild depressive symptoms, although thus far there has been documentation for an antidepressant effect of this drug only at much higher dosages in young or middle-aged patients.

PSYCHOSIS

A variety of psychotic conditions occur in the elderly. Some of these disturbances may be treated by withdrawing rather than prescribing medication. Others may respond to a limited extent to pharmacotherapy, and still others may respond dramatically to judicious pharmacological intervention. The clinician must be able to differentiate these conditions in order to administer proper treatment. An elderly person who develops agitation, paranoid ideation, or delusions may be suffering from a drug-induced delirium. The most common pharmacological property likely to induce a toxic psychosis in an older person is that of cholinergic blockade.[1,19] Since many drugs, including antiparkinsonian agents, quinidine, antihistamines, and psychotropics, can induce an anticholinergic-type psychosis or delirium, it is important to avoid complicating the clinical picture by prescribing additional anticholinergic medications.[1] Withholding all drug therapy for a period of 12 to 48 hours may be the most judicious management for this form of psychotic disturbance. On the other hand, the cautious administration of physostigmine, a cholinesterase inhibitor, may rapidly reverse an anticholinergic behavioral disturbance, thus clarifying the diagnosis.[31] If physostigmine is to be administered to an elderly patient, 1 mg of the drug should be diluted to a total volume of 10 mL with normal saline. The diluted solution is then injected slowly intravenously over a period of five minutes. Prior to the administration of physostigmine, it should be determined that the patient is free of bronchospasm, acute coronary heart disease, and cardiac arrhythmias. Blood pressure and pulse should be monitored prior to and following the administration of physostigmine, and the patient should be observed for a period of 20 to 30 minutes after the drug is administered to determine the physiological effects as well as evidence of reversal of the previous behavioral abnormality.[1] Agitated elderly people who have anticholinergic psychoses may require cautious use of haloperidol (0.25 to 1 mg) or amobarbital in small doses of 30 to 100 mg, orally or intramuscularly. It must be remembered that some elderly people will develop paradoxical agitation in response to barbiturates and this risk must be weighed before such agents are administered.[1] The use of low potency antipsychotic agents with greater anticholinergic action, such as chlorpromazine and thioridazine, is to be avoided in patients presenting evidence of anticholinergic deliria.

Geriatric patients may become agitated, belligerent, paranoid and delusional during the course of organic dementias such as Alzheimer's disease. It is generally not of value to strongly sedate these patients with benzodiazepines or barbiturates. Strongly anticholinergic agents, such as thioridazine and chlorpromazine, may actually worsen the behavioral disturbance.[1] High potency antipsychotic drugs are the agents of choice in managing agitation and psychotic manifestations in patients with nondrug-induced organic psychoses. In such patients the use of haloperidol with gradual dosage titration is generally the preferred treatment. Many such patients will show improvement following the oral or intramuscular administration of this drug in doses as low as 0.25 mg once or twice daily. The individualization of dosage is important since some agitated elderly patients with organic brain disorders will require haloperidol doses as high as 10 to 20 mg daily. The majority, however, can be managed utilizing doses in the 0.5 mg to 5 mg per day range. It must be realized that antipsychotic drugs have no curative value in the treatment of Alzheimer's disease, yet they often allow the patient to be more comfortable and increase the comfort of those who live with the individual.[8] Since agitation and belligerent behavior may make it impossible for some patients with organic brain dysfunction to be maintained in either their family's home or in a nursing home, the appropriate treatment of these symptoms may benefit the quality of life of the patient by allowing him to remain in the best possible living environment.[8]

Since schizophrenia often is a chronic but not fatal illness, it is not surprising that clinicians will frequently encounter elderly persons who are schizophrenic. A history of long-standing psychotic symptoms, or of multiple recurrent episodes of psychosis generally with an onset before the third decade of life, is suggestive of a schizophrenic illness in the absence of a prior history of major affective illness. Use of low dose, high potency antipsychotic agents is preferable in treating the elderly schizophrenic patient. As has already been mentioned, the elderly are particularly sensitive to anticholinergic effects and the low potency drugs that are more strongly anticholinergic are to be avoided.[1] Drugs, such as chlorpromazine and thioridazine, that are more likely to produce hypotension, cardiac effects, and excessive sedation are likely to present greater risk to the geriatric patient.[1] Because cardiovascular homeostasis is more fragile in older people, drugs that produce more pronounced hypotension are likely to induce dizziness, fainting, falling, and the possibility that the patient will sustain physical injuries as the result of these effects.

Elderly patients whose psychotic symptoms periodically worsen may experience dramatic benefit with the administration of haloperidol in doses of 0.25 to 2 mg twice daily. Occasionally, doses of 10 to 15 mg per day may be required and, infrequently, geriatric patients will require haloperidol doses of up to 30 mg per day on a temporary basis. Even these larger doses are generally tolerated without adverse cardiovascular effect. Although the high potency agents are more likely to produce acute extrapyramidal effects, these unwanted effects are generally transitory and respond to dosage reduction, or the administration of small amounts (10 to 25 mg) of diphenhydramine or amantadine in doses of 50 to 100 mg per day.[1,32] Antiparkinsonian drugs, such as trihexyphenidyl or benztropine, should be avoided in elderly patients because of the risk of complications due to their anticholinergic action. In geriatric patients who have had persistent paranoid ideation, hallucinations, and delusions over periods of many years that have failed to respond to conventional doses of antipsychotic agents, it is generally not advantageous to begin a course of aggressive pharmacotherapy using high dose regimens of potent antipsychotic agents.

Affective disorders account for a sizable proportion of the psychotic disturbances encountered in geriatric patients. Elderly people who become severely depressed often exhibit psychotic features including paranoid ideation, delusional thinking and at times hallucinations. Treatment of psychotic depressive disorders in the elderly should begin with the administration of low doses of high potency antipsychotic drugs prior to instituting antidepressant medication.[1] Once there is a dimunition on psychotic symptomatology, appropriate antidepressant drugs can be added to the regimen using the suggestions presented in the previous discussion on the treatment of depression. Many elderly patients with psychotic depressive disorders will require antipsychotic chemotherapy only during the initial phase of treatment and then can be maintained on the antidepressant agent alone. Others will require concurrent administration of both medications throughout the course of treatment.

All too often, clinicians fail to consider manic depressive illness and acute manic psychosis as they evaluate and treat the geriatric patient.

Mania may first appear at virtually any age. Careful review of historical data may provide clues to the existence of manic symptoms on one or more occasions much earlier in the lifetime of the elderly patient. Acute manic episodes in the elderly are best managed by proper dosage titration utilizing high potency antipsychotic agents such as haloperidol. At first, low doses are administered with gradually increased dosage given as tolerated and as required to control symptoms. Elderly manic patients will very likely require somewhat higher doses of antipsychotic agents than will elderly schizophrenic patients. On the other hand, in both cases the dosage administered is likely to be considerably lower than used in younger individuals.

Lithium in the Elderly

Advanced age is not a contraindication to lithium carbonate therapy provided the patient has reasonably normal renal function and is not on a severely salt-restricted diet.[33] It should be kept in mind, however, that although the half-life of lithium is about 24 hours in young adults, it is likely to extend to 36 or 48 hours in the elderly.[1] Since the action of lithium is terminated by renal excretion, the fact that glomerular filtration rate decreases as patients age explains its longer half-life in these patients.[33] Geriatric patients are more likely to show signs of lithium intoxication at serum lithium levels well within the therapeutic range employed in younger patients.[33] The usual therapeutic serum level for lithium is 0.6 to 1.2 mEq/L in young and middle-aged patients, while in the elderly it is preferable to aim for serum lithium concentration in the range of 0.4 to 0.6 mEq/L.[1] Some elderly manic patients require higher serum concentrations of lithium while others will experience confusion, lassitude, and weakness at serum concentrations of 0.6 mEq/L. On occasion, I have seen 70- to 80-year-old patients whose affective symptoms were well controlled by serum lithium concentrations of 0.3 to 0.4 and who had intolerable side effects at concentrations of 0.5 or 0.6 mEq/L.[1] Lithium should never be administered in a single daily dose. A starting dose of 150 mg of lithium carbonate administered twice daily is reasonable in most elderly patients with adequate renal function and normal electrolyte balance. The lithium dosage may then be gradually titrated upward as required to achieve a satisfactory blood level and, more importantly, a satisfactory therapeutic response in the absence of unwanted adverse effects.

Before starting lithium treatment, it is essential to determine serum creatinine in order to assess renal function.[33] If the serum creatinine exceeds 1.5 mg/100 mL and lithium therapy is clearly necessary, it may be best to start with a single dose of 150 mg once daily and repeat the serum creatinine determination and measure the serum lithium level within two days of starting lithium. It is useful to measure serum electrolytes prior to starting lithium and this determination must be made before instituting treatment if the patient has been on a diuretic or salt-restricted diet.[33] The administration of lithium to a patient who continues on a salt-restricted diet is contraindicated. On the other hand, the coadministration of lithium along with a diuretic is generally acceptable provided that renal function is relatively normal and frequent measurements of serum concentration of lithium and electrolytes can be done.[1] Patients who are undernourished and not taking adequate fluids are at a greater risk for lithium intoxication and generally require discontinuation of lithium treatment until adequate fluid intake and urinary output can be established and maintained. Since lithium may suppress thyroid function, it is advisable to obtain baseline thyroid function tests including T_3, T_4, and TSH prior to starting lithium therapy.[33] Likewise, electrocardiographic changes may occur during lithium treatment in the absence of lithium intoxication. Therefore, it is useful to obtain a baseline electrocardiogram prior to starting lithium treatment.[1] Cardiac arrhythmias are not likely to be seen during the course of lithium treatment of elderly patients unless lithium intoxication, hypokalemia, or both occur. The development of hypokalemia increases the risk of lithium intoxication even at otherwise acceptable serum lithium concentrations.[1] Elderly patients receiving diuretics with lithium may well require supplemental potassium administration to avoid or correct this problem.

With the possible exception of confusional states occurring in the elderly lithium-treated patient at acceptable serum lithium concentrations, its side effects are not qualitatively different in geriatric patients. Some persons may experience increased thirst, polydipsia, polyuria, hand tremor, nausea and diarrhea early in the course of lithium treatment or in the presence of excessive serum lithium concentration. These symptoms generally abate as lithium therapy is continued or in some cases in response to a reduction in lithium dose. In the event that unwanted effects occur at the outset of lithium therapy, it of often useful in the elderly patient to discontinue the drug for a week or two and then reinstitute lithium at a reduced dosage and titrate the dosage and blood level upward more slowly than was undertaken during the first attempt at lithium therapy.[1] In spite of the possibility of lithium-induced side effects in the geriatric patient, many older individuals I have treated have achieved a satisfactory response and minimal or nonexistent side effects with this useful therapeutic agent. In the acutely manic geriatric patient, it is often preferable to allow the neuroleptic drug to produce initial behavioral control and then slowly add lithium as the patient's mood begins to normalize.

Although cautious administration of neuroleptic drugs and lithium is not likely to produce any greater risk of adverse reaction than would be produced by either drug individually, certainly the increased physiological frailty that occurs with aging should dictate administration of the lowest dose of any therapeutic agent and the least complicated regimen likely to be therapeutically effective. Once manic symptoms are controlled, the neuroleptic can generally be withdrawn and the patient then maintained on lithium alone. Although some elderly patients with recurrent depressive disorders will require indefinite maintenance with antidepressant drugs, many such individuals will achieve satisfactory prophylaxis against recurrent depression by the administration of lithium carbonate.

ANXIETY AND INSOMNIA

A widely divergent group of chemical substances has been used to induce sedation throughout the history of medicine. Since these drugs exert a generalized central nervous system depressant effect, they should be used with even greater caution in the elderly who are likely to be more sensitive to central nervous system depressant effects.[26,34] In managing anxiety in the aged, the physician must first be aware that as a person becomes older he encounters a variety of realistic life issues which may contribute to feelings of anxiety, worry, and generalized nervousness. Often, supportive psychotherapy and appropriate counseling of the geriatric patient will be more effective than pharmacological intervention to control symptoms whose origins are realistic. It may at times be easier to prescribe medication than to help these patients in other ways, although the complications of pharmacotherapy may in the long run be more difficult to solve than those of psychotherapeutic or social service intervention.

Most psychotropic drugs are strongly lipid soluble. The increased fat to lean body mass ratio and decreased efficiency of drug metabolism in the aging individual contributes to a more persistent action of any drug administered.[5] The drugs most widely used to control anxiety are the benzodiazepines. Of this group, chlordiazepoxide, diazepam, and flurazepam are most often used and have long half-lives in young healthy people. Following a single dose, these drugs or their metabolites may be measured in body fluids for 24 to 72 hours. If one of these compounds is administered to a young person on a daily basis for a week or more, the drug may be measurable for approximately twice that long; if the drug is administered over a period of time to an elderly person, measurable quantities may remain in body fluids for one to two weeks.[1,3,5] If an elderly patient experiences persistent and severe anxiety unresponsive to psychotherapeutic intervention, it may be appropriate to prescribe a short-acting benzodiazepine administered as infrequently as possible for as brief an interval as necessary. The benzodiazepines with shorter duration of action include alprazolam, lorazepam, and oxazepam. These drugs normally have half-lives approximating 12 hours following a single dose administration.[1] Recognizing that in an elderly person the half-life may be much longer and will be further increased, paralleling the duration of administration, caution should be exerted in prescribing these medications to the geriatric patient.[5] If they are prescribed, the doses used should be as low as possible, and generally they should be administered not more than once daily.[1] In some cases the patient may benefit from only two or three doses of the medication during the course of a week. Suggested geriatric doses of benzodiazepines are presented in Table 12-2.

Insomnia is a common complaint in the geriatric population. As people age, they require fewer hours of sleep. It is important not to try to medicate this normal variation in the sleep cycle. Furthermore, a variety of medical conditions common in the elderly may cause insomnia.[35] Diabetes may be associated with hypoglycemia and polyuria, both of which can disturb sleep. Cardiovascular disturbances, including cerebral atherosclerosis and cardiac arrhythmias, may also impair sleep. Decreased pulmonary function, particularly if associated with clinically significant hypoxia, is a fairly common cause of insomnia in the elderly.[35] Elderly patients who have more serious sleep disturbances than those from aging alone must be evaluated for depression, one of the most common causes of insomnia.[1]

If there is evidence of an affective illness, appropriate treatment with antidepressants has greater therapeutic value than any sedative. In the absence of medical or psychiatric causes for insomnia, the elderly patient who has difficulty falling asleep may benefit from chloral hydrate in a dose of 250 to 500 mg. Patients who are being treated with anticoagulants should not receive chloral hydrate because it affects the binding and metabolism of these drugs and may lead to excessive anticoagulant effect.[36] Alprazolam (0.25 mg), lorazepam (0.5 mg), oxazepam (10 mg), temazepam (15 mg), or triazolam (0.125 mg) may be used cautiously to induce sleep. These benzodiazepines do not interact with anticoagulants. If they are administered frequently or over a prolonged time, they may lead to excessive daytime sedation in the elderly. Sedating antihistamines, such as hydroxyzine (25 mg) or diphenhydramine (25 to 50 mg), may help elderly patients fall asleep more quickly.[1] These antihistamines produce no risk of drug dependency, but they do possess anticholinergic actions which may lead to confusion, hallucinations, or nightmares in elderly persons, particularly those with organic brain dysfunction.[1]

REFERENCES

1. Bernstein JG: *Handbook of Drug Therapy in Psychiatry.* Littleton, MA, John Wright • PSG Inc, 1983.
2. Prien RF: Problems and practices in geriatric psychopharmacology. *Psychosomatics* 1980;21:213–223.
3. Ouslander JG: Drug therapy in the elderly. *Ann Intern Med* 1981;95:711–722.
4. Seidl LG, Thornton GF, Smith JW, et al: Studies on the epidemiology of adverse drug reactions on a general medical service. *Bull Johns Hopkins Hospital* 1966;119:299–303.
5. Hicks R, Dysken MW, Davis JM, et al: The pharmacokinetics of psychotropic medication in the elderly: A review. *J Clin Psychiatry* 1981;42:374–385.
6. Greenblatt DJ, Sellers EM, Shader RI: Drug disposition in old age. *N Engl J Med* 1982;306:1081–1088.
7. Thompson PL, Moran MG, Nies AS: Psychotropic drug use in the elderly. *N Engl J Med* 1983;308:134–138, 194–199.
8. Thal LJ: Diagnosing and treating dementia. *Drug Therapy* 1982;12:53–68.
9. Davies P, Malony AJF: Selective loss of central cholinergic neurons in Alzheimer's disease. *Lancet* 1976;2:1403.
10. Kiloh LG; Pseudo-dementia. *Acta Psychiatr Scand* 1961;37:336–340.
11. Drachman DA: Memory, dementia and the cholinergic system, in Katzman R, Terry R, Bick K (eds): *Alzheimer's Disease: Senile Dementia and Related Disorders.* New York, Raven Press, 1978, pp 141–148.
12. Sitaram N, Weingarten H, Gillin J: Human serial learning: Enhancement with arecoline and choline, and impairment with scopolamine. *Science* 1978;201: 274–276.
13. Davis KL, Mohs RC, Tinkelberg JR: Enhancement of memory by physostigmine. *N Engl J Med* 1979;301:946–949.
14. Cohen EL, Wurtman RJ: Brain acetylcholine: Increase after systemic choline administration. *Life Sci* 1975;16:1095–1102.
15. Christie JE, Blackburn IM, Glen AIM, et al: Effects of choline and lecithin on CSF choline levels and on cognitive function in patients with presenile dementia of the Alzheimer type, in Barbeau A, Growdon JH, Wurtman RJ (eds): *Nutrition and the Brain.* New York, Raven Press, 1975, vol 5, pp 377–387.
16. Thal LJ, Fuld PA, Masur D, et al: Oral physostigmine and lecithin improve memory in Alzheimer's disease. *Ann Neurol* 1983;13:491–496.
17. Snyder SH: *Biological Aspects of Mental Disorder.* New York, Oxford University Press, 1980.
18. Schatzberg AF, Cole JO, Blumer DP: Speech blockage: A tricyclic side effect. *Am J Psychiatry* 1978;135:600–601.
19. Tune LE, Strauss ME, Lew MF, et al: Serum levels of anticholinergic drugs and impaired recent memory in chronic schizophrenic patients. *Am J Psychiatry* 1982;139:1460–1462.
20. Snyder SH, Yamamura HI: Antidepressants and the muscarinic cholinergic receptor. *Arch Gen Psychiatry* 1977;34:236–239.
21. Jefferson JW: A review of the cardiovascular effects and toxicity of tricyclic antidepressants. *Psychosom Med* 1975;37:160–179.
22. Bigger JT Jr, Giardina E, Perel J, et al: Cardiac antiarrhythmic effect of imipramine hydrochloride. *N Engl J Med* 1977;296:206–208.
23. Veith RC, Raskind MA, Caldwell JH, et al: Cardiovascular effects of tricyclic antidepressants in depressed patients with chronic heart disease. *N Engl J Med* 1982;306:954–959.

24. Maas JW: Biogenic amines and depression. *Arch Gen Psychiatry* 1975;32: 1357–1361.
25. Shopsin B, Cassano GB, Conti L: An overview of new "Second Generation" antidepressant compounds: Research and treatment implications, in Enna SJ, Malick JB, Richelson E (eds): *Antidepressants: Neurochemical, Behavioral and Clinical Perspective.* New York, Raven Press, 1981, pp 219–251.
26. Bernstein JG: Medical-psychiatric drug interation, in Hackett JP, Cassem NH (eds): *Massachusetts General Hospital Handbook of General Hospital Psychiatry.* St Louis, CV Mosby Company, 1978, pp 483–507.
27. Nies A, Robinson DS, Friedman MJ, et al: Relationship between age and tricyclic plasma levels. *Am J Psychiatry* 1977;134:790–793.
28. Ashford JW, Ford CV: Use of MAO inhibitors in elderly patients. *Am J Psychiatry* 1979;136:1466–1467.
29. White K, Pistole T, Boyd JL: Combined monoamine oxidase inhibitor-tricyclic antidepressant treatment: A pilot study. *Am J Psychiatry* 1980;137: 1422–1425.
30. Tesar GE: The role of stimulants in general medicine. *Drug Therapy* 1982;12: 186–196.
31. Granacher RP, Baldessarini RJ: Physostigmine. *Arch Gen Psychiatry* 1975; 32:375–380.
32. Fann WE, Lake C: Amantadine versus trihexyphenidyl in the treatment of neuroleptic induced Parkinsonism. *Am J Psychiatry* 1976;133:940–943.
33. Roose SP, Bone S, Haidorfer C, et al: Lithium treatment in older patients. *Am J Psychiatry* 1979;136:843–844.
34. Salzman C, Shader RI, Harmatz JS: Psychopharmacologic investigations in elderly volunteers: Effect on diazepam in males. *J Am Geriatr Soc* 1975;23: 451–455.
35. Amin MM: Drug treatment of insomnia in old age. *Psychopharmacology Bull* 1976;12:52–55.
36. Udall JA: Clinical implications of Warfarin interactions with five sedatives. *Am J Cardiol* 1975;35:67–69.

Index